HYPERTENSION
and the
BRAIN

Edited by

Gordon P. Guthrie, Jr., M.D.
Associate Professor of Medicine
Division of Endocrinology and Metabolism
University of Kentucky Medical Center
Lexington, Kentucky

and

Theodore A. Kotchen, M.D.
Professor of Medicine
Chief, Division of Endocrinology and Metabolism
University of Kentucky Medical Center
Lexington, Kentucky

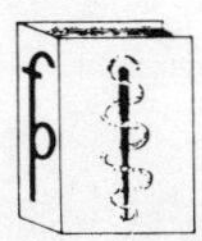

FUTURA PUBLISHING COMPANY
Mount Kisco, New York
1984

Contributors

James I. Ausman, M.D., Ph.D., Chairman, Department of Neurology, Henry Ford Hospital, Detroit, Michigan

Robert M. Berne, Ph.D., Chairman of Physiology, University of Virginia, Charlottesville, Virginia

K. Bridget Brosnihan, Ph.D., Staff Member, Department of Cardiovascular Research, Cleveland Clinic Foundation, Cleveland, Ohio

Franco Calaresu, M.D., Professor, Department of Physiology, University of Western Ontario, London, Ontario, Canada

Robert M. Carey, M.D., Professor of Internal Medicine; Head, Division of Endocrinology and Metabolism, University of Virginia Medical Center, Charlottesville, Virginia

Monica M. Caverson, B.Sc., Department of Physiology, University of Western Ontario, London, Ontario, Canada

David F. Cechetto, M.Sc., Research Associate, Department of Physiology, University of Western Ontario, London, Ontario, Canada

John Ciriello, Ph.D., Assistant Professor, Department of Physiology, University of Western Ontario, London, Ontario, Canada

Fernando G. Diaz, M.D., Ph.D., Staff Neurosurgeon, Department of Neurological Surgery, Henry Ford Hospital, Detroit, Michigan

Gerald F. DiBona, M.D., Professor and Vice Chairman, Department of Internal Medicine, The University of Iowa Hospitals and Clinics, Iowa City, Iowa

Henry Dinsdale, M.D., Professor and Head, Department of Medicine [Neurology], Queens University, Kingston, Ontario, Canada

Brent Egan, M.D., Instructor in Internal Medicine, The University of Michigan, Medical School, Ann Arbor, Michigan

Carlos M. Ferrario, M.D., Chairman, Department of Cardiovascular Research, Cleveland Clinic Foundation, Cleveland, Ohio

M. Andrew Fitzpatrick, M.D., Fellow in Hypertension, The University of Michigan, Medical School, Ann Arbor, Michigan

Jacques Genest, CC, M.D., D.Sc., Professor of Medicine, University of Montreal; Scientific Director, Clinical Research Institute of Montreal, Montreal, Quebec, Canada

Gordon P. Guthrie, Jr., M.D., Associate Professor, Division of Endocrinology and Metabolism, University of Kentucky Medical Center, Lexington, Kentucky

E. Clarke Haley, Jr., M.D., Fellow, Massachusetts General Hospital, Harvard Medical School, Boston, Massachusetts

Hallvard Holdaas, M.D., Ph.D., Visiting Assistant Professor, Department of Internal Medicine, University of Iowa, College of Medicine, Iowa City, Iowa *on leave from:* Institute for Experimental Medical Research, Ullevaal Hospital, University of Oslo, Oslo, Norway

Stevo Julius, M.D., Sc.D., Professor of Internal Medicine and Associate Professor of Physiology; Director, Hypertension Division, The University of Michigan Medical School, Ann Arbor, Michigan

William B. Kannel, M.D., M.P.H., Chairman, Section of Preventive Medicine and Epidemiology, Professor of Medicine, Boston University School of Medicine, Boston, Massachusetts

Walter Kobinger, M.D., Universitätsprofessor; Facharzt für Pharmakologie; Leiter des Pharmakologischen Laboratoriums, Ernst Boehringer Institut für Arzneimittelforschung, Vienna, Austria

Ulla C. Kopp, Ph.D., Assistant Research Scientist, Department of Internal Medicine, University of Iowa, College of Medicine, Iowa City, Iowa

Theodore A. Kotchen, M.D., Professor of Medicine; Chief, Division of Endocrinology and Metabolism, University of Kentucky Medical Center, Lexington, Kentucky

Teresa L. Krukoff, Ph.D., Research Associate, Department of Physiology, University of Western Ontario, London, Ontario, Canada

Jeffrey E. Pearce, M.D., Department of Neurological Surgery, Henry Ford Hospital, Detroit, Michigan

M. Ian Phillips, Ph.D., Professor and Chairman, Department of Physiology, University of Florida, Gainesville, Florida

Mark W. Roy, Ph.D., Division of Neurosurgery, University of Kentucky Medical Center, Lexington, Kentucky

Robert Schneider, M.D., Fellow in Hypertension, The University of Michigan, Medical School, Ann Arbor, Michigan

Terry W. Sherraden, M.D., Fellow in Endocrinology, Division of Endocrinology and Metabolism, University of Kentucky Medical Center, Lexington, Kentucky

Marc Thames, M.D., Professor of Internal Medicine, Medical College of Virginia; Chief of Cardiology, McGuire V.A. Medical Center, Richmond, Virginia

Glen Van Loon, M.D., Ph.D., Professor of Medicine, University of Kentucky Medical Center, Lexington, Kentucky

Joel Verter, Ph.D., National Heart, Lung, and Blood Institute, Mathematical and Applied Statistics Branch, Division of Heart and Vascular Disease, Bethesda, Maryland

H. Richard Winn, M.D., Professor and Chairman, Department of Neurosurgery, University of Washington; Harborview Medical Center V.A., Seattle, Washington

Philip A. Wolf, M.D., Professor of Neurology, Boston University School of Medicine, Boston, Massachusetts

Foreword

The brain plays a most important role in the regulation of blood pressure and in hypertension by its major influence on peripheral resistance and on cardiac output. This book is very timely. With the collaboration of many outstanding experts, Drs. Gordon P. Guthrie and Theodore A. Kotchen have covered almost every aspect of the relationship of the brain and hypertension, both from an experimental and a clinical point of view. Publication is most opportune because the book brings together and clarifies existing knowledge and informs of the very rapid advances linking various parts of the brain to hypertensive disease.

Important advances in methodology, especially affinity chromatography and specific antirenin antibodies, have confirmed the presence of a true renin system in the brain and in other tissues, such as the adrenals and the arteries. The relationships of the baroreflexes and the endogenous opioid peptides to the control of blood pressure and of the nervous system to renin secretion and sodium excretion are well covered. The editors have added an important feature by covering key advances in the clinical relationship of hypertension to the brain, especially in relation to strokes, hypertensive encephalopathy, and the consequences of hypertension.

This book will be most useful to all those interested in the clinical or research aspects of hypertension as well as to clinical neurologists. The editors have done an immense service and must be congratulated warmly for their important contribution.

Jacques Genest

Introduction

The brain has important influences on the circulation. Pain, fear, emotional excitement and mental stress each can elevate blood pressure, whereas sleep, sedation or meditation can lower it. Because of such potent effects on blood pressure control, a role for the brain in the genesis or perpetuation of essential hypertension has long been suspected. This suspicion has been reinforced by experimental models of hypertension in animals involving manipulations of central neural centers, and by abnormalities of central (and peripheral) neural function in some patients with hypertension. This close relationship between the brain and blood pressure has an additional facet. The vascular bed of the brain is damaged by hypertension of all degrees of severity. This pertains to both an increased risk for stroke as well as to alterations in cerebral function. Since much of past and new information about the interplay between blood pressure and the brain is specialized and not well collated, we sought to collect in a single volume separate chapters describing these and other reciprocal relationships between the brain and blood pressure control.

The first section of this book reviews basic mechanisms pertinent to the anatomy and pharmacology of central blood pressure regulation. Drs. Calaresu, Ciriello, Caverson, Cechetto and Krukoff in their chapter describe the anatomy of the multiple neural centers that are now known to interact upon blood pressure control. Dr. Kobinger then describes the related pharmacology of the neurotransmitters known to modulate the function of these neural centers.

The second section describes basic mechanisms involved in the physiology of blood pressure regulation. Dr. Thames discusses the baroreflex and its relation to experimental and clinical hypertension. Dr. Phillips describes the recently appreciated and still evolving knowledge of the brain renin-angiotensin system. Drs. Brosnihan and Ferrario then discuss those central mechanisms that regulate the peripheral renin-angiotensin system. Drs. Kopp, Holdaas and DiBona describe how peripheral neural function directly modulates not only renal renin release but renal sodium excretion, both potentially important for the regulation of blood pressure. Dr. Van Loon discusses the newly described endogenous opioid systems within the brain and their as yet incompletely defined relationships to blood pressure control and hypertension.

The third section contains chapters describing consequences of elevated blood pressure on central nervous function and anatomy. Drs. Winn, Haley and Berne describe the regulation of blood flow to the brain and the effects of hypertension on it. Drs. Kotchen and Roy then present clinical aspects of hypertensive encephalopathy, one of the most severe cerebral consequences of hypertension. Dr. Dinsdale outlines the several anatomic lesions which can be produced by both acute and sustained degrees of hypertension, and Drs. Wolf, Kannel and Verter review the body of evidence directly relating hypertension with stroke risk. Finally Drs. Pearce, Ausman and Diaz discuss the causes and management of acute stroke itself.

The final section contains discussions of those types of hypertension thought to be directly related to central nervous system dysfunction. Dr. Carey reviews models of experimental neurogenic hypertension, and Drs. Julius, Fitzpatrick, Egan and Schneider describe analogous types of neurogenic hypertension occurring in man. Drs. Fitzpatrick and Julius extend these observations to evidence of central causes of the more common disease, essential hypertension. Finally, Drs. Guthrie and Sherraden review the actions of centrally active antihypertensive drugs used to treat these and other hypertensive disorders.

We hope that this volume containing reviews from diverse disciplines, yet all related to the common theme of hypertension and the brain, will bring together information that will be of use to both clinicians and researchers.

Gordon P. Guthrie, Jr.
Theodore A. Kotchen

Abbreviations

ABI	Atherothrombotic Brain Infarction
ACE	Central Nucleus of the Amygdala
ACTH	Adrenocorticotrophic Hormone
ADN	Aortic Depressor Nerve
ATP	Adenosine Triphosphate
AII or Ang II	Angiotensin II
AV3V	Anteroventral Third Ventricle
AVP	Arginine Vasopressin
BBB	Blood Brain Barrier
BP	Blood Pressure
BUN	Blood Urea Nitrogen
CBF	Cerebral Blood Flow
CC	Corpus Callosum
CE	Cerebral Embolism
CEA	Carotid Endarterectomy
CHD	Coronary Heart Disease
CHF	Congestive Heart Failure
CNS	Central Nervous System
CPP	Cerebral Perfusion Pressure
CRF	Corticotropin Releasing Factor
CSF	Cerebrospinal Fluid
CSN	Carotid Sinus Nerve
CT	Computerized Tomographic
CVD	Cardiovascular Disease
DI	Diabetes Insipidus
DM	Dorsal Medulla
DMV	Dorsal Motor Nucleus of the Vagus
DR	Dorsal Region
ECG	Electrocardiogram
EEG	Electroencephalogram
5-HT	5-Hydroxytryptamine (Serotonin)
5-HTP	5-Hydroxytryptophan
5,7-DHT	5,7 Dihydroxytryptamine
FN	Fastigial Nucleus
GH	Growth Hormone

HDFP	Hypertension Detection and Follow-Up Program
HDR	Hypothalamic Defense Response
HR	Heart Rate
ICP	Intracranial Pressure
ICV	Intracerebroventricular
IH	Intraparenchymatous Hemorrhage
IML	Intermediolateral Nucleus
IV	Intravenous
IVT	Intravenous Transfusion
LH	Lateral Hypothalamus
LMFL	Lower Medial Quadrant of the Frontal Lobe
LVH	Left Ventricular Hypertrophy
MABP	Mean Arterial Blood Pressure
MBH	Mediobasal Hypothalamic
MI	Myocardial Infarction
MR	Median Region
NLC	Nucleus Locus Coeruleus
NMR	Nuclear Magnetic Resonance
NSM	Nucleus Septalis Medius
NTS	Nucleus Tractus Solitarius
OVLT	Organum Vasculosum Laminae Terminalis
PAG	Periaqueductal Gray
PB	Parabrachial Nucleus
PCA	Parachloramphetamine
PCPA	Parachlorophenylalanine
PRA	Plasma Renin Activity
PRC	Plasma Renin Concentration
PSWM	Paracingulate Subneocortical White Matter
PVH	Paaraventricular Nucleus of the Hypothalamus
rCBF	Regional Cerebral Blood Flow
RIND	Reversible Ischemic Neurologic Deficit
SFO	Subfornical Organ
SH	Subarachnoid Hemorrhage
SHEP	Systolic Hypertension in the Elderly Program
SHR	Spontaneously Hypertensive Rat
6-OHDA	6-Hydroxydopamine
SN	Sympathetic Nerve Endings
SMN	Supramammillary Nucleus
St 587	2-(2-Chloro-t-Trifluoromethylphenylimino) Imidazolidine
STA-MCA	Superficial Temporal Artery to Middle Cerebral Artery
TIA	Transient Ischemic Attack
TRH	Thyrotropin Releasing Hormone
TSH	Thyroid Stimulating Hormone
VIP	Vasoactive Intestinal Peptide
VLM	Ventrolateral Medulla
WKY	Wistar-Kyoto

Contents

Basic Mechanisms: Anatomy and Pharmacology

Basic Mechanisms: Physiology

Basic Mechanisms: Anatomy and Pharmacology

Chapter 1

Functional Neuroanatomy of Central Pathways Controlling the Circulation

Franco R. Calaresu, John Ciriello, Monica M. Caverson,
David F. Cechetto, and Teresa L. Krukoff

Introduction

The cardiovascular system is controlled by mechanical, chemical, and neural mechanisms whose contribution to circulatory regulation varies in different vascular beds. Neural control of the circulation has certain unique advantages over other mechanisms, such as speed of operation and the ability to redistribute blood quickly to certain vascular beds under different physiological conditions. Central control of the circulation is complex, as the central nervous system (CNS) receives sensory information from many sources and sends out appropriate control signals to effector organs through a central network of neural circuits widely distributed in the CNS. In recent years a large body of literature has suggested that a neural imbalance at the peripheral and/or central level may result in a chronic elevation in systemic arterial pressure.[1-4] It is unlikely that this hypertension, neurogenic in origin, results from destruction of neural tissue. More likely it is related to some subtle alterations in the organization of neural mechanisms involved in the regulation of the circulation or in its neurochemistry.

The aim of this chapter is not to provide a comprehensive and detailed review of neural mechanisms involved in the control of the cardiovascular system, but rather to provide information about some specific neural circuits that play established roles in the control of the circulation and may contribute to the pathogenesis of neurogenic hypertension. These neural circuits will be discussed on the basis of physiological observations indicating their role in the control of arterial pressure, their neuroanatomical con-

3

nections, and the possible chemical substances involved in transmitting information within these circuits.

Although much of our early knowledge has come from physiological and electrophysiological observations, after many decades of neglect the study of central cardiovascular pathways using neuroanatomical methods has begun to flourish and has provided a more complex picture of the circuits controlling cardiovascular function. The primary reason for this increased activity is the development of new methods for tracing neural pathways. These are: 1) the autoradiographic technique, which employs the anterograde axonal transport of radio-labelled proteins from cell bodies to axon terminals; 2) the retrograde axonal transport of horseradish peroxidase and fluorescent dyes from axon terminals or damaged axons to cell bodies; 3) the immunohistochemical methods for identification of transmitter-specific pathways; and 4) the 2-deoxyglucose technique as a marker of metabolic activity of functionally specific pathways. These techniques are described and discussed in detail in a recent monograph.[5]

The neuroanatomy reviewed in this chapter will be presented in three sections: efferent neural systems, afferent neural systems, and central interconnections. Figures 1-1 and 1-2 schematically summarize the neural circuitry to be described in detail in the text. In addition, the functional implications of neuroanatomical circuits and perspectives for future research are discussed.

Efferent Neural Systems

The preganglionic neurons of the efferent pathway of relex arcs influencing the cardiovascular system have been shown to be located in the spinal cord and in the medulla oblongata (Figure 1-1). The origin of sympathetic preganglionic fibers has been well established since 1851.[6] These fibers originate from the intermediolateral nucleus (IML) of the spinal cord between C_8 and L_4[7,8] and innervate both the heart and smooth muscle of vessels. Vagal preganglionic cardioinhibitory axons originate from at least two nuclei in the medulla oblongata: the dorsal motor nucleus of the vagus (DMV) and the nucleus ambiguus.[9,10] These two structures have been shown to influence heart rate. In addition, it has been suggested that the DMV is involved in controlling ventricular contractility.[11] The inputs to the preganglionic neurons in the spinal cord and medulla are described in detail in the next section.

Afferent Neural Systems

The carotid sinus (CSN) and aortic depressor nerves (ADN), known collectively as buffer nerves, have been the subject of considerable attention over the past several decades,[12–14] primarily because these nerves con-

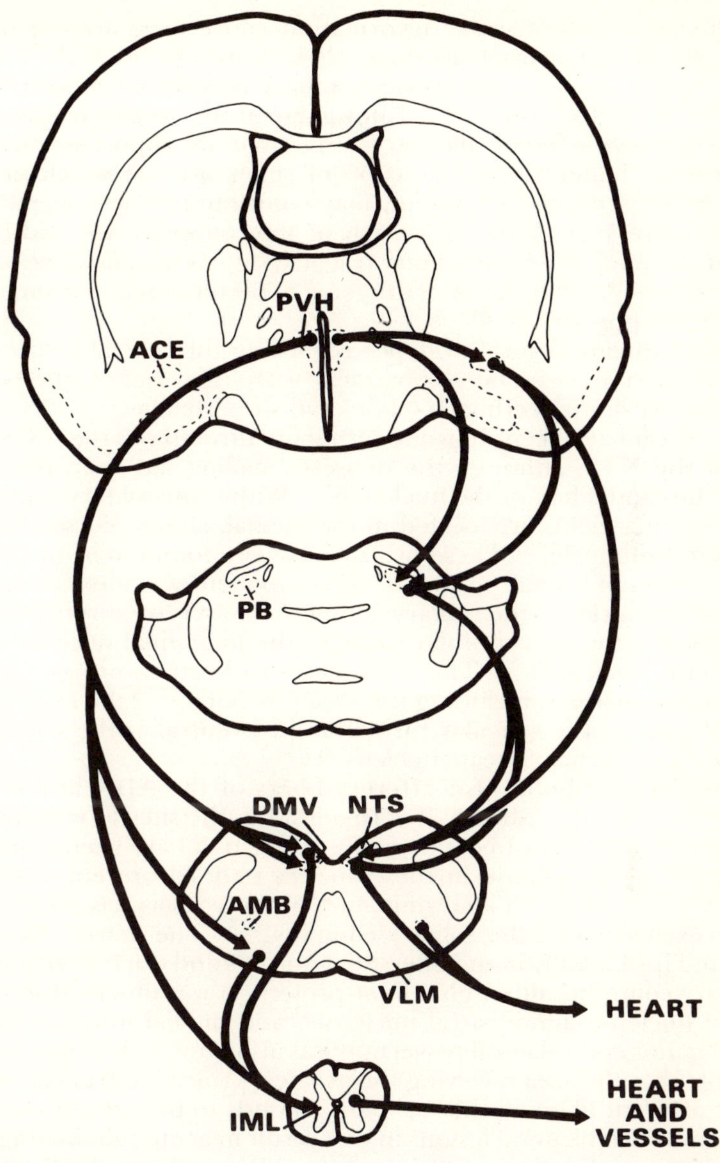

Figure 1-1. Wiring diagram of major descending cardiovascular pathways. Note that only unilateral projections are shown although the pathways are bilateral with an ipsilateral predominance. Abbreviations: ACE = central nucleus of the amygdala; ADN = aortic depressor nerve; AMB = nucleus ambiguus; CSN = carotid sinus nerve; DMV = dorsal motor nucleus of the vagus; NTS = nucleus of the solitary tract; PB = parabrachial nucleus; PVH = paraventricular nucleus of the hypothalamus; VLM = ventrolateral medulla; IML = intermediolateral nucleus.

vey exclusively cardiovascular information concerning arterial pressure (baroreceptors) and arterial blood gases (chemoreceptors) to the CNS, and because their stimulation and transection have been shown to alter the resting level of arterial pressure.[15-19] Knowledge of the precise anatomical termination of these afferent fibers is of fundamental importance in understanding how changes in the function of reflex arcs, of which these two nerves are the sensory component, may contribute to neurogenic hypertension (Figure 1-2). Both transection of the buffer nerves and bilateral lesions of the nucleus of the solitary tract (NTS), the primary site of termination of these fibers, result in neurogenic hypertension or extreme lability of the arterial pressure.[19-20]

Most of the anatomical evidence regarding the central projections of the buffer nerves has been obtained with the use of the sensitive tetramethylbenzidine method for horseradish peroxidase.[21] CSN afferent fibers in the cat have been shown to terminate throughout the rostrocaudal extent of the NTS, although the densest labelling has been reported to occur in the caudal half of the nucleus.[22,24] Within the solitary complex the densest terminal fields are located in the medial, lateral, dorsolateral, and commissural subnuclei.[24] These projections were found to be primarily ipsilateral, although a small contralateral component was identified. Several additional subnuclei of the solitary complex also receive direct projections from the CSN: the parvocellular nucleus, the interstitial nucleus, and the ventrolateral nucleus.[22-26] The CSN has also been shown to project to other brain stem areas, including the area postrema,[25,26] the DMV, the nucleus ambiguus,[25] the reticular formation just ventral to the solitary complex, and the external cuneate nucleus.[24]

A similar distribution for afferent fibers of the ADN in the solitary complex has been described.[23,24,27] In addition, the sites of termination of exclusively baroreceptor fibers from the aortic arch have been described in the rat and rabbit because in these species only baroreceptor fibers are carried in the ADN.[28,29] The termination of these fibers has been reported to occur exclusively in the solitary complex.[30,31] The densest projections were found ipsilaterally in the interstitial nucleus and dorsolateral aspect of the solitary complex, although a light projection was observed to the ventrolateral nucleus, commissural nucleus,[30] and medial nucleus.[31] In both species a minor contralateral projection was also observed.[30,31] It is interesting to note that the area receiving the greatest projection from aortic baroreceptor afferent fibers in the rat[30] corresponds to the area of the solitary complex in which bilateral lesions in cats result in acute fulminating hypertension.[20] Since bilateral transection of the ADN in the rat has been shown to produce a mild chronic elevation in arterial pressure,[15,16,19,24] it is likely that the hypertension that follows lesions of the NTS is due primarily to the destruction of aortic baroreceptor afferent fibers and terminals.

The neurotransmitters released from baroreceptor and chemoreceptor afferent fibers at the first synapse in the NTS have not been identified unequivocally. Several substances have been suggested, including catecholamines, substance P, serotonin, and L-glutamic acid. The NTS is

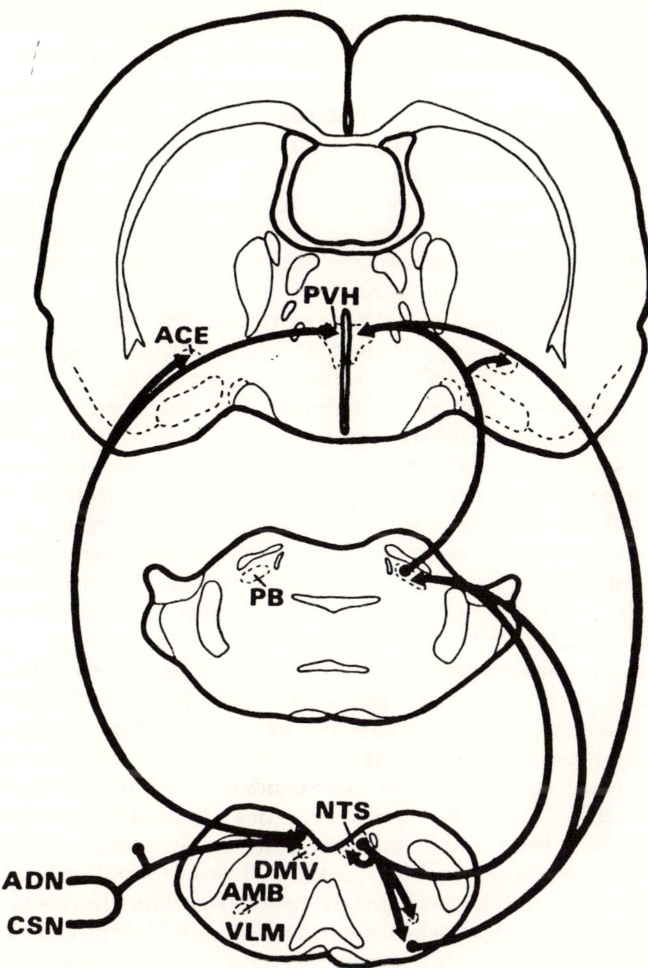

Figure 1-2. Wiring diagram of major ascending cardiovascular pathways. Unilateral projections are shown although these projections are bilateral with an ipsilateral predominance. For abbreviations, refer to Figure 1-1.

richly innervated by varicosities containing catecholamines,[32–34] although the origin of these fibers has not been completely elucidated.[32–34] Microinjection of norepinephrine,[35,36] epinephrine,[35] dopamine,[37] and other adrenergic agonists[35,38] into the region of the NTS has been shown to elicit bradycardia and arterial hypotension not unlike those that occur when the baroreceptor reflex is activated. In addition, destruction of catecholaminergic terminals in the NTS with 6-hydroxydopamine (6-OHDA) results in permanent lability of arterial pressure.[39] Despite this evidence the role of catecholamines as the transmitters of the primary afferent fibers has been questioned because transection of the glossopharyngeal and vagus nerves does not alter the integrity of catecholamine terminals in the nucleus,[32,40,41] and destruction of these terminals with microinjection of 6-OHDA does not abolish the baroreceptor reflex.[39,42–45]

The identification of substance P immunoreactive cell bodies in the petrosal and nodose ganglia—the peripheral ganglia containing the cell bodies of baroreceptor and chemoreceptor afferent fibers—suggests that substance P may be the transmitter of primary afferent cardiovascular fibers.[46–49] This suggestion is further supported by the finding of reduced substance P immunoreactivity in the NTS after transection of the glosso-pharyngeal and vagus nerves[50] and nodose ganglionectomy.[51] In addition, injection of substance P into the region of the NTS elicits cardiovascular responses similar to those observed during activation of the baroreceptor reflex.[47,52,53] However, this latter finding remains controversial as other studies have reported opposite cardiovascular responses[52] or no responses[54] when this peptide is microinjected into the nucleus. A recent study has also shown that neonatal depletion of substance P with capsaicin, a specific toxin for peripheral C fibers, does not alter the baroreceptor reflex,[55] further supporting the view that substance P is not the transmitter in primary baroreceptor afferent fibers.

Another biogenic amine, serotonin, has been suggested as a transmitter in the central projections of the ADN; this suggestion is based on the observation that approximately 75% of the cell bodies of ADN fibers in the nodose ganglion contain serotonin.[56]

At present, L-glutamic acid is considered the most likely putative neurotransmitter of primary afferent cardiovascular fibers.[45,54,57] Microinjection of either L-glutamate or kainic acid, an analog of glutamate, into the NTS elicits dose-dependent cardiac slowing and arterial hypotension.[45,54,57] In addition, nodose ganglionectomy results in the reduction of the high-affinity uptake mechanism of glutamate in the NTS.[45] Finally, glutamate levels in the solitary complex have been shown to be reduced after section of the glossopharyngeal and vagus nerves.[58]

Central Interconnections

The neuroanatomy of the projections of baroreceptor and chemoreceptor reflex arcs from the NTS remains mostly unexplored. Although several medullary and supramedullary structures have been shown to receive afferent inputs from the CSN and ADN using electrophysiological techniques, it cannot be unequivocally concluded that the afferent fibers projecting to these central areas are baroreceptor or chemoreceptor. This is because in all species studied both baroreceptor and chemoreceptor afferent fibers are found in the CSN and, with the notable exceptions of the rat and rabbit, in the ADN, and it is not possible to selectively activate one group of afferent fibers by electrical stimulation. Nevertheless, using autoradiographic and retrograde transport techniques, direct anatomical projections have been demonstrated from the solitary complex to the ventrolateral medulla (VLM), the parabrachial nucleus (PB), the paraventricular nucleus of the hypothalamus (PVH), the central nucleus of the amygdala (ACE), and the IML of the spinal cord. These efferent connections of the NTS, and the efferent connections of the structures receiving projections from the NTS will be described next.

In addition, two recent studies have provided a comprehensive functional map of CNS areas which receive aortic baroreceptor afferent information using the 2-deoxyglucose method.[59,60] Brain stem structures that increased their uptake of deoxyglucose during selective activation of aortic baroreceptors included the NTS, DMV, nucleus ambiguus, inferior olivary nucleus, the PB, and the VLM. In the hypothalamus, the PVH and supraoptic nuclei and the anterior, posterior, and periventricular hypothalamic areas increased their metabolic activity. In addition, increased activity was observed in the suprachiasmatic nucleus and the amygdala. Finally, sympathetic sites in the thoracolumbar cord previously shown to be involved in the control of circulation increased their activity after activation of aortic baroreceptors.[60]

Ventrolateral Medulla

The VLM has been shown to play an important role in the regulation of vasomotor tone, and the catecholamine cell groups in this region of the brain stem (divided into the A1 noradrenergic and C1 adrenergic groups; 33) have been suggested to be involved in the pathogenesis of hypertension.[61,62]

The NTS has been shown to project directly to the ventral surface of the brain stem near the exiting rootlets of the hypoglossal nerve and to the region of the A1 and C1 catecholamine cell groups.[63] These regions of the VLM in turn have been shown to contain neurons that project directly to several central areas known to be involved in cardiovascular regulation, including the PB and the PVH.[64–66] The IML has been shown to receive a dense catecholaminergic innervation originally assumed to descend from the A1 catecholamine cells in the VLM.[33] Although combined catecholamine-horseradish peroxidase studies have identified a small number of doubly labelled cell bodies in the region of the VLM, recent evidence suggests that the A1 neurons do not project to the spinal cord but the descending pathway arises from the C1 neurons in the rostral VLM and is most likely adrenergic.[67] It is now thought that the descending noradrenergic pathway to the IML originates in another group of noradrenergic neurons, the A5 region in the rostral VLM.[68] Substance P may also be involved in this descending pathway from the VLM to the IML as lesions of the VLM decrease substance P immunoreactivity in the IML.[69] In addition, intrathecal administration of a substance P antagonist attenuates the pressor effects of application of kainic acid to the VLM.[70]

The VLM has also been shown to project directly to the PVH (for a review, see Ref. 65). Autoradiographic studies have demonstrated that labelled fibers from the VLM terminate in virtually all parts of the PVH.[64–66] The densest projections have been ascribed to cell bodies of the dorsal and medial parvocellular part, which in turn have been shown to project directly to the spinal cord[71] and to the median eminence,[72,73] respectively. An additional projection from the VLM has been shown to the posterior magnocellular part where vasopressin cells have been identified.[74] The ascending pathways from the VLM to the PVH are thought to be catecholaminergic on the basis of immunocytochemistry.[65] Evidence for a serotonergic pathway from neurons in the VLM to the PVH has also been presented.[64,66] On the other hand, the neurotransmitter in the ascending pathway from the VLM to the PB is not known, although a catecholaminergic pathway has been suggested.[64,65]

Parabrachial Nucleus

In addition to receiving projections from medullary nuclei involved in cardiovascular control as indicated, the PB has been demonstrated to project to areas in the hypothalamus, amygdala, and cortex,[75] which are also thought to be involved in cardiovascular control.

The results of an autoradiographic study in the rat[75] suggest that a major input to the PVH originates primarily from the lateral part of the PB. These results can be contrasted with those of another autoradiographic study in which the injection sites were confined to the medial portion of the PB; this projection was seen to pass through the lateral hypothalamus with little labelling in the region of the PVH.[76] The dense labelling seen in the PVH as a result of depositing ^{3}H-amino acids in the lateral PB is found primarily in the medial and posterior parvocellular portions of the PVH.[75] The results obtained by autoradiography have been confirmed by horseradish peroxidase injections in the PVH, which resulted in retrograde labelling of many cells in the lateral PB.[77,78] The neurotransmitters involved in this pathway from the PB to the PVH are not known, but cells staining for both enkephalin[79] and neurotensin[80] have been found in the PB. The PVH has also been shown to have reciprocal descending connections with the PB.[81]

Many neuroanatomical studies have demonstrated a direct projection from the PB to the region of the ACE in the rat, cat, and monkey.[75,76,82–88] Injections of horseradish peroxidase in the ACE in the rat and cat have shown that retrograde labeling is observed primarily in the ventrolateral portion of the PB,[82,84,85] and injections of ^{3}H-amino acids in the PB have suggested a topographical organization. Both the lateral and medial PB have been demonstrated to project to the ACE; the lateral PB also projects to the medial nucleus of the amygdala, while the medial PB projects to parts of the basolateral nucleus of the amygdala.[75] In addition, reciprocal descending projections to the PB have been demonstrated using the autoradiographic and horseradish peroxidase techniques.[89] Of particular interest are the results of injections of horseradish peroxidase in the amygdala in which it was demonstrated that terminals labelled by anterograde transport of horseradish peroxidase made contacts with cells labelled by retrograde transport.[86]

High concentrations of both enkephalin and neurotensin are found in fibers in the ACE[90,91] suggesting that these fibers may originate from the cell bodies in the PB shown to contain enkephalin and neurotensin.[92,93]

In addition to its ascending pathways, the PB has been shown to send projections to the NTS; the lateral PB projects to the ventral part of the nucleus whereas the medial PB projects to the commissural nucleus.[75] Horseradish peroxidase injections into the region of the NTS have revealed retrogradely labelled neurons in the PB.[94]

Descending fibers from the PB have been shown to course through the VLM and through the region of the nucleus ambiguus, but it has not been demonstrated that they make synaptic contacts with neurons in these regions.[75] In addition, a direct pathway from neurons in the ventrolateral aspect of the PB to the region of the IML has been shown.[95]

Paraventricular Nucleus

In addition to its well established role in the control of posterior pituitary hormones,[96] the PVH has recently been shown to play a major role in the regulation of the cardiovascular system.[97] Furthermore, this nucleus has been implicated in hypertension as lesions of this structure prevent and/or reverse the elevation in arterial pressure due to aortic baroreceptor deafferentation and alter the development of hypertension in the spontaneously hypertensive rat.[98–101] The cardiovascular pathways most likely responsible for these effects are described next.

The connections of the PVH have been the subject of an extensive review.[65] The PVH has been shown to receive direct projections from the PB,[75] dorsal vagal complex,[65] and the VLM[64–66] and these projections have been shown to relay cardiovascular afferent information.[102,103] In addition, the PVH maintains direct reciprocal connections with these structures[65] and also projects directly to the DMV[65,104] and the IML,[65,104] the site of origin of vagal and sympathetic preganglionic neurons, respectively. Although there is no direct anatomical evidence suggesting that the PVH projects to neurons in the VLM, fibers from the PVH have been shown to course throughout this region.[81] In addition, neurons in the VLM that project directly to the IML have been shown electrophysiologically to alter their firing rates during stimulation of the PVH.[105]

The descending pathways from the PVH to the dorsal vagal complex and thoracic spinal cord have been shown to be primarily oxytocinergic, although vasopressinergic[104] pathways have also been described. These peptides have been shown to elicit cardiovascular responses when injected into the NTS, and to alter the activity of sympathetic preganglionic neurons when administered microiontophoretically.[106] In addition, several other possible neurotransmitters have been shown to be contained within these descending pathways. After injections of fluorescent dyes in the dorsal vagal complex and thoracic spinal cord, retrogradely labelled neurons in the PVH have been shown to be immunoreactive to somatostatin, leucine-enkephalin, methionine-enkephalin, and dopamine.[107,108]

Central Nucleus of the Amygdala

The ACE has been shown to receive afferent cardiovascular information from the CSN and ADN,[109] and its stimulation elicits changes in arterial pressure and heart rate.[110,111]

Ricardo and Koh,[112] using both horseradish peroxidase and autoradiographic methods, have demonstrated in the rat that the NTS projects directly to the ACE, a projection confirmed by others.[84,113] This projection cannot be demonstrated in other species such as the cat and monkey.[82–85] However, a descending projection, primarily ipsilateral, from the medial ACE to the NTS and DMV has been demonstrated in the rabbit, rat, cat, and monkey.[89,114–118] It has been demonstrated that neurotensin, metenkephalin, and somatostatin-containing cell bodies can be found in the ACE, suggesting that one of these cell types may give rise to the descending projection to the region of the NTS-DMV.[91] Recently, evidence has been presented demonstrating a long, descending, somatostatin-containing neuron system from the amygdala to the medulla.[119]

The ACE also receives a projection from the PVH, demonstrated by depositing horseradish peroxidase in the ACE[82,85] and injection of ^{3}H-amino acids in the PVH.[120] Swanson[121] has demonstrated that neurophysin-I stained fibers from the PVH could be followed to the amygdala, suggesting that the pathway may be oxytocinergic.

Conclusions and Perspectives

It is clear from the evidence reviewed here that the most significant advances in the last few years have provided information about the complex connections between clearly identified sensory nuclei receiving cardiovascular information and motor nuclei sending control signals to cardiovascular effector organs. Two important general conclusions may be drawn from the recent neuroanatomical evidence. First, that supramedullary structures that commonly control either integrated physiological responses or behavioral events must be aware of the current status of the circulation before sending out the control signals that alter circulatory variables in a way that is appropriate for the particular behavior. It may then be suggested that the functional significance of these distributed neural circuits is that sensory information from the cardiovascular system is made available to a large portion of the CNS and therefore is an important component of the mechanisms responsible for integrated physiological responses.

The second conclusion is that many of the CNS sites in neuronal circuits between the primary sensory input and the effector neurons appear to have reciprocal connections (Figure 1-3). This can be interpreted to indicate that cell assemblies that receive sensory information from primary sensory nuclei can in turn affect the flow of sensory information from the cardiovascular system. This feature may function as an override mechanism that can disable lower-order reflexes when necessary. An example of a mechanism of this kind is the relative insensitivity of the baroreceptor reflex in physiological conditions in which maintaining a high level of arterial pressure is desirable.

Progress has been made in recent years not only in establishing connections of central cardiovascular pathways by using the new tracing techniques, but also in assigning functional significance to these connections by physiological and electrophysiological experiments. The technique most likely to make the most significant contributions in this area is the 2-deoxyglucose autoradiographic method, which displays levels of metabolic activity in specific regions of the CNS, corresponding to functional states in an experimental animal. Before the introduction of this method the available neuroanatomical and electrophysiological techniques allowed the study of only one synapse at a time in specific cardiovascular pathways. The development of the 2-deoxyglucose method offers the opportunity to visualize simultaneously all the neuronal circuitry associated with the activation of specific receptors, whether the input is excitatory or inhibitory.[59,60]

The possibility that long-term alterations in the physiological range of regulation of cardiovascular variables, such as arterial hypertension, may be related to dysfunctions in the CNS has prompted a flurry of experimental activities attempting to demonstrate a neurogenic component in different models of hypertension. These studies are likely to contribute significantly to a better understanding of normal mechanisms controlling cardiovascular variables.

Another exciting new area is that of the chemical messengers involved in transmitting information from one CNS area to another. There have been developments suggesting a role for a variety of chemical substances in either altering ionic permeabilities of neurons or changing their metabolism, although the problem that is largely unsolved is to determine the physiological function of these substances. It is clear that we will witness great developments in this area, and that one of the final outcomes of this approach will be the ability to identify functional flaws in neural systems involved in central cardiovascular control as the primary cause of certain

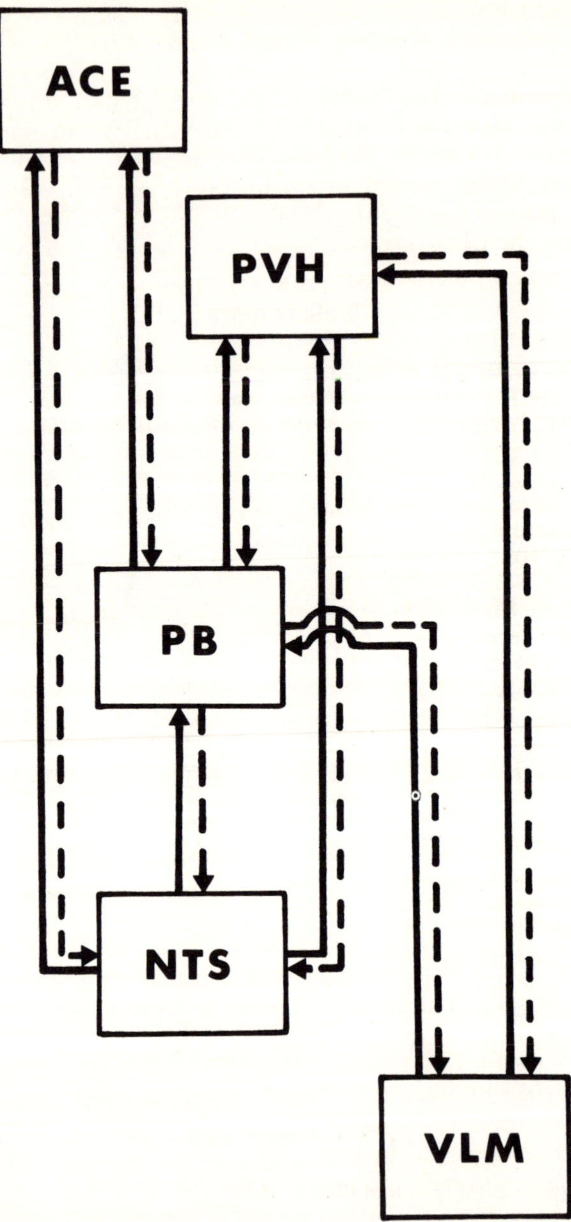

Figure 1-3. Diagrammatic representation of direct reciprocal connections between central nervous system sites demonstrated to be involved in cardiovascular control. Ascending projections are represented by solid lines and the reciprocal descending projections are shown as dashed lines. For abbreviations, refer to Figure 1-1.

forms of hypertension. It may then be possible to correct these functional derangements by using selective drugs known to affect neurochemical transmission.

Acknowledgements: The work by the authors quoted here has been supported by the Medical Research Council of Canada and the Ontario Heart Foundation. J. Ciriello is a Canadian Heart Foundation Scholar and M. M. Caverson is the holder of an Ontario Graduate Scholarship. We thank Mrs. N. Wilson for typing the manuscript and Miss Rebecca Woodside for drawing the illustrations.

References

1. Reis DJ: The brain and arterial hypertension: evidence for a neural-imbalance hypothesis. *In* Disturbances in Neurogenic Control of Circulation, edited by Abboud FM, Fozzard HA, Gilmore JP, Reis DJ. Bethesda, Am Physiol Soc, 1981, p 87
2. Brody MJ, Johnson AK: Role of forebrain structures in models of experimental hypertension. *In* Disturbances in Neurogenic Control of Circulation, edited by Abboud FM, Fozzard HA, Gilmore JP, Reis DJ. Bethesda, Am Physiol Soc, 1981, p 105
3. Abboud FM, Fozzard HA, Gilmore JP, Reis DJ: Disurbances in Neurogenic Control of the Circulation. Bethesda, Am Physiol Soc, 1981
4. Buckley JP, Ferrario CM: Central Nervous Mechanisms in Hypertension. New York, Raven Press, 1981
5. Heimer L, Robards MJ: Neuroanatomical Tract-Tracing Methods. New York, Plenum Press, 1982
6. Clarke JL: Researches into the structure of the spinal cord. Phil Trans R Soc Lond, Part 1, **141:**607, 1851
7. Henry JL, Calaresu FR: Topography and numerical distribution of neurons of the thoracolumbar intermediolateral nucleus in the cat. J Comp Neurol **144:**205, 1972
8. Oldfield BJ, McLachlan EM: An analysis of the sympathetic preganglionic neurons projecting from the upper thoracic spinal roots of the cat. J Comp Neurol **196:**329, 1981
9. Ciriello J, Calaresu FR: Distribution of vagal cardio-inhibitory neurons in the medulla of the cat. Am J Physiol **138:**R57, 1980
10. Ciriello J, Calaresu FR: Medullary origin of vagal preganglionic axons to the heart of the cat. J Auton Nerv Syst **5:**9, 1982
11. Geis GS, Wurster RD: Cardiac responses during stimulation of the dorsal motor nucleus and nucleus ambiguus in the cat. Circulat Res **46:**606, 1980
12. Calaresu FR, Faiers AA, Mogenson GJ: Central neural regulation of heart and blood vessels in mammals. Prog Neurobiol **5:**1, 1975
13. Spyer KM: Neural organisation and control of the baroreceptor reflex. Rev Physiol Biochem Pharmacol **88:**23, 1981
14. Spyer KM: Central nervous integration of cardiovascular control. J Exp Biol **100:**109, 1982
15. Fink GD, Kennedy F, Bryan WJ, Werber A: Pathogenesis of hypertension in rats with chronic aortic baroreceptor deafferentation. Hypertension **2:**319, 1980

16. Patel KP, Ciriello J, Kline RL: Noradrenergic mechanisms in brain and peripheral organs after aortic depressor nerve transection in the rat. Am J Physiol **240**:H481, 1981
17. Ciriello J, Calaresu FR: Separate medullary pathways mediating reflex vagal bradycardia to stimulation of buffer nerves in the cat. J Auton Nerv Syst **1**:13, 1979
18. Kirchheim HR: Systemic arterial baroreceptor reflexes. Physiol Rev **56**:100, 1976
19. Krieger EM: Neurogenic hypertension in the rat. Circulat Res **15**:511, 1964
20. Doba N, Reis DJ: Acute fulminating neurogenic hypertension produced by brainstem lesions in the rat. Circulat Res **32**:584, 1973
21. Mesulam M-M: Tetramethyl benzidine for horseradish peroxidase neurochemistry: a non-carcinogenic blue reaction product with superior sensitivity for visualizing neural afferents and efferents. J Histochem Cytochem **26**:106, 1978
22. Berger AJ: Distribution of carotid sinus nerve afferent fibres to solitary tract nuclei of the cat using transganglionic transport of horseradish peroxidase. Neurosci Lett **14**:153, 1979
23. Ciriello J, Calaresu FR: Projections from buffer nerves to the nucleus of the solitary tract: an anatomical and electrophysiological study in the cat. J Auton Nerv Syst **3**:299, 1981
24. Ciriello J, Hrycyshyn AW, Calaresu FR: Horseradish peroxidase study of brainstem projections of carotid sinus and aortic depressor nerves in the cat. J Auton Nerv Syst **4**:43, 1981
25. Davies RO, Kalia M: Carotid sinus nerve projections to the brain stem of the cat. Brain Res Bull **6**:531, 1981
26. Panneton WM, Loewy AD: Projections of the carotid sinus nerve to the nucleus of the solitary tract in the cat. Brain Res **191**:239, 1980
27. Kalia M, Welles RV: Brain stem projections of the aortic nerve in the cat: a study using tetramethyl benzidine as the substrate for horseradish peroxidase. Brain Res **188**:23, 1980
28. Sapru HN, Gonzalez E, Krieger AJ: Aortic nerve stimulation in the rat: cardiovascular and respiratory responses. Brain Res Bull **6**:393, 1981
29. Chalmers JP, Korner PI, White SW: The relative roles of the aortic and carotid sinus nerves in the rabbit in the control of respiration and circulation during arterial hypoxia and hypercapnia. J Physiol (Lond) **188**:435, 1967
30. Ciriello J: Brainstem projections of aortic baroreceptor afferent fibres in the rat. Neurosci Lett **36**:37, 1983
31. Wallach JH, Loewy AD: Projections of the aortic nerves to the nucleus tractus solitarius in the rabbit. Brain Res **188**:247, 1980
32. Chiba J, Kato M: Synaptic structures and quantification of catecholaminergic axons in the nucleus tractus solitarius of the rat: possible modulatory roles of catecholamines in baroreceptor reflexes. Brain Res **151**:323, 1978
33. Dahlström A, Fuxe K: Evidence for the existence of monoamine-containing neurons in the central nervous system. I. Demonstration of monoamines in the cell bodies of brain stem neurons. Acta Physiol Scand **62** (suppl 232):1, 1964
34. Fuxe K: The distribution of monoamine terminals in the central nervous system. Acta Physiol Scand **63** (suppl 247):38, 1965

35. de Jong W, Nijkamp FP: Centrally induced hypertension and bradycardia after administration of α-methylnoradrenaline into the area of the nucleus tractus solitarii of the rat. Br J Pharmacol **58**:593, 1976

36. de Jong W, Zandberg P, Versteeg DHG, Palkovits M: Brain stem structures and catecholamines in the control of arterial blood pressure in the rat. Clin Sci Molec Med **51**:3815, 1976

37. Zandberg P, de Jong W, DeWied D: Effect of catecholamine-receptor agents on blood pressure after local application in the nucleus tractus solitarii of the medulla oblongata. Eur J Pharmacol **55**:43, 1979

38. de Jong W, Nijkamp FP: Hypotensive action of noradrenaline and α-methylnoradrenaline in the area of the nucleus tractus solitarii in the rat brain stem. *In* Central Action of Drugs in Blood Pressure Regulation, edited by Davies DS, Reid JL. London, Pitman, 1975, p 179

39. Talman WT, Synder D, Reis DJ: Chronic lability of arterial pressure produced by destruction of A_2 catecholaminergic neurons in rat brain stems. Circulat Res **46**:842, 1980

40. Chiba T, Doba N: The synaptic structure of catecholaminergic axon varicosities in the dorso-medial portion of the nucleus tractus solitarius of the cat: possible role in the regulation of cardiovascular reflexes. Brain Res **84**:31, 1975

41. Chiba T, Doba N: Catecholaminergic axo-axonic synapses in the nucleus of the tractus solitarius (pars commissuralis) of the cat: possible relation to presynaptic regulation of baroreceptor reflexes. Brain Res **102**:255, 1976

42. Kobinger W, Walland A: Modulating effect of central adrenergic neurones on a vagally mediated cardioinhibitory reflex. Eur J Pharmacol **22**:344, 1973

43. Haeusler G: Organization of central cardiovascular pathways in the cat and the question of an involvement of adrenergic neurones. Naunyn-Schmiedeberg's Arch Pharmacol **285**:R28, 1974

44. Haeusler G: Cardiovascular regulation by central adrenergic mechanisms and its alteration by hypotensive drugs. Circulat Res Suppl 1, 36–37:223, 1975

45. Talman WT, Perrone UH, Reis DJ: Evidence for L-glutamate as the neurotransmitter of baroreceptor afferent nerve fibres. Science **209**:813, 1980

46. Gamse R, Lembeck F, Cuello AC: Substance P in the vagus nerve. Naunyn-Schmiedeberg's Arch Pharmacol **306**:37, 1979

47. Haeusler G, Osterwalder R: Evidence suggesting a transmitter or neuromodulatory role for substance P at the first synapse of the baroreceptor reflex. Naunyn-Schmiedeberg's Arch Pharmacol **314**:111, 1980

48. Lundberg JM, Hökfelt T, Nilsson G, Terenius L, Rehfeld J, Elde R, Said S: Peptide neurons in the vagus, splanchnic and sciatic nerves. Acta Physiol Scand **104**:499, 1978

49. Lundberg JM, Hökfelt T, Fahrenkrug J, Nilsson G, Terenius L: Peptides in the cat carotid body (glomus coroticum): VIP-, enkephalin-, and substance P-life immunoreactivity. Acta Physiol Scand **107**:279, 1979

50. Gillis RA, Helke CJ, Hamilton BL, Norman WP, Jacobowitz DM: Evidence that substance P is a neurotransmitter of baro- and chemoreceptor afferents in nucleus tractus solitarius. Brain Res **181**:476, 1980

51. Helke CJ, Muth EA, Jacobowitz DM: Changes in central cholinergic neurons in the spontaneously hypertensive rat. Brain Res **188**:425, 1980

52. Granata AR, Woodruff GN: A central hypertensive action of substance P in rats. IRCS Med Sci **8**:205, 1980

53. Haeusler G, Osterwalder R: Is substance P the transmitter at the first synapse of the baroreceptor reflex in rats and cats? Clin Sci **59**:2955, 1980
54. Talman WT, Reis DJ: Baroreflex actions of substance P microinjected into the nucleus tractus solitarius in rat: a consequence of local distortion. Brain Res **220**:402, 1981
55. Lorez HP, Haeusler G, Aeppli L: Substance P neurones in medullary baroreflex areas and baroreflex function of capsaicin treated rats. Comparison with other primary afferent systems. Neurosci **8**:507, 1983
56. Gaudin-Chazai G, Portalier P, Puizillout JJ, Vigier D: Simultaneous visualizations of aortic and [^{3}H]-5-hydroxytryptamine-accumulating cell bodies in the nodose ganglion of the cat. J. Physiol (Lond) **337**:321, 1983
57. Talman WT, Perrone MH, Reis DJ: Acute hypertension after the local injection of kainic acid into the nucleus tractus solitarius of rats. Circulat Res **48**:292, 1981
58. Dietrich WD, Lowry OH, Loewy AD: The distribution of glutamate, GABA and aspartate in the nucleus tractus solitarius of the cat. Brain Res **231**:254, 1982
59. Ciriello J, Rohlicek CV, Polosa C: Aortic baroreceptor reflex pathway: a functional mapping using [^{3}H]-2-deoxyglucose autoradiography in the rat. J Auton Nerv Syst **8**:111, 1983
60. Ciriello J, Rohlicek CV, Poulsen RS, Polosa C: Deoxyglucose uptake in the rat thoracolumbar cord during activation of aortic baroreceptor afferent fibers. Brain Res **231**:240, 1982
61. Versteeg DHG, Palkovits M, Van der Gugten J, Wijnen HLJM, Smeets GWM, de Jong W: Catecholamine content of individual brain regions of spontaneously hypertensive rats (SH-rats). Brain Res **112**:429, 1976
62. Wijnen HJ, Versteeg D, Palkovits M, de Jong W: Increased adrenaline content of individual nuclei of the hypothalamus and the medulla oblongata of genetically hypertensive rats. Brain Res **135**:180, 1977
63. Loewy AD, Burton H: Nuclei of the solitary tract: efferent projections to the lower brain stem and spinal cord of the cat. J Comp Neurol **181**:421, 1978
64. Loewy AD, Wallach JH, McKellar S: Efferent connections of the ventral medulla oblongata in the rat. Brain Res Rev **3**:63, 1981
65. Sawchenko PE and Swanson LW: The organization of noradrenergic pathways from the brainstem to the paraventricular and supraoptic nuclei in the rat. Brain Res Rev **4**:275, 1982
66. McKellar S and Loewy AD: Organization of some brain stem afferents to the paraventricular nucleus of the hypothalamus in the rat. Brain Res **217**:351, 1981
67. Ross CA, Armstrong DM, Ruggiero DA, Pickel VM, Joh TH, Reis DJ: Adrenaline neurons in the rostral ventrolateral medulla innervate thoracic spinal cord: a combined immunocytochemical and retrograde transport demonstration. Neurosci Lett **25**:257, 1981
68. Loewy AD, McKellar S, Saper CB: Direct projections from the A5 catecholamine cell group to the intermediolateral cell column. Brain Res **174**:309, 1979
69. Helke CJ, Neil JL, Massari VJ, Loewy AD: Substance P neurones project from the ventral medulla to the intermediolateral cell column and ventral horn in the rat. Brain Res **243**:147, 1982
70. Loewy AD, Sawyer WB: Substance P antagonist inhibits vasomotor responses elicited from ventral medulla in the rat. Brain Res **245**:379, 1982
71. Swanson LW, Kuypers HGJM: The paraventricular nucleus of the hypo-

thalamus: cytoarchitectonic subdivisions and the organization of projections to the pituitary, dorsal vagal complex and spinal cord as demonstrated by retrograde fluorescence double labelling methods. J Comp Neurol **194:**555, 1980

72. Swanson LW, Sawchenko PE, Wiegand SJ, Price JL: Separate neurons in the paraventricular nucleus project to the median eminence and to the medulla or spinal cord. Brain Res **198:**140, 1980
73. Weigand SJ, Price JL: The cells of origin of the afferent fibers to the median eminence in the rat. J. Comp Neurol **192:**1, 1980
74. Rhodes CH, Morel JI, Pfaff DW: Immunohistochemical analysis of magnocellular elements in rat hypothalamus: distribution and numbers of cells containing neurophysin, oxytocin and vasopressin. J Comp Neurol **198:**45, 1981
75. Saper CB, Loewy AD: Efferent connections of the parabrachial nucleus in the rat. Brain Res **197:**291, 1980
76. Norgren R: Taste pathways to hypothalamus and amygdala. J Comp Neurol **166:**17, 1976
77. Berk ML, Finkelstein JA: Afferent projections to the preoptic area and hypothalamic regions in the rat brain. Neurosci **6:**1601, 1981
78. Tribollet E, Dreifuss JJ: Localization of neurones projecting to the hypothalamic paraventricular nucleus area of the rat: a horseradish peroxidase study. Neurosci **6:**1315, 1981
79. Hökfelt T, Elde R, Johansson O, Terenius L, Stein L: The distribution of enkephalin-immunoreactive cell bodies in the rat central nervous system. Neurosci Lett **5:**25, 1977
80. Uhl GR, Goodman RR, Snyder SH: Neurotensin-containing cell bodies, fibers and nerve terminals in the brain stem of the rat: immunohistochemical mapping. Brain Res **167:**77, 1979
81. Saper C, Loewy AD, Swanson LW, Cowan WN: Direct hypothalamo-autonomic connections. Brain Res **117:**305, 1976
82. Cechetto DF, Ciriello J, Calaresu FR: Afferent connections to cardiovascular sites in the amygdala: a horseradish peroxidase study in the cat. J Auton Nerv Syst **8:**97, 1983
83. Mehler WR: Subcortical afferent connections to the amygdala in the monkey. J Comp Neurol **190:**733, 1980
84. Otterson OP: Afferent connections to the amygdaloid complex of the rat with some observations in the cat. III. Afferents from the lower brain stem. J Comp Neurol **202:**335, 1981
85. Russchen FT: Amygdalopetal projections in the cat: II. Subcortical afferent connections. A study with retrograde tracing techniques. J Comp Neurol **207:**157, 1982
86. Takeuchi Y, McLean JH, Hopkins DA: Reciprocal connections between the amygdala and parabrachial nuclei: ultrastructural demonstration by degeneration and axonal transport of horseradish peroxidase in the cat. Brain Res **239:**583, 1982
87. Veening JG: Subcortical afferents of the amygdaloid complex in the rat: an HRP study. Neurosci Lett **8:**196, 1978
88. Voshart K, Van der Kooy D: The organization of the efferent projections of the parabrachial nucleus to the forebrain in the rat: a retrograde fluorescent double labeling study. Brain Res **212:**271, 1981
89. Hopkins DA, Holstege G: Amygdaloid projections to the mesencephalon pons and medulla oblongata in the cat. Exp Brain Res **32:**529, 1978

90. Ben-Ari Y: Transmittors and modulators in the amygdaloid complex: A review. *In* Amygdaloid Complex, edited by Ben-Ari Y. Amsterdam, Elsevier, 1981, p 163
91. Roberts GW, Woodhams PL, Polak JM, Crow TJ: Distribution of neuropeptides in the limbic system of the rat: The amygdaloid complex. Neuroscience **7**:99, 1982
92. Elde R, Hökfelt T, Johansson O, Ljungdahl A, Nilsson G, Jeffcoate SL: Immunohistochemical localization of peptides in the nervous system. *In* Centrally Acting Peptides, edited by Hughes J. London, Macmillan, 1978, p 17
93. Simantov R, Kuhar MJ, Uhl GR, Snyder SH: Opioid peptide enkephalin: immunohistochemical mapping in rat central nervous system. Proc Natl Acad Sci **74**:2167, 1977
94. Gutman MB, Ciriello J, Calarcsu FR: Brain stem projections to cardiovascular areas in the nucleus of the solitary tract in the cat. Proc Can Fed Biol Soc **26**:63, 1983
95. Miura M, Onai T, Takayama K: Projections of upper structure to the spinal cardioacceleratory center in cats: an HRP study using a new microinjection method. J Auton Nerv Syst **7**:119, 1983
96. Hayward JN: Functional and morphological aspects of hypothalamic neurons. Physiol Rev **57**:574, 1977
97. Ciriello J, Calaresu FR: The role of the paraventricular and supraoptic nuclei in central cardiovascular regulation in the cat. Am J Physiol **239**:R137, 1980
98. Zhang TX, Ciriello J: Lesions of paraventricular nucleus reverse the elevated arterial pressure after aortic baroreceptor denervation in the rat. Soc Neurosci Abst **8**:434, 1982
99. Ciriello J, Kline RL, Zhang TX, Caverson MM: Paraventricular nucleus (PVH) lesions alter the development of spontaneous hypertension. Fed Proc **42**:495, 1983
100. Zhang TX, Ciriello J, Caverson MM: Lesions of the paraventricular nucleus (PVH) prevent the elevated arterial pressure and heart rate after aortic baroreceptor denervation in the rat. Fed Proc **42**:495, 1983
101. Zhang TX, Ciriello J: Reversal of the hypertension due to aortic baroreceptor denervation by kainic acid lesions of paraventricular nucleus neurons. Proc Can Fed Biol Soc **26**:84, 1983
102. Ciriello J, Calaresu FR: Monosynaptic pathway from cardiovascular neurons in the nucleus tractus solitarii to the paraventricular nucleus in the cat. Brain Res **193**:529, 1980
103. Ciriello J, Caverson MM, Zhang TX: Direct pathway from cardiovascular neurons in the ventrolateral medulla to the paraventricular nucleus in the cat. Soc Neurosci Abstr **8**:721, 1982
104. Swanson LW, McKellar S: The distribution of oxytocin- and neurophysin-stained fibers in the spinal cord of the rat and monkey. J Comp Neurol **188**:87, 1979
105. Caverson MM, Ciriello J, Calaresu FR: Neurons in the ventrolateral medulla projecting directly to thoracic spinal sympathetic areas receive cardiovascular afferent input. Soc Neurosci Abstr **8**:722, 1982
106. Gilbey MP, Coote JH, Fleetwood-Walker S, Peterson DF: The influence of the paraventricular-spinal pathway, and oxytocin and vasopressin on sympathetic preganglionic neurones. Brain Res **251**:283, 1982

107. Swanson LW, Sawchenko PE, Bérod A, Hartman BK, Helle KB, Vanorden DE: An immunohistochemical study of the organization of catecholaminergic cells and terminal fields in the paraventricular and supraoptic nuclei of the hypothalamus. J Comp Neurol **196:**271, 1981

108. Sawchenko PE, Swanson LW: Immunohistochemical identification of neurons in the paraventricular nucleus of the hypothalamus that project to the medulla or to the spinal cord in the rat. J Comp Neurol **205:**260, 1982

109. Cechetto DF, Calaresu FR: Response of single units in the amygdala to stimulation of buffer nerves in the cat. Am J Physiol **244:**R646, 1983

110. Kapp BS, Gallagher M, Underwood MD, McNall CL, Whitehorn D: Cardiovascular responses elicited by electrical stimulation of the amygdala central nucleus in the rabbit. Brain Res **234:**251, 1982

111. Morin G, Naquet R, Badier M: Stimulation electrique de la region amygdalienne et pression arterielle chez le chat. J Physiol (Paris) **44:**305, 1952

112. Ricardo JA, Koh ET: Anatomical evidence of direct projections from the nucleus of the solitary tract to the hypothalamus, amygdala and other forebrain structures in the rat. Brain Res **153:**1, 1978

113. Pretorius JK, Phelan KD, Mehler WR: Afferent connections of the amygdala in rat. Anat Rec **193:**367,1979

114. Hopkins DA: Amygdalotegmental projections in the rat, cat and rhesus monkey. Neurosci Lett **1:**263, 1975

115. Hopkins DA, McLean JH, Takeuchi Y: Amygdalotegmental projections: light and electron microscope studies utilizing anterograde degeneration and the anterograde and retrograde transport of horseradish peroxidase (HRP). *In* The Amygdaloid Complex, edited by Ben-Ari Y, Amsterdam, Elsevier, 1981, p 133

116. Price JL, Amaral DG: An autoradiographic study of the projections of the central nucleus of the monkey amygdala. J Neurosci **1:**1242, 1981

117. Schwaber JS, Kapp BS, Higgins G: The origin and extent of direct amygdala projections to the region of the dorsal motor nucleus of the vagus and the nucleus of the solitary tract. Neurosci Lett **20:**15, 1980

118. Schwaber JS, Kapp BS, Higgins GA, Rapp PR: Amygdaloid and basal forebrain direct connections with the nucleus of the solitary tract and the dorsal motor nucleus. J Neurosci **2:**1424, 1982

119. Kawai Y, Inagaki S, Shiosaka S, Senba E, Hara Y, Sakanaka M, Takatsuki K, Tohyama M: Long descending projections from amygdaloid somatostatin-containing cells to the lower brain stem. Brain Res **239:**603, 1982

120. Conrad LCA, Pfaff DW: Efferents from the medial basal forebrain and hypothalamus in the rat. II. An autoradiographic study of the anterior hypothalamus. J Comp Neurol **169:**221, 1976

121. Swanson LW: Immunohistochemical evidence for a neurophysin-containing autonomic pathway arising in the paraventricular nucleus of the hypothalamus. Brain Res **123:**356, 1977

Chapter 2

The Pharmacology of Central Adrenergic Mechanisms for Blood Pressure Control

Walter Kobinger

Adrenergic Systems in the Central Nervous System

The presence of the adrenergic transmitters epinephrine and norepinephrine in the brain were described by Vogt in 1954.[1] Subsequently, more detailed studies using modern biochemical and histofluorescence methods have shown a concentration of adrenergic neurons (containing epinephrine, norepinephrine, and dopamine) at those sites in the brainstem known to be important for cardiovascular regulation. Dense networks of adrenergic nerve endings have been demonstrated in the nucleus tractus, solitarii, the nucleus dorsalis of the vagus nerve, and the hypothalamus.[2–5] These findings are strong evidence that adrenergic systems may play a role in central cardiovascular regulation under physiological conditions.

Changes in catecholamine concentrations and turnover in some brain areas have been reported in various forms of spontaneous and experimental hypertension in animals.[6,7] For example, Table 2-1 depicts results from Saavedra et al.[8,91] showing the smaller concentrations of norepinephrine and the enzyme dopamine-β-hydroxylase in discrete areas of the brain of spontaneous hypertensive rats when compared with normotensive Sprague Dawley rats. The enzyme dopamine-β-hydroxylase catalyzes the last step in the biosynthesis of norepinephrine. Such results raise the possibility that adrenergic neurons in the brain participate in the development and maintenance of different hypertensive states. Some of these changes might be causally related to the high blood pressure, whereas others might represent adaptive mechanisms.

Table 2-1
**Norepinephrine Levels and Dopamine-β-Hydroxylase Activity in
Hypothalamic Nuclei of Adult (14-Week-Old) Spontaneously
Hypertensive Rats (SHR) and Normotensive Wistar-Kyoto Rats (WKY)**

Hypothalamic Nuclei	Norepinephrine (ng/mg protein)		Dopamine-β-Hydroxylase (nmol/mg protein/hour)	
	WKY	SHR	WKY	SHR
Nucleus anterior	19 ± 2	9 ± 1[a]	2.0 ± 0.1	1.4 ± 0.2[a]
Nucleus periventricularis	34 ± 3	20 ± 4[a]	4.7 ± 0.2	3.0 ± 0.3[a]
Nucleus paraventricularis	20 ± 2	13 ± 2[a]	2.9 ± 0.2	2.1 ± 0.2[a]
Nucleus dorsomedialis	21 ± 3	13 ± 1[a]	4.2 ± 0.4	3.7 ± 0.3[a]

Results represent $\bar{x}$ ± SEM for groups of eight animals, assayed individually.
[a]Statistically significant ($p < 0.05$) SHR vs. WKY rats. From Saavedra.[91]

At this stage, morphological and biochemical findings do not allow a correlation between central system and defined cardiovascular effects at peripheral sites. Support for central adrenergic mechanisms is provided by the use of drugs, which are specifically effective at adrenergic receptors and moreover are able to penetrate easily into the central nervous system (CNS). Ahlquist[9] proposed two types of adrenoceptors—α and β—based on results with various organs and various drugs. With respect to central cardiovascular control, much information has been gained in recent years on the role and importance of α-adrenoceptors.

The following sections review evidence that stimulation of central medullary α-adrenoceptors leads to cardiovascular depression and that both adrenergic and cholinergic parts of the autonomic nervous system are involved in transmitting the message from brain to periphery (Figure 2-1).

Alpha-Adrenoceptor Stimulation in the Central Nervous System

In the minds of many researchers and physicians, stimulation of α-adrenoceptors is primarily associated with vasoconstriction and blood presssure rise. The idea that stimulation of adrenoceptors within the CNS may induce a decrease in blood pressure was therefore suprising, even though some experimental indications for such a hypothesis can be found in the older literature.[10,11] The antihypertensive agent clonidine served as an important tool to put this idea forward. This imidazoline compound (Table 2-2) was originally designed as a vasoconstricting and decongesting agent, and its sedative and hypotensive properties were discovered by chance.[12,13]

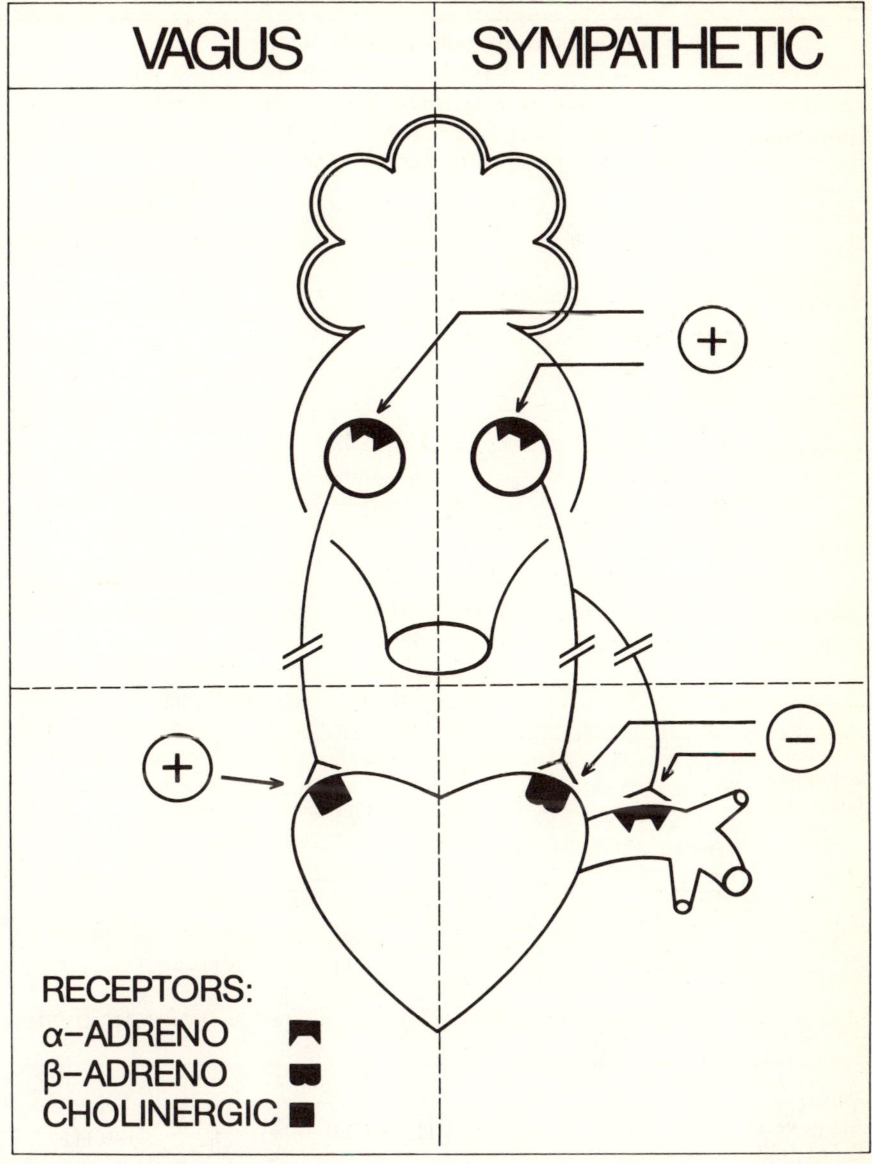

Figure 2-1. Schematic representative of the medullary autonomic nervous sytem (upper part) and the cardiovascular system (lower part). Stimulation (+) of central α-adrenoceptors decreases (−) the activity at peripheral sympathetic sites and increases (+) the activity at peripheral vagal sites.

Table 2-2
Some Drugs of the Clonidine Type

Chemical Group, Substance, Structure	
Iminoimidazolidines: Clonidine	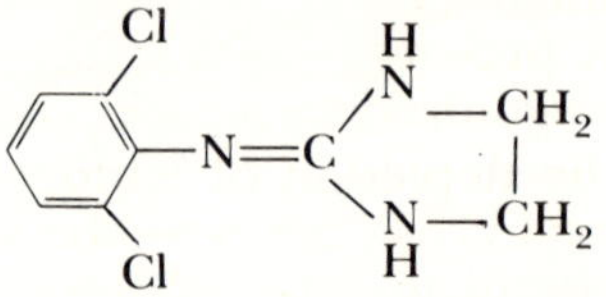
Flutonidine ST 600	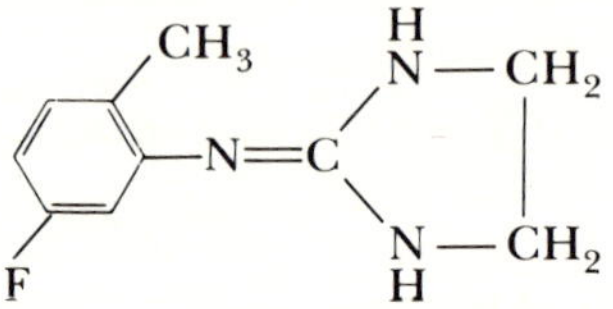
Tiamenidine	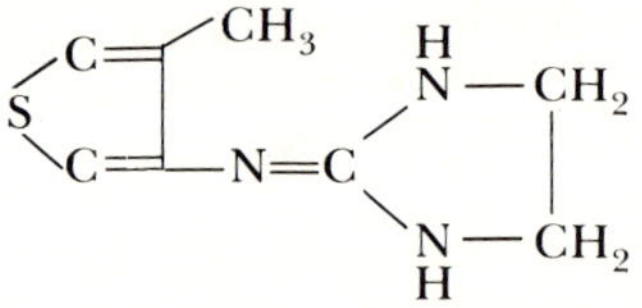
Amino-Dihydrothiazine: Xylazine	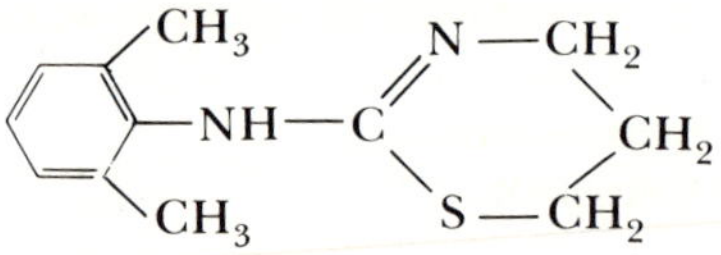
Guanidines: Guanabenz	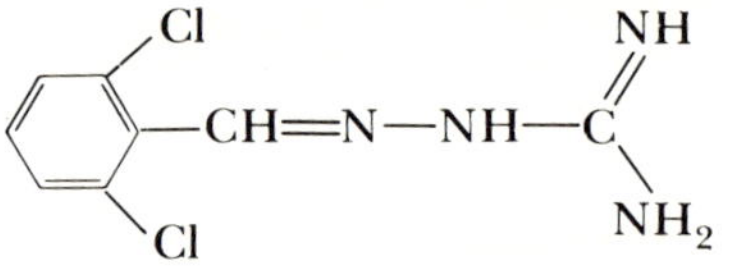
Guanfacine	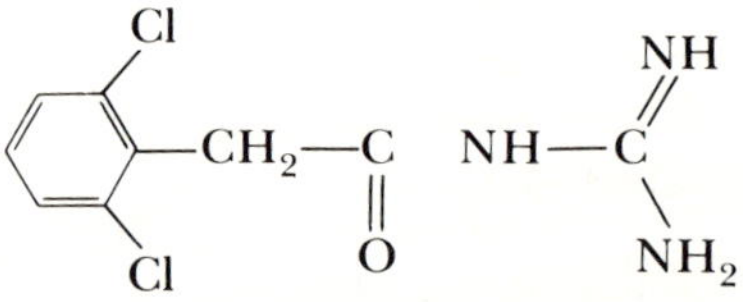
Azepines: Azepexole B-HT 933	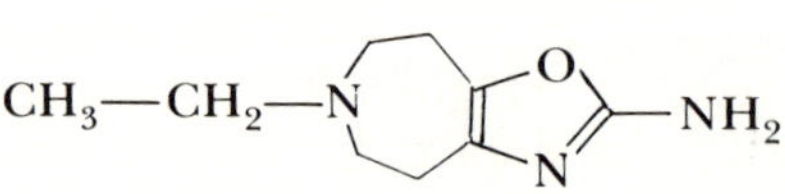
B-HT 920	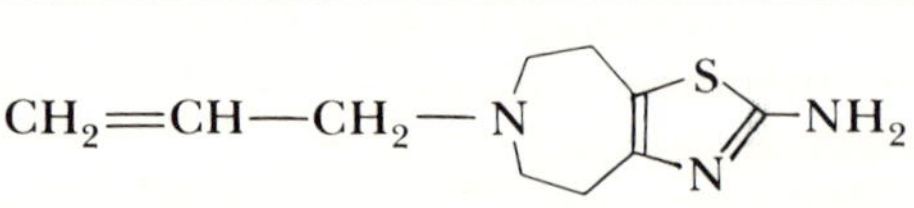

(For references, see Kobinger[92] and text)

In animal experiments, clonidine exerted adrenergic effects—for example, vasoconstriction—following arterial injections and contraction of the nictitating membrane or isolated vascular strips[14,15] (see section later in this chapter on pre- and postsynaptic adrenoceptors). These peripheral effects were antagonized by α-adrenoceptor blocking agents and were still present after the depletion of endogenous catecholamines by reserpine, indicating a direct effect upon α-adrenoceptors.[16,17] There is no evidence that clonidine stimulates β-adrenoceptors.[15]

Clonidine: Central Sympathetic Inhibition and Vagal Activation

The decrease in blood pressure induced by clonidine is due to an effect on the CNS. This was first shown in experiments where intracisternal (cisterna magna cerebellomedullaris) injections of the drug in very small doses decreased blood pressure to a similar extent as much higher doses given intravenously to cats and dogs[18–20] (Figure 2-2).

Analogous results were obtained after injection of the drug into the vertebral artery or in cross-perfusion experiments.[21–23] Figure 2-2 also shows the small, initial blood pressure rise and the increase in total peripheral vascular resistance after intravenous injection, which was not seen after intracisternal injection. This difference is due to the peripheral α-adrenoceptor stimulating effect of the drug, observed only after rapid, systemic application.

The decrease in blood pressure, heart rate, and cardiac output in response to clonidine suggests a decrease of sympathetic activity[16,19] (Figure 2-2; also compare clonidine and the ganglionic blocker trimethidinium). Direct proof of a centrally induced sympathoinhibition is provided by experiments where the electrical discharges of various sympathetic nerves are measured. Clonidine reduces the spontaneous activity in pre- and postganglionic nerves of renal, cardiac, and splanchnic nerves. This effect grossly parallels the cardiovascular depression.[24–27]

In addition to sympathoinhibition, clonidine activates central vagal activity. Facilitation of the vagally mediated baroreceptor reflex has been shown in dogs, rabbits, and rats.[28–31] In β-adrenoceptor-blocked dogs the reflex bradycardia in response to the pressor effect of angiotensin II injected intravenously was facilitated by the intracisternal injection of 1 μg/kg of clonidine, whereas the same dose of clonidine injected intravenously had no effect;[28,29] (Figure 2-3, where this action of the clonidine-like drug B-HT 933 is depicted). An extensive study of the relationship between baroreceptor activity and heart rate response was carried out by Korner et al.[31] in conscious rabbits. Graded changes in blood pressure were produced by inflatable balloons around the abdominal aorta and the inferior vena cava. Figure 2-4 depicts the relationship between blood pressure and heart period (reciprocal value of heart rate) in the control state and during clonidine treatment. The facilitation of the reflex by the drug is seen by the

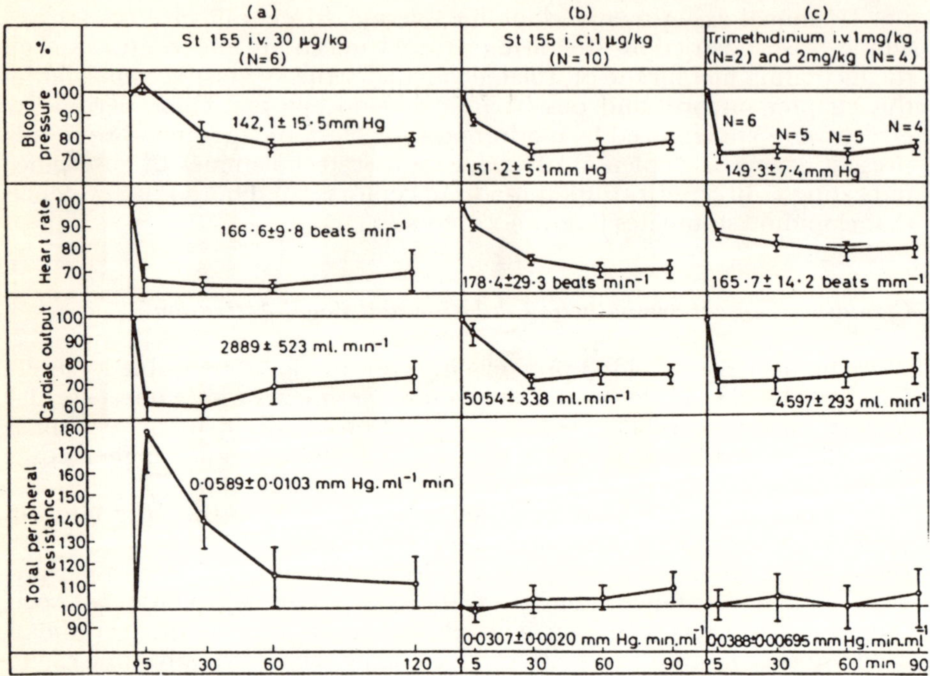

Figure 2-2. Changes in cardiovascular parameters after injection of clonidine (St 155) or the ganglionic blocking agent trimethidinium. (Anesthetized dogs). i.ci. = intracisternal injection (cisterna magna). Abscissae: time in minutes after injection of the drug. Ordinates: values in percent of control (mean ± S.E.M.). Numbers: absolute control values (mean ± S.E.M.). Note the similar cardiovascular response pattern in all experiments. An initial increase in peripheral resistance is only seen after i.v. injection of clonidine. The cardiovascular parameters are lowered to approximately the same extent after 1 µg/kg, i.ci., and 30 µg/kg, i.v. From Kobinger.[15]

shift of the curves to the left, an increase in steepness, and in maximal response. For a detailed analysis of the "resetting" of the reflex the reader is referred to the original paper,[31] which also offers evidence that clonidine affected the central baroreceptor-sensitive neurons by enhancing both vagal excitation and, to a lesser extent, sympathetic inhibition.

Cardiovascular depressor effects of clonidine originate mainly from the medulla oblongata. Sympathoinhibition as well as vagal reflex activation by the drug has been observed after transection of animals' brains rostral to the medulla.[26,32,27,33,34] In addition, depressor effects induced from spinal medullary or supramedullary sites and pressor effects from hypothalamic sites have been proposed.[15,35]

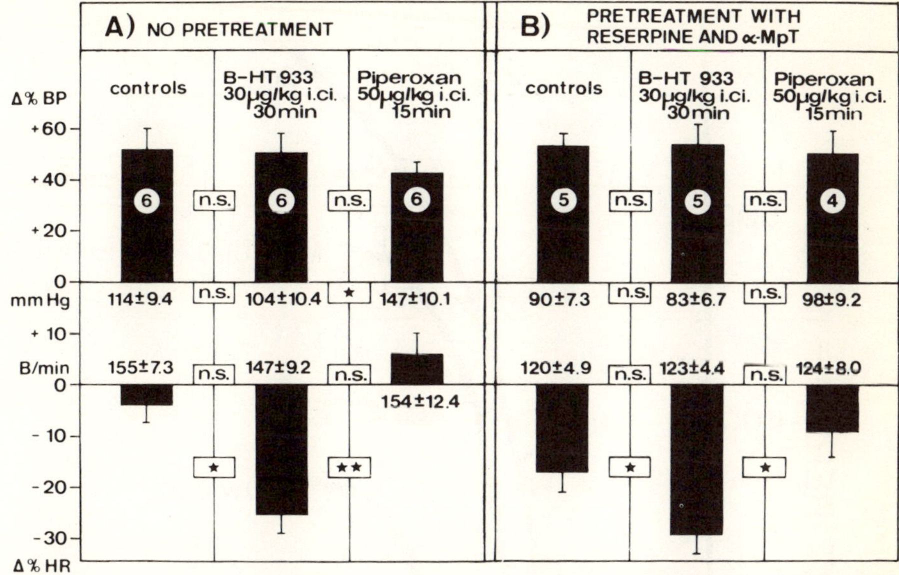

Figure 2-3. Facilitation of the baroreceptor reflex by B-HT 933 (azepexole). Anesthetized dogs with spontaneous respiration and β-adrenoceptor blockade with toliprolol. Mean blood pressure and mean heart rate (B = beats) are given between the columns (± S.E.M.). The baroreceptor reflex was elicited by i.v. injections of angiotensin (0.025–0.3 μg/kg). The resulting maximal changes are expressed as the % of the values before angiotensin and are given by the columns as mean ± S.E.M. BP = blood pressure, HR = heart rate.

Following control injection of angiotensin i.v., B-HT 933 was injected intracisternally (i.ci.) and angiotensin was given 30 minutes later i.v. Then the α-adrenoceptor blocking drug piperoxan was injected i.ci., and 15 min later angiotensin was given i.v. Numbers of dogs are indicated within columns. The significance of differences is indicated between those groups that have been compared: xx, $p <$ 0.01; x, $p <$ 0.05; n.s., not significant ($p >$ 0.05). In A, dogs received no pretreatment. In B, dogs were pretreated with reserpine (5 mg/kg, i.p.) and α-methyl-p-tyrosine (α-Mpt) (300 mg/kg i.p.) 18 hours before the experiment. From Kobinger and Pichler,[84] Pichler et al.[54]

Clonidine and α-Adrenoceptor Blocking Drugs

The conclusion that central cardiovascular effects of clonidine are mediated by the stimulation of central α-adrenoceptors was first drawn from results showing that clonidine's effects can be antagonized by α-adrenoceptor blocking drugs. Schmitt et al.[36,37] reported that treatment with yohimbine or piperoxan prevented the decrease in sympathetic nerve activity (electrical discharges) usually caused by clonidine. Likewise, the vagally mediated baroreceptor reflex, as enhanced by clonidine, was antag-

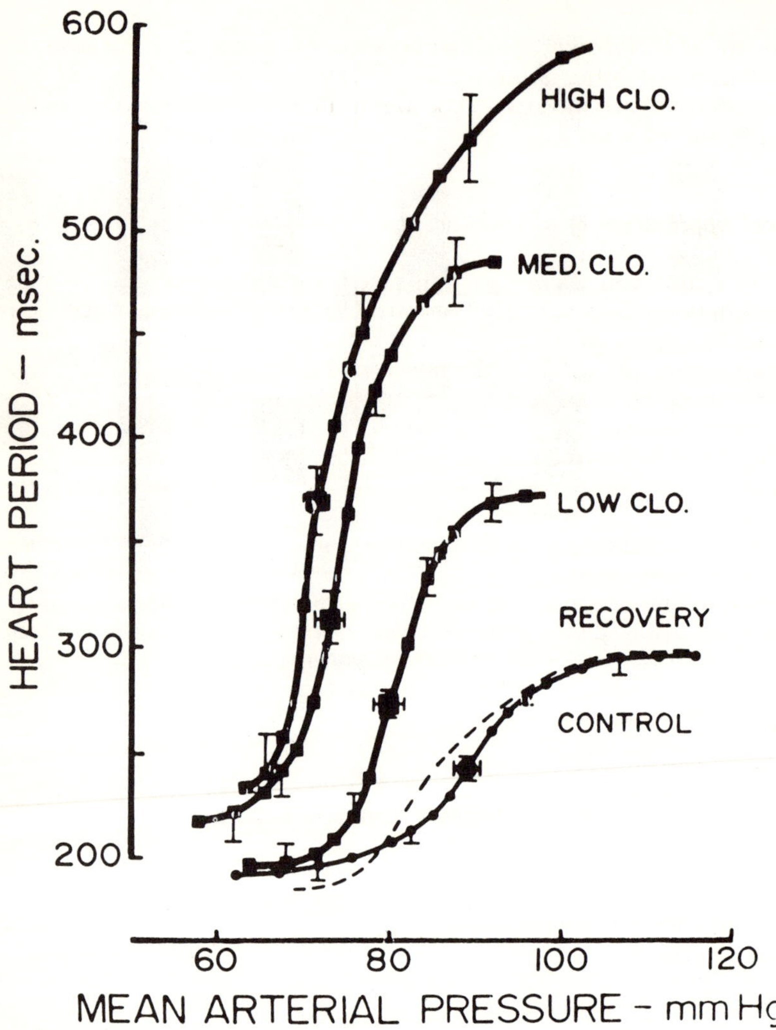

Figure 2-4. Effect of clonidine on baroreceptor reflex response. In conscious rabbits (n = 5), blood pressure was changed by brief inflation of perivascular balloons around aorta and inferior vena cava. Abscissa: mean arterial blood pressure, mm Hg. Ordinate: heart period = pulse interval in msec. Control, after 30 min of continous i.v. infusion of clonidine at 0.5 µg/kg/min (LOW CLO.), 1.0 µg/min (MED CLO.) or 1.5 µg/kg/min (HIGH CLO.), and 1 hr after stopping infusion (RECOVERY). From Korner et al.[31]

onized by the subsequent intravenous or intracisternal injections of phentolamine or other antagonists.[28,38] In both experimental designs, no α-adrenoceptors are interposed between the CNS and the effector systems. Thus, the site of interaction must be located in the CNS.

Cerebral Application of α-Adrenoceptor Stimulating Drugs

Hoyer and van Zwieten[39,40] infused amphetamine and related sympathomimetic amines into the vertebral artery of cats and recorded a decrease of blood pressure.

High doses of norepinephrine injected intracisternally into cats have been shown to decrease blood pressure, heart rate, and electrical activity of sympathetic nerves.[41] A decrease in blood pressure and heart rate has also been reported following microinjection of catecholamines (noradrenaline, adrenaline, α-methylnoradrenaline) into the lower brainstem and the area of the nucleus of the solitary tract.[42-44]

The intracisternal injection of three imidazolines—naphazoline, oxymetazoline, and St 91 [2-(2,6-diethylphenylamino)-2-imidazoline]—that penetrate the blood brain barrier poorly and increase blood pressure after intravenous application produces the cardiovascular and autonomic response pattern as described for clonidine. Following central application, these drugs decrease blood pressure and heart rate in vagotomized cats and dogs, decrease splanchnic nerve activity in cats, and facilitate the vagally mediated baroreceptor reflex after inhibition of β-adrenoceptors in dogs.[45,46] These findings strongly indicate that stimulation of central α-adrenoceptors causes the cardiovascular depression of the clonidine type (Figure 2-1).

The Possible Role of Endogenous Norepinephrine on Central Cardiovascular Regulation

The demonstration of central α-adrenoceptors led to the assumption that under physiological conditions endogenous norepinephrine (or epinephrine) is liberated from distinct neurons in the CNS and triggers responses similar to those described for the α-adrenoceptor agonists clonidine or similar drugs following cerebral administration. This assumption seems even more plausible if one considers the "physiological" response pattern following central α-adrenoceptor stimulation, as shown by the reciprocal action of both parts of the autonomic nervous system (Figure 2-1). A decrease in sympathetic activity and an increase in vagal activity are known to occur during electrical stimulation of the sympathoinhibitory areas of the anterior hypothalamus, of the depressor areas of the anterior cingulate gyrus, and of certain parts of the medulla (depressor areas of the vasomotor center) and afferent baroreceptor nerves.[47-49]

A depressor effect of liberated endogenous norepinephrine on medullary structures was also suggested by Korner and Head[50] using the neurotoxin, 6-hydroxydopamine. This drug has been used for selective destruction of catecholamine-containing neurons;[51] however, release of the transmitter from nerve terminals precedes the stage of neuronal block.[52] Following intracisternal injection into midbrain-sectioned rabbits, 6-hydroxydopamine produced a decrease in blood pressure and heart rate during the first few hours, as well as facilitation of the vagally mediated baroreceptor reflex activity.[50] These results are in accordance with the hypothesis that endogenous catecholamines mediate cardiovascular depression.

The early observations that clonidine facilitates the cardiodepressor reflex by a central effect led to the assumption that these drugs mimic endogenous norepinephrine and that the latter is an essential link in the central part of the reflex loop.[53] To evaluate this hypothesis, dogs were pretreated with a β-adrenoceptor blocking agent (to exclude peripheral adrenergic influences on the heart). By means of intravenous injections of angiotensin II, blood pressure was increased to stimulate baroreceptors, and a resulting reflex bradycardia was observed. Under the experimental conditions this reflex response can be assumed to be mediated by the efferent part of the vagus nerve. No adrenergic transmitter is involved in the peripheral part of the reflex. The α-adrenoceptor blocking drug phentolamine was then injected intracisternally and markedly reduced the cardiodepressor reflex, a result in accordance with the hypothesis that noradrenaline is an essential transmitter in the reflex chain.

This hypothesis, however, had to be discarded in the next experimental step, where the dogs were pretreated with reserpine in order to deplete their endogenous noradrenaline stores. These animals still exerted a marked reflex bradycardia, and this result practically excluded the hypothesis of norepinephrine as a transmitter. In these reserpine-treated dogs, clonidine effectively facilitated the baroreceptor reflex as in controls, and this was antagonized by phentolamine.[53] The results were interpreted as follows: α-adrenoceptors within the brain mediate a facilitation of the baroreceptor reflex; they do not constitute an essential link within the reflex chain but serve a modulatory (facilitatory) function.

Similar results were obtained in later studies where animals (rats, dogs) were pretreated with reserpine and α-methyl-p-tyrosine to exclude not only stores but also the synthesis of catecholamines and where the α_2-selective agonist B-HT 933 (azepexole; see section on pre- and postsynaptic adrenoreceptors; and Figure 2-3) was used instead of clonidine.[33,54]

Clonidine-like Drugs

From the foregoing sections it seems logical to assume that each α-adrenoceptor agonist might exert cardiovascular depressor activities like clonidine provided the drug penetrates from the bloodstream to cardiovascular centers in the brain. The lipid solubility of a drug is an important factor for penetration. A number of imidazolines, closely related chemically to clonidine, were tested in two studies[55,56] with respect to blood pressure increase in spinal or pithed rats (i.e., preparations where the brain was destroyed; test models for peripheral α-adrenoceptor stimulation), and decreases in heart rate or blood pressure were observed in vagotomized or intact rats, respectively (test models for central cardiovascular depression). The central and peripheral effects were highly correlated, provided the partition coefficient octanol/buffer at pH 7.4 was considered for each drug.[57]

In recent years a number of substances have been described that fulfill the criteria for α-adrenoceptor agonists and penetrate the blood brain barrier. These agents have been classified as "clonidine-like drugs."[15] Some of these drugs are chemically close congeners of clonidine, whereas others are chemically quite different (Table 2-2).

Alpha-Adrenoceptor Subtypes

Definition at Peripheral Sites: Pre- and Postsynaptic, α_1 and α_2-Adrenoceptors

Alpha adrenoceptors can be classified on a morphological basis as pre- and postsynaptic.[58,59] The "classical" postsynaptic receptor is localized on the effector organ and mediates the response via muscular, secretory, or biochemical systems. The presynaptic receptor is located on nerve terminals of neurons and modifies the release process of the natural transmitter. In the case of adrenergic neurons, stimulation of presynaptic α-adrenoceptors inhibits the release of catecholamines. The conclusion that pre- and postsynaptic α-adrenoceptors are different is based on the different activity ratios of drugs. Within a series of agonists, clonidine, oxymetazoline, and α-methylnoradrenaline preferentially act presynaptically, whereas phenylephrine and methoxamine preferentially act postsynaptically.[60] Among antagonists, yohimbine preferentially acts presynaptically, but phenoxybenzamine and prazosin act postsynaptically.[59,61,62]

Alpha adrenoceptors can also be classified on an entirely pharmacological basis.[62a–64] The subclass α_1 was proposed for receptor sites where phenylephrine is more potent as an agonist than clonidine, and α_2 for those receptor sites where clonidine is more effective than phenylephrine.

Both subtypes, α_1 and α_2 respectively, might be present post- as well as presynaptically, and both pharmacological types have even been observed at the same morphological site (Figure 2-5;[65–67a]). Evidence is primarily based on the "differential antagonism" of one α-adrenoceptor blocker against two different agonists. For example, in pithed rats, the blood pres-

SYNAPTIC LOCATION

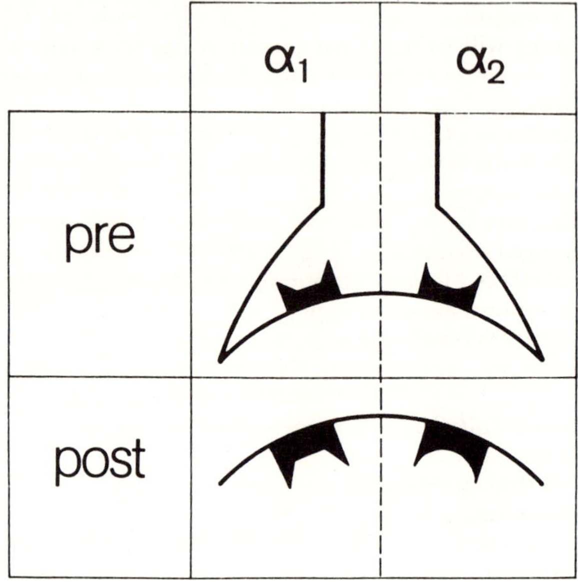

Figure 2-5. α-adrenoceptors at adrenergic neurone terminals (presynaptic = pre) and target tissues (postsynaptic = post). The classification into the subtypes pre- and postsynaptic is morphological. The classification α_1 and α_2 is pharmacological, based on different responses to different drugs (agonists and antagonists). As shown in the figure, the subtypes α_1 as well as α_2 might be present pre- as well as postsynaptically. From Kobinger.[93]

sure increasing effects of clonidine and methoxamine were determined. The dose-response curve of clonidine was shifted by a given dose of yohimbine much more to the right along the abscissa (i.e., to higher agonist doses) than was the dose-response curve of methoxamine. Conversely, prazosin was a more effective antagonist against methoxamine than against clonidine.[67] The best explanation for these results is the assumption of two receptor types at the postsynaptic, vasoconstrictor effector sites: one type, α_1, with high affinity for methoxamine and prazosin, and another type, α_2, with high affinity for clonidine and yohimbine.

From analogous experiments the presence of two receptor subtypes has also been proposed at presynaptic sites. In pithed rats, electrical stimulation with low frequency impulses within the spinal channel at C_7-T_1 stimulates sympathetic fibers, which increases the heart rate, the ultimate responses being mediated by β-adrenoceptors. Injection of α-adrenergic drugs inhibits this tachycardic response by a presynaptic effect; the inhibition is antagonized by α-adrenergic blocking agents. Prazosin proved more effective in antagonizing methoxamine than clonidine, and yohimbine proved more effective in antagonizing clonidine than methoxamine.[67,68]

From the foregoing it appears as a general concept that the response of a target system will depend on (1) the α_1/α_2-selectivity ratio of a given substance (agonist or antagonist), and (2) the α_1/α_2-adrenoceptor ratio in the target system.

For determination of the α_1/α_2-selectivity ratios of various agonists, the method of the "differential antagonism" has been further developed.[69] Pithed rats were treated with a β-adrenoceptor blocker. This made it possible to test α-agonists with additional β-adrenoceptor activity, which might interfere with vasoconstriction. Dose-response curves for the blood pressure increasing effect of various α-adrenoceptor agonists were determined without treatment and after treatment with various doses of the antagonists prazosin (α_1-selective) and rauwolscine (α_2-selective). The shift of the dose-response curve of an agonist along the abscissa was determined by the ratio (f) of the agonist doses with or without antagonist, which caused an equi-effective response (blood pressure increase of 50 mm Hg). In a double logarithmic system, f was plotted against the antagonist dose, and the dose was determined that produced a yield of f = 10 (D10). Table 2-3 shows the different D10 for rauwolscine (R) and prazosin (P) respectively, as determined for various agonists. The ratio D10R/D10P has been proposed as a measure of the α_1/α_2-selectivity ratio for a given agonist. As can be seen from Table 2-3, methoxamine and phenylephrine exert the highest α_1/α_2 selectivity ratio and B-HT 920 and B-HT 933 the lowest—i.e., the highest relative selectivity for α_2; α-methyl norepinephrine and clonidine take an intermediate position.

For an estimation of the α_1/α_2-adrenoceptor ratio of various peripheral target organs the two drugs methoxamine and B-HT 920 have been used, based on their selective α_1 and α_2 agonistic effect respectively (Table 2-3). Equieffective doses of both drugs were evaluated, and the dose ratio B-HT 920/methoxamine has been proposed as a relative measure of the α_1/α_2-adrenoceptor ratio in the target organ.[69] This ratio (termed the ratio of α_1/α_2 "importance") also involves the steps between receptor interaction and biological response, and thus is not identical but might parallel the ratio of the number α_1/α_2-receptors. Inspection of Figure 2-6 reveals approximately equal "importance" of both receptor types in the peripheral vascular system (blood pressure rise in pithed rats).

The low α_1/α_2 (i.e., high α_2/α_1) adrenoceptor ratio at presynaptic sites deserves some comment. It is obvious that drugs that are primarily active at α_2-adrenoceptors will exert a higher pre/postsynaptic activity ratio than drugs that are primarily active at α_1-adrenoceptors, provided the postsynaptic sites have a higher α_1/α_2-receptor ratio than the presynaptic site. This is the case in most vascular preparations, as in pithed rats or isolated artery strips. In Table 2-3 (last column), the post/presynaptic activity ratios

Table 2-3

Agonist	D_{10} (mg/kg i.v.)		$\dfrac{D_{10R}}{D_{10P}}$	$\dfrac{ID_{50}}{PD_{30}}$
	Rauwolscine	Prazosin		
B-HT 920	1.25	100.0	0.012	0.09
B-HT 933 (Azepexole)	0.7	9.0	0.08	0.22
α-m-Norepinephrine	1.9	10.0	0.19	/
Xylazine	3.6	2.8	1.28	0.46
Clonidine	5.5	0.7	7.86	0.45
Norepinephrine	4.8	0.55	8.73	/
Epinephrine	3.7	0.12	30.83	/
St 91	14.0	0.36	38.89	1.45
Phenylephrine	9.5	0.06	158.33	/
Methoxamine	15.0	0.07	214.28	5.88

α_1/α_2 adrenoceptor selectivity and post/presynaptic α-adrenoceptor potency ratio of various agonists. The blood pressure increasing effect of the agonists was determined in pithed rats by means of dose-response curves. The α-adrenoceptor antagonists rauwolscine and prazosin shifted the dose-response curves to the right. Those antagonist doses were evaluated that caused a tenfold shift of agonist dose-response curves to the right (D_{10}). The ratio D_{10}rauwolscine/D_{10}prazosin (D_{10R}/D_{10P}) was proposed as a measure of the α_1/α_2-selectivity for the agonists tested. In these experiments, animals were treated with a β-adrenoceptor blocking agent. The post/presynaptic activity ratio is expressed by the ratio ID_{50}/PD_{30}, where ID_{50} = dose that inhibited electrically induced tachycardia in pithed rats by 50% (presynaptic effect); PD_{30} = dose that increased blood pressure in spinal rats by 30 mm Hg (postsynaptic effect). The ratios D_{10R}/D_{10P} and ID_{50}/PD_{30} are significantly correlated ($r = 0.998$; $P < 0.001$; $n = 6$). From Kobinger and Pichler.[69]

for some agonists are given (ID50/PD30), and among two substances, significantly correlate with the α_1/α_2-activity ratio ($P < 0.001$).

Alpha-Adrenoceptor Subtypes at Central Cardiovascular Sites

Pre- or Postsynaptic α-Adrenoceptors? Presynaptic α-adrenoceptors in the CNS might be located on neuron endings and also on cell bodies (soma-dendritic receptors, autoreceptors).[70,71] There is no doubt that presynaptic α-adrenoceptors exist within the CNS, and their stimulation decreases adrenergic neuron activity. Thus, clonidine or oxymetazoline inhibits the liberation of norepinephrine from rat brain slices, induced by electrical field stimulation.[72,73] The spontaneous firing rate of adrenergic cells in the locus coeruleus of rats is also inhibited by the local application of clonidine.[71]

It has been proposed that the cardiovascular depressor effects of centrally active α-adrenoceptor agonists are caused by stimulation of such pre-

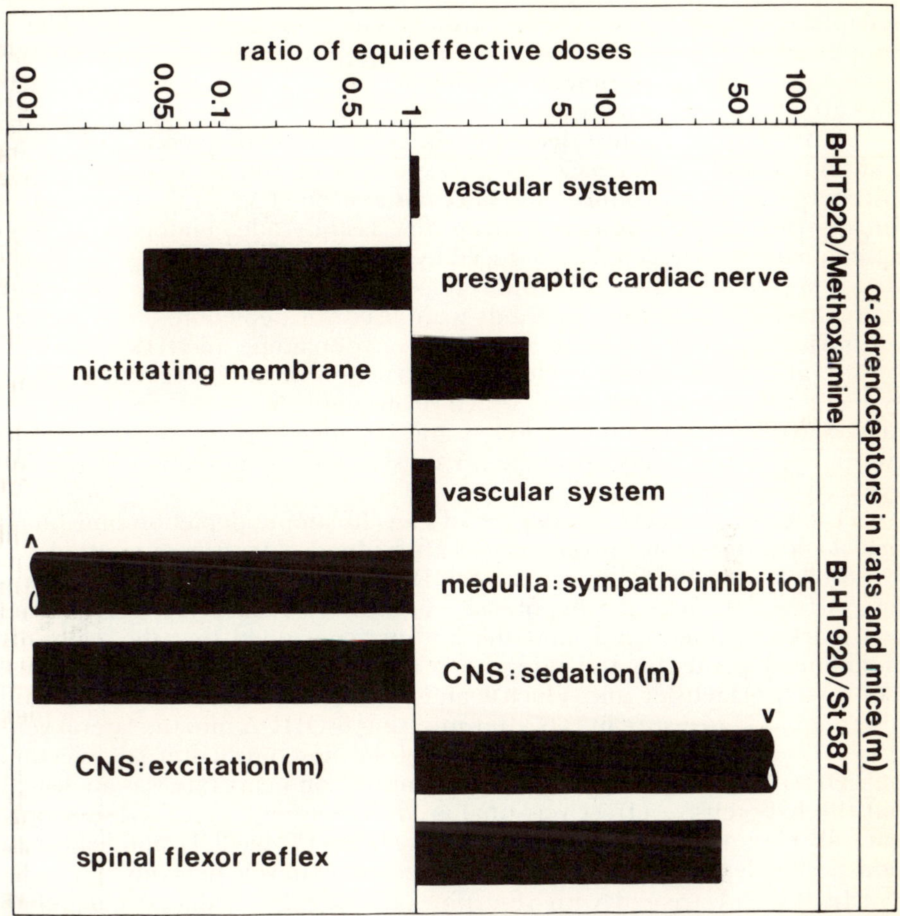

Figure 2-6. Ratios of equipotent doses (ordinate) of two selective agonists: B-HT 920 (α_2) and methoxamine (α_1) or St 587 (α_1, easily penetrates the blood brain barrier) in different test-systems at peripheral and CNS sites. The dose ratio B-HT 920/methoxamine or St 587 respectively is proposed as an expression of the relative distribution of α_1/α_2 adrenoceptors ("receptor importance").

From dose response curves the following parameters were determined: Vascular system: increase in blood pressure of 50 mm Hg, pithed rats. Presynaptic cardiac nerve: 50% inhibition of tachycardia as induced by electrical stimulation of the cardiac nerves in pithed rats. Nictitating membrane: 50% contraction, pithed rats. Medulla sympathoinhibition: 50% decrease of heart rate in vagotomized rats. CNS sedation: 50% decrease of motility, mice. CNS excitation: 100% increase in motility of mice previously treated with reserpine + apomorphine. Spinal flexor reflex: in spinal cord transected rats (midthoracic level), increase in reflex response to an arbitrarity given level. From Kobinger and Pichler.[88]

synaptic α-adrenoceptors within cardiovascular regulatory centers. This is supported by the observation that those agonists (such as clonidine) and antagonists (such as yohimbine), which are active at central cardiovascular sites are also preferentially active at peripheral presynaptic sites.[73,74]

A presynaptic agonist decreases the release of endogenous adrenergic transmitter and a pharmacological response can only be expected if the adrenergic neuron produces and liberates a certain level of the transmitter. In a series of experiments during the last decade, endogenous norepinephrine was depleted or reduced by pharmacological means, assuming that a presynaptically acting α-adrenoceptor agonist would be ineffective thereafter. The following methods were used for depletion: intracisternal or intraventricular injection of 6-hydroxydopamine (6-OHDA), which causes, after some days, a selective destruction of adrenergic neurons;[51] systemic injection of reserpine, which profoundly decreases catecholamine (and 5-hydroxytryptamine) stores;[75] and systemic injection of α-methyl-p-tyrosine, which inhibits norepinephrine synthesis by inhibition of the enzyme tyrosine hydroxylase.[76]

Table 2-4 presents the degree of catecholamine depletion and pharmacological results in various species after identical treatment methods.

Dollery and Reid[77] injected 6-OHDA into the cisterna magna of rabbits. A few days later the hypotensive and bradycardic effect of clonidine was markedly attenuated, and the authors concluded that the action of clonidine depends on the integrity of central monoaminergic neurons. Conversely, Haeusler and Finch[78] and Finch[79] found that clonidine still lowered blood pressure in rats after injecting 6-OHDA into the lateral ventricle. Reynoldson et al.[80] found that following intracisternal injection of 6-OHDA into rabbits the effect of clonidine on heart rate was abolished but the hypotensive effect was unaltered. Treatment with 6-OHDA only partially eliminates norepinephrine in the brain (Table 2-4), and leads to a nonspecific destruction of other, noncatecholaminergic neurons.[81]

In dogs pretreated with reserpine, the vagally mediated baroreflex bradycardia is facilitated by clonidine as it is in controls.[53] Analogous results were obtained in rats pretreated with reserpine or with α-methyl-p-tyrosine.[30,33] Haeusler[82] pretreated cats with reserpine and α-methyl-p-tyrosine; intravenous injection of clonidine (30–300 μg/kg) reduced electrical activity of the splanchnic nerve, but somewhat less than in controls. Intracisternal injection of clonidine (1 μg/kg), oxymetazoline, azepine derivatives B-HT 933 (azepexole), or B-HT 920 decreased splanchnic nerve discharges in reserpine + α-methyl-p-tyrosine pretreated cats similar to that in controls.[46,54,83] In dogs pretreated with reserpine and α-methyl-p-tyrosine, the intracisternal injection of B-HT 933 (azepexole) facilitated the vagally mediated baroreflex bradycardia, similar to controls (Figure 2-3).[54]

Treatment with reserpine and with reserpine + α-methyl-p-tyrosine

Table 2-4

Decrease of Brain Norepinephrine Concentrations (Analytical Results) and Pharmacological Actions of α-Adrenoceptor Stimulation in the CNS Following Various Treatments. α-mpt = Alpha-methylparatyrosine, 6-OHDA = 6-OH Dopamine, BP = Blood Pressure, HR = Heart Rate, i.ci. = Intracisternal

| | Determination of Norepinephrine in Brain | | | | Pharmacology of CNS α-Adrenoceptor Stimulation | |
| | | Concentration ng/g | | | | |
Treatment	Species	Control	Treatment	References	Results	References
6-OHDA i.ci. 500 µg/kg 10 days before	rabbits*	261 ± 10	58 ± 8	10	Effect of i.v. clonidine on BP and HR significantly reduced; effect of i.ci. clonidine abolished	10
6-OHDA i.ci. 600 µg/kg 7 days before	rabbits‡	466 ± 20§	276 ± 34‡	80	Effect of i.c v. clonidine on HR abolished or reduced, on BP unchanged	80
Reserpine 7.5 mg/kg† α-mpt 250 mg/kg	rats*	590 ± 20	<8	94	i.v. clonidine facilitated vagal reflex bradycardia as in controls	30, 33
Reserpine 5 mg/kg† α-mpt 300 mg/kg	dogs†	396 ± 47	2.3 ± 0.6	54	i.ci. B-HT 933 facilitated vagal reflex bradycardia as in controls	54
Reserpine 5 mg/kg† α-mpt 2 × 300 mg/kg	cats†	223 ± 39	<5	82	i.v. clonidine reduced or abolished spontaneous sympathetic nerve activity but less than in controls	82
					i.ci. clonidine, i.ci. oxymetazoline, i.ci. B-HT 933 or i.ci. B-HT 920 decreased spontaneous sympathetic nerve activity as in controls	46, 54, 83

*whole brain
†medulla
‡pons + medulla
§total catecholamines determined

efficiently depletes the brain of endogenous norepinephrine (Table 2-4). The ability of clonidine and other centrally active α-adrenoceptor agonists to elicit comparable cardiovascular depression in these treated animals as in controls practically excludes the presynaptic mode of action, and it strongly suggests the effect is on α-adrenoceptors, which act upon cells that are nonadrenergic. The complete or partial inhibition of the effect of clonidine, following pretreatment with 6-OHDA, as reported by some authors (Table 2-4 and preceding), can hardly be explained by the removal of endogenous norepinephrine, which is considerably less than following pretreatment with reserpine + α-methyl-p-tyrosine (Table 2-4). It may be explained by the destruction of other, non-catecholaminergic neurons.[81]

α_1- or α_2-Adrenoceptors? There are a number of arguments indicating that the α_2-type of adrenoceptors triggers cardiovascular depression within the CNS. All clonidine-like drugs are agonists with high α_2/α_1 (i.e., low α_1/α_2) selectivity ratio, and some of these are given in Table 2-3. The two drugs with the highest selectivity toward α_2-adrenoceptors and nearly no effect at α_1-adrenoceptors, B-HT 920 and B-HT 933 (azepexole), exert the typical signs of central sympathoinhibition and vagal reflex activation, which characterize the cardiovascular pattern of central α-adrenoceptor stimulation[83,84] (Figure 2-6). An interesting detail is the high α_2/α_1 ratio of α-methyl norepinephrine (Table 2-3), structurally more related to phenylephrine (which has a high α_1/α_2 ratio) than to any of the "clonidine-like" drugs. This drug is the active metabolite of the antihypertensive agent, α-methyldopa, and within the CNS exerts effects similar to clonidine.[85,86]

de Jong et al.[87] described a congener of clonidine, St 587 [2-(2-chloro-5-trifluoromethylphenylimino)imidazolidine], a highly selective α_1 agonist, which after intravenous injection increases blood pressure but does not induce a secondary pressure fall or hypotension after injection into the vertebral artery of cats. These results suggest that α_1-adrenoceptors in the brain are not involved in hypotensive activities of clonidine-like drugs. Contrary to methoxamine, St 587 easily penetrates from bloodstream to brain.

Activity ratios for B-HT 920/St 587 have now been determined for various central nervous effects to estimate the α_1/α_2 receptor ratios (Figure 2-5). The central sympathoinhibitory effects of clonidine-like drugs have been investigated in urethane anesthetized, vagotomized rats by the decrease in heart rate following intravenous injection. In this test, B-HT 920 proved effective but St 587 practically ineffective. The indefinable small dose ratio B-HT 920/St 587 from Figure 2-5 (medulla: sympathoinhibition) is the quantitative expression of the indefinable high α_2/α_1-adrenoceptor ratio, responsible for central sympathoinhibition.[88]

Alpha 2-adrenoceptors as mediators of the blood pressure lowering effect of clonidine were also suggested by experiments with α-adrenoceptor antagonists. The α_2-selective drug rauwolscine was more effective in antagonizing the hypotensive effect of clonidine than the stereoisomer corynanthine, which is α_1-selective.[89]

Alpha-Adrenoceptor Subtypes at Central Sites Not Involved in Cardiovascular Regulation

It is of interest to compare the central α-adrenoceptors responsible for cardiovascular functions with those that mediate other, non-cardiovascular events. Therefore the method to determine α_1/α_2-adrenoceptor ratios in various target tissues in the periphery and at central sympathoregulatory sites was extended (see preceding sections).[88] Dose ratios for B-HT 920/St 587 were determined and the results summarized in Figure 2-5. Sedation was tested by the 50% decrease in motility of mice during the exploratory phase—i.e., immediately after placing the animals into the cages where motility was measured. The small dose ratio B-HT 920/St 587 indicates the high α_2/α_1 (i.e., small α_1/α_2) receptor ratio responsible for sedation (Figure 2-5, CNS sedation).

Clonidine has also been reported to exert stimulating effects in the CNS. After treatment with reserpine, mice are practically motionless. Following stimulation of dopaminergic receptors by apomorphine, some activity can be achieved, and additional injection of clonidine further stimulates motility.[90]

B-HT 920 is practically ineffective but St 587 is active when used instead of clonidine (Figure 2-5). Thus an indefinable high α_1/α_2-adrenoceptor ratio was calculated as being responsible for this CNS stimulating quality. In rats with spinal cord transection in the mid-thoracic region, the hind limb flexor reflex can be activated by clonidine.[90] The high dose ratio B-HT 920/St 587 in Figure 2-5 "spinal flexor reflex" reveals the importance of the α_1-adrenoceptor subgroup.

In conclusion and from inspection of Figure 2-5 it can be said that a great variety of α_1/α_2-adrenoceptor ratios are involved in responses of various target systems—centrally as well as peripherally. The α_2-subtype seems mainly responsible for central cardiovascular depression as well as for sedation and peripheral presynaptic nerve inhibition.

References

1. Vogt M: The concentration of sympathin in different parts of the central nervous system under normal conditions and after the administration of drugs. J Physiol **123**:451, 1954
2. Fuxe K: The distribution of monoamine terminals in the central nervous system. Acta Physiol Scand **64**(Suppl 247):1965
3. Andén NE, Dahlström A, Fuxe K, Larsson K, Olson L, Ungerstedt U: Ascending monoamine neurons to the telencephalon and diencephalon. Acta Physiol Scand **67**:313, 1966
4. Ungerstedt U: Stereotaxic mapping of the monoamine pathways in the rat brain. Acta Physiol Scand **367**(Suppl):1, 1971
5. Palkovits M: The anatomy of central cardiovascular neurons. *In* Central Adrenaline Neurons, edited by Fuxe K, Goldstein M, Hökfelt B, Hökfelt T. Oxford, Pergamon Press, 1980, p 3

6. Fuxe K, Ganten D, Bolme P, Agnati LF, Hökfelt T, Andersson K, Goldstein M, Härfenstrand A, Unger T, Rascher W: The role of central catecholamine pathways in spontaneous and renal hypertension. *In* Central Adrenaline Neurons, edited by Fuxe K, Goldstein M, Hökfelt B, Hökfelt T. Oxford, Pergamon Press, 1980, p 259

7. Saavedra JM: Brain stem adrenergic neurons participate in the regulation of the stress response and in genetic and experimental hyptertension. *In* Central Adrenaline Neurons, edited by Fuxe K, Goldstein M, Hökfelt B, Hökfelt T. Oxford, Pergamon Press, 1980, p 235

8. Saavedra JM, Grobecker H, Axelrod J: Changes in central catecholamines neurons in the spontaneously (genetic) hypertensive rat. Circ Res **42**:529, 1978

9. Ahlquist RP: A study of the adrenergic receptors. Amer J Physiol **153**:586, 1948

10. Heller H: Über die zentrale Blutdruckwirkung des Adrenalins. Naunyn Schmiedeberg's Arch Pharmacol **173**:291, 1933

11. McCubbin JW, Kaneko Y, Page IH: Ability of serotonin and norepinephrine to mimic the central effects of reserpine on vasomotor activity. Circ Res **8**:849, 1960

12. Stähle H: Clonidine. *In* Chronicles of Drug Discovery 1, edited by Bindra JS, Lednicer D. New York, Wiley, 1982, p 87

13. Kobinger W: Central Antihypertensives. *In* Discoveries in Pharmacology, Vol 2, edited by Parnham MJ, Bruinvels J. Amsterdam, Elsevier Biomedical Press, in press

14. Schmitt H: The pharmacology of clonidine and related products. *In* Handbook of Experimental Pharmacology, edited by Gross F. New York, Springer, 1977, p 299

15. Kobinger W: Central α-adrenergic systems as targets for hypotensive drugs. Rev Physiol Biochem Pharmacol **81**:40, 1978

16. Kobinger W, Walland A: Kreislaufuntersuchungen mit 2-(2,6-dichlorphenyl-amino)-2-imidazolinhydrochloride. Arzneim Forsch **17**:292, 1967

17. Boissier JR, Giudicelli JF, Fichelle J, Schmitt H, Schmitt H: Cardiovascular effects of 2-(2,6-dichlorphenylamino)-2-imidazoline-hydrochloride (St 155). I. Peripheral sympathetic system. Eur J Pharmacol **2**:333, 1968

18. Kobinger W: Über den Wirkungsmechanismus einer neuen anti-hypertensiven Substanz mit Imidazolinstruktur. Naunyn Schmiedeberg's Arch Pharmacol **258**:48, 1967

19. Kobinger W, Walland A: Investigations into the mechanism of the hypotensive effect of 2-(2,6-dichlorphenylamino)-2-imidazoline HCl. Eur J Pharmacol **2**:155, 1967

20. Onesti G, Schwartz AB, Kim KE, Paz-Martinez V, Swartz CH: Antihypertensive effect of clonidine. Circ Res **28** (Suppl 2):53, 1971

21. Sattler RW, van Zwieten PA: Acute hypotensive action of 2-(2,6-dichlor-phenylamino)-2-imidazoline hydrochloride (St 155) after infusion into the cat's vertebral artery. Eur J Pharmacol **2**:9, 1967

22. Constantine JW, McShane WK: Analysis of the cardiovascular effects of 2-(2,6-dichlorphenylamino)-2-imidazoline hydrochloride (catapresan). Eur J Pharmacol **4**:109, 1968

23. Sherman GP, Grega GJ, Woods RJ, Buckley JP: Evidence for a central hypotensive mechanism of 2-(2,6-dichlorphenylamino)-2-imidazoline (catapresan, St 155). Eur J Pharmacol **2**:326, 1969

24. Schmitt H, Schmitt H, Boissier JR, Giudicelli JF: Centrally mediated decrease in sympathetic tone induced by 2-(2,6-dichlorphenylamino)-2-imidazoline (St 155, catapresan). Eur J Pharmacol **2:**147, 1967

25. Schmitt H, Schmitt H, Boissier JR, Giudicelli JF, Fichelle J: Cardiovascular effects of 2-(2,6-dichlorphenylamino)-2-imidazoline hydrochloride (St 155). II. Central sympathetic structures. Eur J Pharmacol **2:**340, 1968

26. Hukuhara T Jr, Otsuka Y, Takeda R, Sakai F: Die zentralen Wirkungen des 2-(2,6-dichlorphenylamino)-2-imidazoline Hydrochlorides. Arzneim Forsch **18:**1147, 1968

27. Klupp H, Knappen F, Otsuka Y, Streller J, Teichmann H: Effects of clonidine on central sympathetic tone. Eur J Pharmacol **10:**225, 1970

28. Kobinger W, Walland A: Involvement of adrenergic receptors in central vagus activity. Eur J Pharmacol **16:**120, 1971

29. Kobinger W, Walland A: Evidence for a central activation of a vagal cardiodepressor reflex by clonidine. Eur J Pharmacol **19:**203, 1971

30. Kobinger W, Pichler L: Evidence for direct α-adrenoceptor stimulation of effector neurons in cardiovascular centers by clonidine. Eur J Pharmacol **27:**151, 1974

31. Korner PI, Oliver JR, Sleight P, Chalmers JP, Robinson JS: Effects of clonidine on the baroreceptor-heart rate reflex and on single aortic baroreceptor fibre discharge. Eur J Pharmacol **28:**189, 1974

32. Schmitt H, Schmitt H: Localization of the hypotensive effect of 2-(2,6-dichlorphenylamino)-2-imidazoline hydrochloride (St 155, catapresan), Eur J Pharmacol **6:**8, 1969

33. Kobinger W, Pichler L: The central modulatory effect of clonidine on the cardiodepressor reflex after suppression of synthesis and storage of noradrenaline. Eur J Pharmacol **30:**56, 1975

34. Kobinger W, Pichler L: Localization in the CNS of adrenoceptors which facilitate a cardioinhibitory reflex. Naunyn Schmiedeberg's Arch Pharmacol **286:**371, 1975

35. Przuntek H, Guimarez A: Importance of adrenergic neurons of the brain for the rise of blood pressure evoked by hypothalamic stimulation. Naunyn Schmiedeberg's Arch Pharmacol **271:**311, 1971

36. Schmitt H, Schmitt H, Fenard S: Evidence for an α-sympathomimetic component in the effects of catapresan on vasomotor centres: antagonism by piperoxane. Eur J Pharmacol **14:**98, 1971

37. Schmitt H, Schmitt H, Fenard S: Action of α-adrenergic blocking drugs on the sympathetic centres and their interactions with the central sympatho-inhibitory effect of clonidine. Arzneim Forsch **23:**40, 1973

38. Kobinger W, Walland A: Facilitation of vagal reflex bradycardia by an action of clonidine on central α-receptors. Eur J Pharmacol **19:**210, 1972

39. Hoyer J, van Zwieten PA: The centrally induced fall in blood pressure after the infusion of amphetamine and related drugs into the vertebral artery of the cat. J Pharm Pharmacol **23:**892, 1971

40. Hoyer J, van Zwieten PA: The central hypotensive action of amphetamine, ephedrine, phentermine, chlorphentermine and fenfluramine. J Pharm Pharmacol **24:**452, 1972

41. Sinha JN, Schmitt H: Central sympatho-inhibitory effects of intracisternal and intravenous administrations of noradrenaline in high doses. Eur J Pharmacol **28:**217, 1974

42. de Jong W: Noradrenaline: central inhibitory control of blood pressure and heart rate. Eur J Pharmacol **29:**179, 1974
43. de Jong W, Nijhamp FP, Bolms B: Role of noradrenaline and serotonin in the central control of blood pressure in normotensive and spontaneously hypertensive rats. Arch Int Pharmacodyn **213:**272, 1975
44. Struyker Boudier HAJ, van Rossum JM, De Schaepdryzer AF (eds): Essays on blood pressure control. Proceedings of an International Symposium on Hypertension, Nijmegen, 1974. Published by Arch Int Pharmacodyn, 1975
45. Kobinger W, Pichler L: Investigation into some imidazoline compounds, with respect to peripheral α-adrenoceptor stimulation and depression of cardiovascular centers. Naunyn Schmiedeberg's Arch Pharmacol **291:**175, 1975
46. Kobinger W, Pichler L: Centrally induced reduction in sympathetic tone—a postsynaptic α-adrenoceptor stimulating action of imidazolines. Eur J Pharmacol **40:**311, 1976
47. Uvnäs B: Central cardiovascular control. *In* Handbook of Physiology, Section 1: Neurophysiology. Washington, American Physiological Society, Vol II, 1960, p 1131
48. Löfwing B: Cardiovascular adjustments induced from the rostral cingulate gyrus. With special reference to sympathoinhibitory mechanisms. Acta Physiol Scand **53**(Suppl 184):1, 1961
49. Folkow B, Neil E: Circulation. New York, Oxford University Press, 1971
50. Korner PI, Head GA: Effects of noradrenergic and serotonergic neurons on blood pressure, heart rate and the baroreceptor-heart rate reflex of the conscious rabbit. J Autonom Nerv Syst **3:**511, 1981
51. Uretsky NY, Iverson LL: Effects of 6-hydroxydopamine on catecholamine-containing neurons in the rat brain. J Neurochem **17:**269, 1970
52. Haeusler G: Early pre- and post-junctional effects of 6-hydroxydopamine. J Pharmac Exp Ther **178:**49, 1971
53. Kobinger W, Walland A: Modulating effect of central adrenergic neurons on a vagally mediated cardioinhibitory reflex. Eur J Pharmacol **22:**344, 1973
54. Pichler L, Placheta P, Kobinger W: Effect of azepexole (B-HT 933) on pre- and postsynaptic α-adrenoceptors at peripheral and central nervous sites. Eur J Pharmacol **65:**233, 1980
55. Hoefke W, Kobinger W, Walland A: Relationship between activity and structure in derivatives of clonidine. Arzneim Forsch **25:**786, 1975
56. Timmermans PBMWM, van Zwieten PA: Central and peripheral α-adrenergic effects of some imidazolines. Eur J Pharmacol **45:**229, 1977
57. Timmermans PBMWM, Hoefke W, Stähle H, van Zwieten PA: Structure-activity relationship in clonidine-like imidazolidines and related compounds. Progr Pharmac **3:**1, 1980
58. Langer SZ: Presynaptic receptors and their role in the regulation of transmitter release. Br J Pharmacol **60:**481, 1977
59. Starke K: Regulation of noradrenaline release by presynaptic receptor systems. Rev Physiol Biochem Pharmacol **77:**1, 1977
60. Starke K, Endo T, Taube HD: Relative pre- and postsynaptic potencies of α-adrenoceptor agonists in the rabbit pulmonary artery. Naunyn Schmiedeberg's Arch Pharmacol **291:**55, 1975
61. Weitzell R, Tanaka T, Starke K: Pre- and postsynaptic effects of yohimbine stereoisomers on noradrenergic transmission in the pulmonary artery of the rabbit. Naunyn Schmiedeberg's Arch Pharmacol **308:**127, 1979

62. Cavero I, Roach AG: The pharmacology of prazosin, a novel antihypertensive agent. Life Sci **27:**1525, 1980.
62a. Berthelsen S, Pettinger WA: A functional basis for classification of α-adrenergic receptors. Life Sci **21:**595, 1977
63. Wikberg JES: The pharmacological classification of adrengergic α_1 and α_2 receptors and their mechanisms of action. Acta Physiol Scand **468**(Suppl):1, 1979
64. Starke K, Langer SZ: A note on terminology for presynaptic receptors. *In* Presynaptic Receptors, Advances in the Biosciences, edited by Langer SZ, Starke K, Dubocovich ML. Oxford, Pergamon Press, Vol 18, 1979, p 1
65. Drew GM, Whiting SB: Evidences for two distinct types of postsynaptic α-adrenoceptors in vascular smooth muscle in vivo. Br J Pharmacol **67:**207, 1979
66. Docherty JR, McGrath JC: A comparison of pre- and postjunctional potencies of several alpha-adrenoceptor agonists in the cardiovascular system and anococcygens muscle of the rat. Evidence of two types of postjunctional α-adrenoceptor. Naunyn Schmiedeberg's Arch Pharmacol **312:**107, 1980
67. Kobinger W, Pichler L: Investigation into different types of post- and presynaptic α-adrenoceptors at cardiovascular sites in rats. Eur J Pharmacol **65:**393, 1980
67a. Timmermans PBMWM, van Zwieten PA: Postsynaptic α_1 and α_2 adrenoceptors in the circulatory system of the pithed rat. Selective stimulation of the α_2-type by B-HT 933. Eur J Pharmacol **63:**199, 1980
68. Kobinger W, Pichler L: α-Adrenoceptor subtypes in cardiovascular regulation. J Cardiovasc Pharmacol **4:**S81, 1982
69. Kobinger W, Pichler L: α_1- and α_2-Adrenoceptor subtypes: selectivity of various agonists and relative distribution of receptors as determined in rats. Eur J Pharmacol **73:**313, 1981
70. Starke K: Presynaptic modulation of catecholamine release in the central nervous system. Some open questions. *In* Presynaptic Receptors, Advances in the Biosciences, edited by Langer SZ, Starke K, Dubocovich ML. Oxford, Pergamon Press, Vol 18, 1979, p 129
71. Svensson TH, Bunney BS, Aghajanian GK: Inhibition of both noradrenergic and serotonergic neurons in brain by the α-adrenergic agonist clonidine. Brain Res **92:**291, 1975
72. Farneboe LD, Hamberger B: Drug-induced changes in the release of ³H-monoamines from field stimulated rat brain slices. Acta Physiol Scand Suppl **371:**35, 1971
73. Starke K, Montel H: Involvement of alpha-receptors in clonidine-induced inhibition of transmitter release from central monoamine neurons. Neuropharmacology **12:**1073, 1973
74. Andén NE, Grabowska M, Strömbom U: Different alpha-adrenoceptors in the central nervous system mediating biochemical and functional effects of clonidine and receptor blocking agents. Naunyn Schmiedeberg's Arch Pharmacol **292:**143, 1976
75. Pletscher AH, Besendorf H, Bächtold HP: Benzo-a-chinolizine, eine neue Körperklasse mit Wirkung auf den 5-Hydroxy-tryptamin- und Noradrenalin-Stoffwechsel des Gehirns. Naunyn Schmiedeberg's Arch Pharmacol **232:**499, 1958
76. Spector S, Sjoerdsma A, Udenfriend S: Blockade of endogenous norepinephrine synthesis by α-methyltyrosine, an inhibitor of tyrosine hydroxylase. J Pharmacol Exp Therap **147:**86, 1965

77. Dollery CT, Reid JL: Central noradrenergic neurons and the cardiovascular actions of clonidine in the rabbit. Br J Pharmacol **47:**206, 1973
78. Haeusler G, Finch L: On the nature of the central hypotensive effect of clonidine and alpha-methyldopa. Reunion Commune de la Deutsche Pharmakologische Gesellschaft et de l'Association Francaise des Pharmacologistes, Paris, Abstracts, 1972, p 16
79. Finch L: The central hypotensive action of clonidine and Bay 1470 in cats and rats. Clin Sci Mol Med **48:**273s, 1975
80. Reynoldson JA, Head GA, Korner PI: Effect of 6-hydroxydopamine on blood pressure and heart rate responses to intracisternal clonidine in conscious rabbits. Eur J Pharmacol **55:**257, 1979
81. Butcher LL, Eastgate SM, Hodge GK: Evidence that punctate intracerebral administration of 6-hydroxydopamine fails to produce selective neuronal degeneration. Comparison with copper sulfate and factors governing the deportment of fluids injected into brain. Naunyn Schmiedeberg's Arch Pharmacol **285:**31, 1974
82. Haeusler G: Clonidine induced inhibition of sympathetic nerve activity: no indication for a central presynaptic or an indirect sympathomimetic mode of action. Naunyn Schmiedeberg's Arch Pharmacol **286:**97, 1974
83. Pichler L, Kobinger W: Centrally mediated cardiovascular effects of B-HT 920 (6-allyl-2-amino-5,6,7,8-tetrahydro-4H-thiazolo-[4,5-d]-azepine dihydrochloride), a hypotensive agent of the "clonidine type." J Cardiovasc Pharmacol **3:**269, 1981
84. Kobinger W, Pichler L: Pharmacological characterization of B-HT 933 (2-amino-6-ethyl-4,5,7,8-tetrahydro-6H-oxazolo-[5,4-d]-azepin dihydrochloride) as a hypotensive agent of the "clonidine-type." Naunyn Schmiedeberg's Arch Pharmacol **300:**39, 1977
85. Henning M, van Zwieten PA: Central hypotensive effect of α-methyl-DOPA. J Pharm Pharmacol **19:**403, 1967
86. Henning M, van Zwieten PA: Central hypotensive action of α-methyl-DOPA. J Pharm Pharmacol **20:**409, 1968
87. de Jong W, van Meel JCA, Timmermans PBMWM, van Zwieten PA: A lipophilic, selective α_1-adrenoceptor agonist: 2-(2-chloro-5-trifluoromethyl-phenylimino) imidazolidine (St 587). Life Sci **28:**2009, 1981
88. Kobinger W, Pichler L: Subgroups of a-adrenoceptors: selectivity of drugs and receptor importance in various target systems. Drug Res, in press
89. Timmermans PBMWM, Schoop AMC, Kwa HY, van Zwieten PA: Characterization of α-adrenoceptors participating in the central hypotensive and sedative effects of clonidine using yohimbine, rauwolscine and corynanthine. Eur J Pharmacol **70:**7, 1981
90. Andén NE, Corrodi H, Fuxe K, Hökfelt T, Rydin C, Svensson T: Evidence for a central noradrenaline receptor stimulation by clonidine. Life Sci **9:**513, 1970
91. Saavedra JM: Central biogenic amines and neuropeptides in genetic hypertension. *In* Central Nervous System Mechanism in Hypertension, edited by Buckley JP, Ferrario CM. New York, Raven Press, 1981, p 129
92. Kobinger W: Central and peripheral alpha adrenergic receptors: are they the same? *In* Trends in Autonomic Pharmacology, Vol 2, edited by Kalsner S. Baltimore, Urban & Schwarzenberg, 1982, p 363
93. Kobinger W: The role of α-adrenoceptors in central nervous and peripheral vascular regulation. Jap J Pharmacol **31**(Suppl):13P, 1981
94. Scheel-Krüger J: Comparative studies of various amphetamine analogues demonstrating different interactions with the metabolism of the catecholamines in the brain. Eur J Pharmacol **14:**47, 1971

Basic Mechanisms: Physiology

Chapter 3

Arterial Baroreflexes in Hypertension

Marc D. Thames

Stimulation of sensory endings in the carotid sinus and aortic arch cause powerful reflex responses.[23] The sensory information originating from these endings travels to the central nervous system via branches of the glossopharyngeal nerve (carotid baroreceptors) and vagus nerve (aortic baroreceptors). The primary afferent neurons synapse with second order neurons in the nucleus of the tractus solitarius in the medulla, and the input from these sensory endings ultimately affects the outflow of sympathetic nerve activity to the heart and peripheral circulation and of parasympathetic or vagal efferent outflow to the heart (Figure 3-1).

The sensory endings themselves are called arterial baroreceptors because they are pressure sensitive. They are mechanoreceptors and respond to changes in vessel wall distention, and their activity is related to changes in blood pressure because of concomitant changes in vessel stretch and thus in the deformation of the endings that occur in association with changes in arterial pressure. When arterial pressure is increased, the discharge of the arterial baroreceptors also is increased. This results in a reflex excitation of parasympathetic cholinergic fibers passing to the heart via the vagal nerves and an inhibition of sympathetic outflow to the heart and to virtually every peripheral vascular bed examined. These nervous responses result in bradycardia and withdrawal of neurogenic vasoconstrictor tone. Conversely, decreases in arterial pressure result in decreases in baroreceptor discharge and augmented sympathetic outflow to the heart and peripheral circulation, and decreased parasympathetic cholinergic outflow to the heart—i.e., tachycardia and increased neurogenic vasoconstrictor tone.

Supported by HL 30506 and by the Veterans Administration.

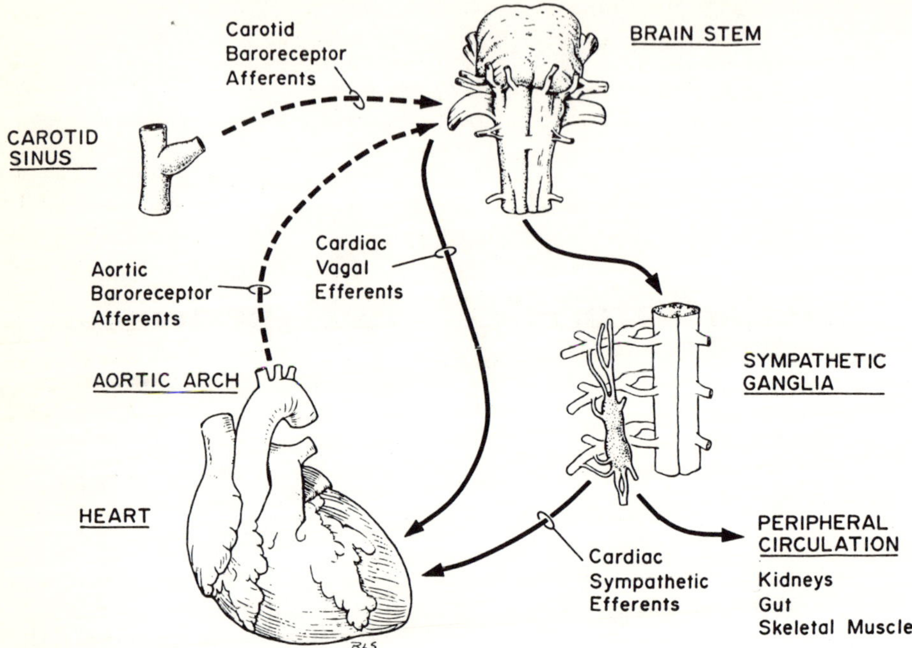

Figure 3-1. Schematic illustrating afferent and efferent limbs of arterial baro-reflexes. The afferent limbs are represented by broken lines and the efferent limbs by solid lines.

Under normal resting conditions, the arterial baroreflexes exert a tonic inhibitory influence on sympathetic outflow and a tonic excitatory influence on vagal parasympathetic outflow. These tonic influences are reduced when arterial pressure is decreased and become augmented during increases in arterial pressure.

Many investigators have been interested in the relationship between the baroreceptor reflexes and hypertension.[1,31] A number of early studies showed that acute interruption of sinoaortic baroreceptor input resulted in large acute increases in arterial pressure, heart rate, and peripheral resistance. Other studies suggested that such denervations could exacerbate renal hypertension. However, more recent studies indicate that chronic denervation of the baroreceptor afferent pathways in normal animals results in modest hypertension[21] in the hands of some investigators and no hypertension in the experience of others.[13] It is probably fair to conclude that chronic arterial baroreceptor denervation does not result in chronic large increases in average arterial pressure recorded over a 24-hour period, although there is a dramatic increase in blood pressure variability around the mean following such denervation.[13,21] Thus, it seems unlikely that abnormalities in baroreceptor function per se result in hypertension.

In recent years, interest regarding the arterial baroreceptor reflexes has turned to the manner in which these reflexes control the heart and peripheral circulation in a variety of animal models of hypertension and in human essential hypertension. There is evidence that there are abnormalities in the baroreflex control of the heart and of portions of the peripheral circulation, although these abnormalities appear to be nonuniform.

The purpose of this chapter is to summarize the mechanisms of arterial baroreflex control of the heart and circulation in normotension and in hypertension. Abnormalities in the receptors, in the central nervous system, and in neuroeffector mechanisms that may contribute to abnormal or preserved baroreflex control in hypertension will be discussed. It is not the intent here to provide an exhaustive review of this area but rather to provide a conceptual framework that is current and that will provide a general understanding of baroreflex control of the circulation in hypertension. The influence of vagal cardiopulmonary baroreflexes in hypertension will not be reviewed.

Baroreflex Control in Normotension

A great deal is known about the arterial baroreflex control of the heart and peripheral circulation in normotension. Much of this information has been reviewed by Kirchheim.[23] In addition, the reader is referred to a forthcoming volume of the *Handbook of Physiology*.[32]

Stimulation of arterial baroreceptors results in reflex bradycardia and peripheral vasodilatation. The bradycardia is the result of a simultaneous activation of vagal parasympathetic fibers passing to the heart and a withdrawal of sympathetic activity passing to the heart, although the former is more important. The peripheral vasodilatation is the result of a reflex withdrawal of sympathetic nerve activity passing to virtually every organ evaluated. Decreases in cardiac, renal, splenic, splanchnic, and lumbar sympathetic nerve activity have been observed. Activation of arterial baroreceptor afferent pathways can decrease myocardial contractility in anesthetized dogs by withdrawal of sympathetic influences and by concomitant activation of efferent vagal fibers passing to the ventricles. As indicated, the first synapse for the primary afferent neurons in the baroreceptor reflex is in the nucleus of the tractus solitarius. Second-order neurons in this nucleus synapse with higher-order neurons that pass in turn to a variety of areas in the brain stem and to higher centers. The influence of this baroreceptor input spreads to the nucleus ambiguus, where it alters the discharge of cardiac vagal motor neurons, and to regions in the hypothalamus and brain stem involved in the control of sympathetic preganglionic neurons.

There are important differences in the way in which cardiac vagal motor neurons and sympathetic neurons are controlled by the arterial baroreflexes. We recently showed that denervation of carotid or aortic baroreceptors impaired baroreflex control of heart rate but not baroreflex control of sympathetic outflow in the lumbar[20] or renal nerves.[5] In contrast, if the vagal nerves are sectioned first, then denervation of either aortic or carotid baroreceptors fails to alter the baroreflex control of heart rate or of hindlimb vascular resistance.[20] Thus, it appears that both sets of baroreceptors are required for full control of cardiac vagal motor neurons and thus of heart rate. In contrast, the preservation of baroreflex control of sympathetic outflow to hindlimb[20] and kidney[5] following partial arterial baroreceptor denervation is evidence that the control of these sympathetic nerves by the baroreflexes is redundant.

This pattern of summation of baroreflexes has been referred to as occlusive or mutual inhibitory summation and is illustrated in Figure 3-1. Thus, the baroreflex control of the heart is quite different from control of the peripheral circulation, and abnormalities in the baroreflex control of heart rate should not be taken as evidence of a generalized impairment of baroreflex control of the circulation.

Baroreflex Control in Hypertension

It has been known for many years that baroreflex control of heart rate is impaired in human essential hypertension. Bristow and colleagues[7] determined the relationship between changes in blood pressure and changes in RR interval and defined the slope of the regression relationship between these changes as the baroreflex sensitivity. They found that baroreflex sensitivity is impaired in human essential hypertension. This finding has been confirmed in a number of other investigations in humans and has also been confirmed in virtually every animal model of hypertension investigated, including renal hypertension,[2] spontaneous hypertension, and Dahl salt-sensitive hypertension.[16] Recent experiments by Thames and colleagues[29] in conscious renal hypertensive dogs have shown that abnormal baroreflex control of heart rate is due primarily to an abnormality in the control of cardiac vagal motor neurons and is not the result of abnormal control of sympathetic outflow to the heart.

Few studies have evaluated the arterial baroreflex control of sympathetic outflow to the peripheral circulation in hypertension. Obviously, reflex control of peripheral resistance plays an important role in the control of blood pressure in hypertensive as well as normotensive states. Because of the well-known impairment in the arterial baroreflex control of heart rate in hypertension,[1] it has been suggested that there may be a generalized impairment in baroreflex control of the peripheral circulation. Results of recent studies that will be reviewed indicate that baroreflex control of the peripheral circulation may be preserved for selected vascular beds and impaired for others. Moreover, the duration of the hypertension may have an important impact on the types of abnormalities detected in specific parts of the circulation.

Thames and colleagues recently found that the baroreflex control of hindlimb vascular resistance and lumbar sympathetic nerve activity is preserved in rabbits with renal hypertension even though heart rate control was abnormal in these animals.[19] As suggested from experiments in dogs,[29] it appears that this abnormal heart rate control is largely the result of impaired control of cardiac vagal motor neurons. Although control of sympathetic outflow to the hindlimb is preserved in rabbits with renal hypertension when all arterial baroreceptor reflexes are intact,[19] baroreflex control of hindlimb vascular resistance and of lumbar sympathetic nerve activity is impaired following partial arterial (carotid or aortic) baroreceptor denervation in these hypertensive animals.[19] This suggests that the redundancy in the baroreflex control of sympathetic outflow to the hindlimb present in normotensive rabbits[20] is not present in hypertensive rabbits (Figures 3-2, and 3-3).

In contrast to the baroreflex control of the sympathetic outflow to the hindlimb, which is preserved in renal hypertensive rabbits with baroreflexes intact, baroreflex control of *renal* sympathetic nerve activity is impaired[30] even with all arterial baroreflexes intact. Thus, one cannot generalize from impaired heart rate control to impaired control of sympathetic outflow to the peripheral circulation, and it is also not possible to conclude that preserved control of sympathetic outflow to one vascular bed implies preservation of sympathetic outflow to all vascular beds.

The abnormalities in the arterial baroreflex control of the circulation could be localized to the afferent limb of the reflex, to the central nervous system, to neuroeffector mechanisms, or to a combination of these.

Additionally, changes in vascular reactivity and/or structural changes in the vessel wall in hypertension (hypertrophy, altered wall-to-lumen ratio) may modify the responses of resistance vessels to changes in sympathetic drive. Thus, the responses of blood pressure and of resistance of specific vascular beds may not necessarily indicate impaired baroreflexes.

A number of investigators have shown that hypertension results in a shift to higher pressures along the pressure axis of the stimulus-response curve for the arterial baroreceptors.[4,9,28] In these animals the receptors behave early[28] in hypertension in a fashion similar to those in normotensive animals, except that the threshold pressure for stimulation of these receptors is higher, the linear portion of the stimulus response curve is shifted to the right (Figure 3-4), and the saturation pressure for these endings also is shifted to the right.

With an increase in arterial pressure of greater duration, the sensitivity of the endings becomes reduced, so that for comparable increases in arterial pressure there are smaller increases in arterial baroreceptor discharge in animals with relatively longstanding hypertension[4,9] than in those with hypertension of shorter duration. There may also be reductions in the maximum firing frequencies of these afferent nerve endings.

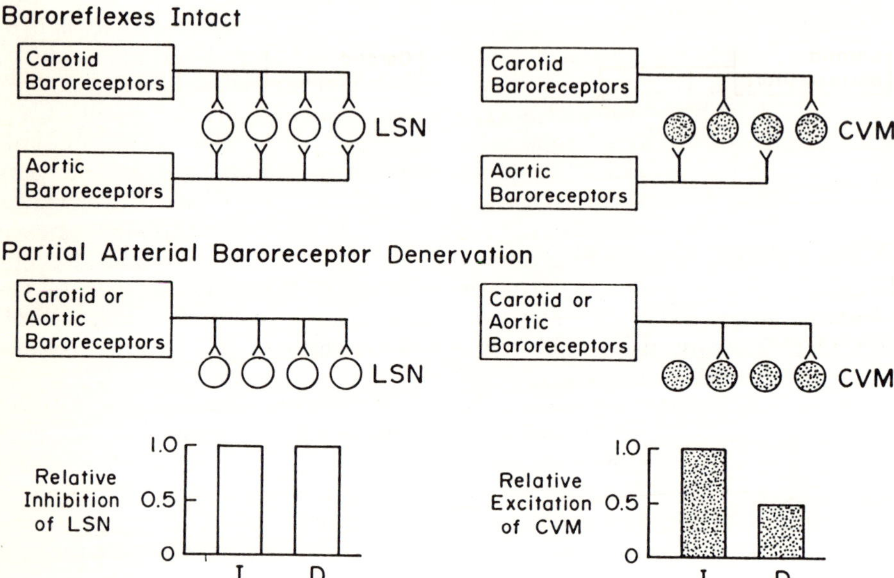

Figure 3-2. Relative influence of arterial baroreceptors on lumbar sympathetic nerves (LSN) and cardiac vagal motor neurons (CVM) in *normotensive* rabbits with baroreflexes intact (I) and after partial arterial baroreceptor denervation (D). This figure illustrates relative *influence* and should not be interpreted to indicate direct connections between baroreceptor afferent fibers and LSN or CVM. The graphs at the lower part of the figure illustrate the relationships presented above. With all baroreflexes intact, all LSN are controlled by both carotid and aortic baroreflexes. After carotid or aortic baroreceptor denervation, all LSN are still controlled by the remaining set of baroreflexes. By contrast, both carotid and aortic baroreflexes are needed to control all CVM. After carotid or aortic baroreceptor denervation, only half of CVM are controlled by the remaining set of baroreflexes, and heart rate control is impaired.

Andresen and colleagues[3] and Angell-James[4] have assessed the physiological basis for the resetting of baroreceptors in two different animal models of hypertension. Angell-James found that the vessels in renal hypertensive rabbits were stiffer than in normotensive rabbits, and attributed the resetting of these baroreceptors to a splinting effect of the hypertrophied vessel wall on vessel wall mechanics and thus on the receptors. Put another way, for a given stress the resulting change in vessel diameter (strain) would be smaller, and thus presumably the baroreceptors them-

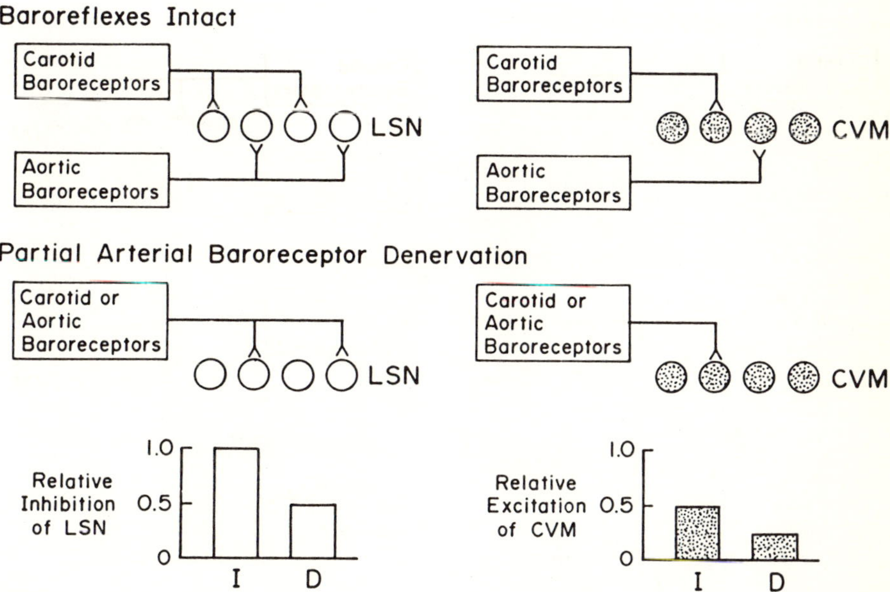

Figure 3-3. Relative influence of arterial baroreceptors on lumbar sympathetic nerves (LSN) and cardiac vagal motor neurons (CVM) in *hypertensive* rabbits with baroreflexes intact (I) and after partial arterial baroreceptor denervation (D). The graphs at the lower part of the figure illustrate the relationships presented above. In hypertension, aortic and carotid baroreflexes are needed to control all LSN. After carotid or aortic baroreceptor denervation, only part of LSN are controlled by the remaining baroreflexes. Note the difference in effect of partial arterial baroreceptor denervation on baroreflex control of LSN in hypertension (this figure) and normotension (Figure 3-1). In hypertension, both carotid and aortic baroreflexes control only part of CVM, resulting in impaired baroreflex control of heart rate. After carotid or aortic baroreceptor denervation, this abnormality is even greater. The influence of baroreflexes on CVMs in hypertension (this figure) should be contrasted with normotension (Figure 3-1).

selves would be stimulated to a smaller degree in these stiff vessels for comparable changes in pressure.

Recent experiments by Andresen and colleagues[3] carried out in spontaneously hypertensive rats indicate that the impairment in the baroreceptors is due largely to a mismatch between the strain sensitivity of the vessel wall and the strain sensitivity of the baroreceptors themselves. Early in hypertension the strain sensitivity of the baroreceptors is decreased compared with normotensive animals. Later in hypertension, strain sensitivity

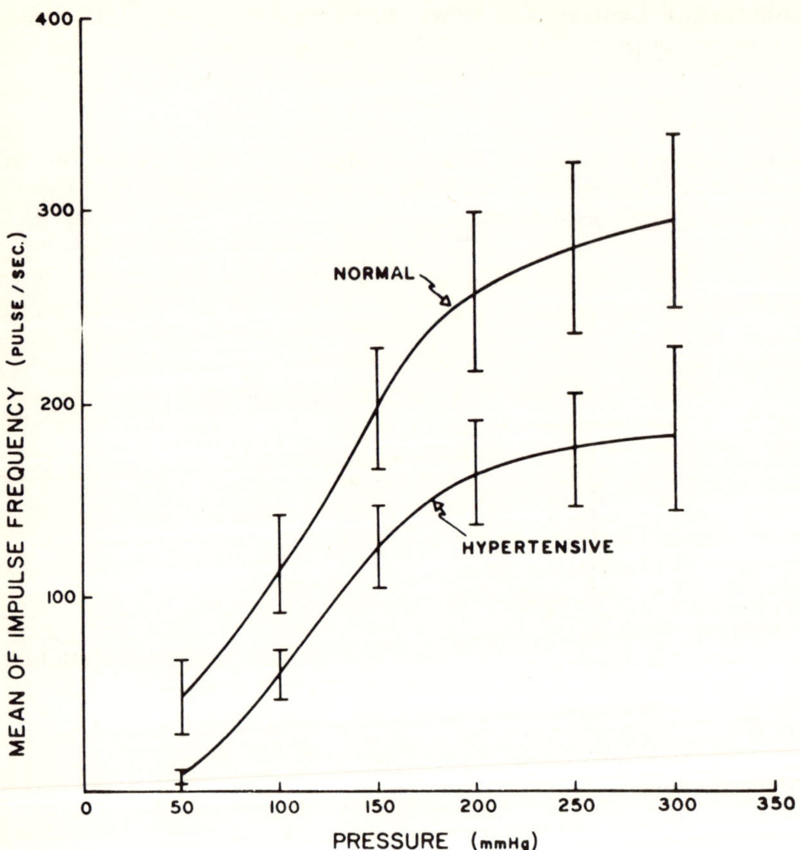

Figure 3-4. Relationship between isolated perfused carotid sinus baroreceptor discharge and carotid sinus pressure in normotensive and hypertensive dogs. Data was obtained by using pulsatile pressure stimulation of the receptors around the mean pressures shown on the pressure axis. The curve for the hypertensive dogs is shifted to the right along the pressure axis. (From P. Kezdi. Resetting of the carotid sinus in experimental renal hypertension. In *Baroreceptors and Hypertension,* edited by P. Kezdi. New York, Pergamon Press, 1967; with permission.)

of the endings may actually be increased, but this increase is not sufficient to compensate for the reduced strain sensitivity of the vessel wall in these hypertensive animals.[9] Thus, abnormalities in the receptors themselves could contribute to impaired baroreflex control of the heart and circulation.

There are a number of indirect lines of evidence pointing to central nervous system abnormalities in arterial baroreflexes in hypertension. The central nervous system may be involved in renal hypertension since depletion of central norepinephrine by intracisternal administration of 6-hydroxydopamine prevents or normalizes it.[10] It also has been suggested that the integrity of the central noradrenergic system, including that in the hypothalamus, is crucial for the prevention of renal hypertension.[6,26] Baroreflex control of heart rate may be selectively suppressed during stimulation of the hypothalamic defense area.[11,15] Mild excitation of the hypothalamic defense area has been postulated to explain the dissociation of baroreflex control of heart rate and splanchnic nerve activity in spontaneously hypertensive rats or blood pressure in humans.[27]

Finally, recent studies by Brody and colleagues[8] indicate that the region of the anteroventral third ventricle (AV3V) of the rat plays an important role in the development of several models of hypertension in rats. They found that AV3V lesions prevented the development of renal hypertension as well as hypertension produced by administration of the sodium-retaining steroid deoxycorticosterone and 1% NaCl for drinking fluid. AV3V lesions also reduced the severity of salt-induced hypertension in the Dahl strain of rats, which become hypertensive when fed a normal or high salt diet. Application of angiotensin to the AV3V region results in increased arterial pressure, increased drinking, and augmented release of vasopressin.[33] Thus, it seems likely that the central nervous system could participate in the genesis of impaired baroreflex control in hypertension.

Abnormalities in the receptors themselves may also contribute to impaired baroreflex control. As noted, baroreflex control of hindlimb vascular resistance and lumbar sympathetic nerve activity is preserved in normotensive animals after partial arterial baroreceptor denervation.[20] In contrast, baroreflex control of hindlimb vascular resistance and lumbar sympathetic nerve activity is impaired in renal hypertension[19] following partial arterial baroreceptor denervation (Figures 3-2 and 3-3). It can be argued that this is either the result of a central abnormality in the integration of carotid and aortic baroreflexes or of an abnormality in the receptors themselves, which in turn alters the inputs from these two receptor groups. We recently found[18] that raising arterial pressure, which induced increases in input over one aortic nerve (both carotid sinus nerves and the remaining aortic nerve sectioned), resulted in strikingly impaired reflex bradycardia and decreases in lumbar sympathetic nerve traffic in renal hypertensive compared to normotensive rabbits. The sensitivity of the reflex responses to changes in arterial pressure was markedly reduced.

Such experiments make an important assumption regarding the comparability of the changes in baroreceptor input during blood pressure changes. We reasoned that if the responses to the same input (electrical stimulation of one aortic nerve with all baroreceptor afferent pathways interrupted) were reduced in hypertensive rabbits compared with normotensive rabbits, it would strongly suggest a central abnormality. However, we found[18] that there were no differences in the responses of blood pressure, heart rate, and *lumbar sympathetic nerve traffic* in normotensive and renal hypertensive rabbits over a wide range of stimulus frequencies when only the large, rapidly conducting myelinated fibers or both myelinated and the fine, slowly conducting nonmyelinated fibers were stimulated.

Since the responses to electrical stimulation and therefore to comparable levels of input were similar, yet the responses to physiological activation (acute increases in arterial pressure) of one aortic nerve were impaired in hypertension, this strongly suggests an abnormality in the baroreceptors per se, which accounts for the impaired heart rate control with all baroreflexes intact and the impaired control of lumbar sympathetic nerve activity following partial arterial baroreceptor denervation. Since intact heart rate control required normally functioning aortic and carotid baroreceptors,[20] the abnormal heart rate control in hypertension seems to be due mainly to abnormalities in the baroreceptors—that is, hypertensive animals behave as if they have some degree of arterial baroreceptor denervation (Figure 3-2).

Similarly, although removal of carotid or aortic baroreceptors does not impair control of lumbar sympathetic nerve activity in normotensive animals (Figure 4-1), control of lumbar nerve activity in hypertension is abnormal after partial arterial baroreceptor denervation (Figure 3-2). Thus, in hypertension, denervation of the aortic or carotid baroreceptors is more than equivalent to removing either the carotid or aortic baroreceptor input in normotension. Abnormalities in arterial baroreceptors and in baroreflex control may even precede the development of hypertension.

Gordon and colleagues[16] recently reported that Dahl genetically salt-sensitive rats, which remain normotensive on a low salt diet but become hypertensive when fed a high salt diet, have impaired baroreflex control of heart rate, even while normotensive on low salt. Baroreflex buffering of phenylephrine-induced increases in arterial pressure also was impaired in the pre-hypertensive phase. These abnormalities in baroreflex control are due, at least in part, to an abnormality in the baroreceptors (A. Farrari and A. Mark, personal communication) since their recorded sensitivity is reduced in the pre-hypertensive phase.

In contrast to the preserved baroreflex control of *lumbar* sympathetic nerve activity in renal hypertensive rabbits with arterial baroreflexes intact, baroreflex control of *renal* sympathetic nerve activity is impaired both in spontaneously hypertensive rats[12,22] and in renal hypertensive rabbits.[30] The latter abnormality appears to be due largely to a central nervous system abnormality in the baroreflex. We recently found that for comparable increases in aortic baroreceptor discharge there were smaller decreases in renal sympathetic nerve activity in hypertensive rabbits than in normotensive rabbits.[30] These data were suggestive of a central nervous system abnormality.

In additional experiments the aortic and carotid sinus nerves were sectioned and one aortic nerve stimulated electrically over a wide range of frequencies in normotensive and hypertensive rabbits. We found that the reflex inhibition of renal sympathetic nerve activity during electrical stimulation of the left aortic nerve was impaired in hypertensive rabbits, particularly during selective activation of myelinated afferent fibers. This points to a central impairment in baroreflex control of renal nerve activity in renal hypertension. In spontaneously hypertensive rats, baroreflex control of splanchnic nerve activity appears to be preserved, just as lumbar sympathetic outflow is preserved in renal hypertensive rabbits.

Thus, baroreflex control of sympathetic outflow to specific vascular beds may be preserved (hindlimb and splanchnic circulation) or impaired (renal circulation). Abnormalities in the receptors appear to be responsible in large part for impaired heart rate control and the reduced redundancy in the baroreflex control of lumbar sympathetic nerve activity in hypertension. A central nervous system abnormality appears to account for impaired control of renal nerve activity in hypertension. Abnormalities in both arterial baroreceptors and the central nervous system appear to play an important role in baroreflex abnormalities present in hypertension, and the relative contribution of abnormalities in the receptors and the central nervous system may change with time.

Even though there appears to be no central nervous system abnormality in the baroreflex control of lumbar sympathetic nerve activity early in renal hypertension, recent preliminary data[17] suggest that the baroreflex control of lumbar nerve activity is impaired (with all baroreflexes intact) later in the course of renal hypertension, and this impairment is the result of a central nervous system abnormality.

Baroreflexes in Human Essential Hypertension

Arterial baroreflex control of heart rate is abnormal in human essential hypertension.[1,7,14] The severity of this impairment appears to be related to the severity of the hypertension.[14] Patients with minimal hypertension have minimal impairment of baroreflex control of heart rate, whereas subjects with greater hypertension have a more significant impairment of heart rate control.

Although studies on reflex regulation and human hypertension have consistently shown impaired baroreflex control of heart rate, the results of studies on the baroreflex control of the peripheral circulation have yielded divergent results. Since the sensitivity of the baroreceptors to changes in arterial pressure is reduced in experimental hypertension and since baroreflex control of heart rate is impaired in hypertension, it has generally been assumed that baroreflex control of the peripheral circulation also is abnormal. However, the available evidence in this area has not settled the question. There is no apparent reduction in the sensitivity of carotid sinus baroreflex control of blood pressure in human essential hypertension[24] although there is the expected rightward shift of the baroreceptor stimulus-response curve. However, hypertensive subjects appear to be positioned on the upper part of this sigmoid relationship, while normotensive subjects appear to be positioned on the lower part of the curve.

In contrast, Mark and Kerber[25] have reported that young subjects with borderline hypertension have impaired carotid baroreflex control of forearm vascular resistance. One possible explanation for preserved baroreflex control of arterial pressure but abnormal control of sympathetic outflow to selected vascular beds is that augmented vascular responses in some beds may compensate for decreased responses in other beds, resulting in no net differences in reflex control of blood pressure or total peripheral resistance. Clearly, there is still a great deal to be learned about baroreflex control of the circulation in human essential hypertension.

Summary and Conclusions

The circulation is controlled by arterial baroreflexes, which include an afferent limb (the arterial baroreceptor sensory endings and their primary afferent fibers), the central nervous integrative components of the reflex, and neuroeffector mechanisms.

There are important differences in the way in which cardiac vagal motor neurons and sympathetic neurons are controlled by arterial baroreflexes. Hypertension alters the control of these effector mechanisms in a nonuniform way that cannot be predicted from the baroreflex control of a specific effector mechanism. Abnormalities in the receptors themselves as well as in the central nervous system appear to play an important role in the establishment of impaired baroreflex control of the heart and peripheral circulation in experimental hypertension. These abnormalities may contribute to a worsening of hypertension, to the pathogenesis of hypertension in selected animal models, and may increase the resistance to normalization of arterial pressure in the treatment of patients with hypertension.

Although we have come to know a great deal about the arterial baroreflex control of the heart and peripheral circulation in hypertension, there is still a great deal to be learned.

References

1. Aars H: The baroreflex in arterial hypertension. Scand J Clin Lab Invest **35:** 97–102, 1975
2. Alexander N, Decuir M: Loss of baroreflex bradycardia in renal hypertensive rabbits. Circ Res **19:**18, 1966
3. Andresen MC, Kuraoka S, Brown AM: Baroreceptor function and changes in strain sensitivity in normotensive and spontaneously hypertensive rats. Circ Res **47:**821–828, 1980
4. Angell-James JC: Characteristics of single aortic and right subclavian baroreceptors fiber activity in rabbits with chronic renal hypertension. Circ Res **31:** 149–161, 1973
5. Ballon BJ, Thames MD: Mutual inhibitory summation of carotid and aortic baroreflexes in control of renal nerve activity. Clin Res **31:**167A, 1983

6. Boslant MD, Versteeg DHG, VanPut J, deJong W: Effect of depletion of spinal noradrenaline by 6-hydroxydopamine on the development of renal hypertension in rats. Clin Exp Pharmacol Physiol **8:**67–77, 1981

7. Bristow JD, Honour AJ, Pickering GW, Sleight P, Smyth HS: Diminished baroreflex sensitivity in high blood pressure. Circulation **39:**48–54, 1969

8. Brody MJ, Johnson AK: Role of anteroventral third ventricle region in fluid and electrolyte balance, arterial pressure regulation, and hypertension. *In* Frontiers in Neuroendocrinology, Vol 6, edited by Martini L, Ganong WF. New York, Raven Press, 1980, pp 249–292

9. Brown AM: Receptors under pressure: an update on baroreceptors. Circ Res **46:**1–10, 1980

10. Chalmer JP, Dollery CT, Lewis PJ, Reid JL: The importance of central adrenergic neurons in renal hypertension in rabbits. J Physiol London **238:**403–411, 1974

11. Coote JH, Perez-Gonzalez JF: Baroreceptor-reflex during stimulation of the hypothalamic defense region. J Physiol London **224:**74P-75P, 1972

12. Coote JH, Sato Y: Reflex regulation of sympathetic activity in the spontaneously hypertensive rat. Circ Res **40:**571–577, 1977

13. Cowley AW Jr, Liard JF, Guyton AC: Role of the baroreceptor reflex in daily control of arterial blood pressure and other variables in dogs. Circ Res **32:**564–576, 1973

14. Eckberg DL: Carotid baroreflex function in young men with borderline blood pressure elevation. Circ **59:**632–636, 1979

15. Gebber GL, Snyder DW: Hypothalamic control of baroreceptor reflexes. Am J Physiol **218:**124–131, 1970

16. Gordon FJ, Matsuguchi H, Mark AL: Abnormal baroreflex control of heart rate in prehypertensive and hypertensive Dahl genetically salt-sensitive rats. Hypertension **3**(Supp I):I-135–I-141, 1981

17. Guo GB, Abboud FM: Temporal sequence of impairment of baroreflex control of heart rate and lumbar sympathetic nerve activity in renal hypertensive rabbits. Fed Proc **42:**481, 1983

18. Guo GB, Thames MD: Differential baroreflex control of heart rate and lumbar sympathetic traffic in hypertension. Am J Physiol, in press

19. Guo GB, Thames MD, Abboud FM: Arterial baroreflexes in renal hypertensive rabbits: Selectivity and redundancy of baroreceptor influence on heart rate, vascular resistance, and lumbar sympathetic nerve activity. Circ Res **53:**223–234, 1983

20. Guo GB, Thames MD, Abboud FM: Differential baroreflex control of heart rate and vascular resistance in rabbits: relative role of carotid, aortic and cardiopulmonary baroreceptors. Circ Res **50:**554–565, 1982

21. Ito CS, Scher AM: Hypertension following arterial baroreceptor denervation in the unanesthetized dog. Circ Res **48:**576–586, 1981

22. Judy WV, Farrell SK: Arterial baroreceptor reflex control of sympathetic nerve activity in the spontaneosuly hypertensive rat. Hypertension **1:**605–614, 1979

23. Kirchheim H: Systemic arterial baroreceptor reflexes. Physiol Rev **56:**100–176, 1976

24. Mancia G, Ludbrook J, Ferrari A, Gregogini L, Zanchetti A: Baroreceptor reflexes in human hypertension. Circ Res **43:**170–177, 1978

25. Mark AL, Kerber RE: Augmentation of cardiac baroreflexes in borderline hypertension. Clin Res **28:**500A, 1980

26. Petty MA, Reid JL: Changes in noradrenaline concentration in the brain stem

and hypothalamic nuclei during the development of renovascular hypertension. Brain Res **136:**376–380, 1977

27. Ricksten SE, Thoreu P: Reflex inhibition of sympathetic activity during volume load in awake normotensive and spontaneously hypertensive rats. Acta Physiol Scand **110:**77–82, 1980

28. Sleight P, Robinson JL, Brooks DE, Rees PM: Characteristics of single carotid sinus baroreceptor fibers and whole nerve activity in the normotensive and the renal hypertensive dog. Circ Res **41:**750–758, 1977

29. Thames MD, Eastman CL, Marcus ML: Baroreflex control of heart interval in conscious renal hypertensive dogs. Am J Physiol **241:**H332–H336, 1981

30. Thames MD, Gupta BN, Ballon BJ: Central abnormality in baroreflex control of renal nerve in hypertension. Am J Physiol, in press

31. Zanchetti A: Overview of cardiovascular reflexes in hypertension. Am J Cardiol **44:**912–918, 1979

32. Handbook of Physiology, Washington DC, American Physiological Society, in press

33. Phillips MI: New evidence for brain angiotensin and its role in hypertension. Fed Proc **42:**2667–2672, 1983

Chapter 4

Brain Renin-Angiotensin and Hypertension

M. Ian Phillips

Introduction

Hypertension is a multiple disease state. The causes of hypertension are those that increase blood pressure, and as every medical student learns, blood pressure is the product of cardiac output and peripheral resistance. However, the numerous factors that go into this equation are not all obvious. Laragh[1] has described a useful continuum from causes due to direct vasoconstriction such as pheochromocytoma, high renin, and unilateral renovascular disease states to hypertension largely involving increased volume states such as hyperaldosteronism and bilateral renovascular states. In between are those states where there is both vasoconstriction and excess volume but where there is no obvious excess of vasoconstrictive agents such as angiotensin or catecholamines or overt volume-causing agents such as aldosterone.

Several different organs are involved in the control of blood pressure. The heart controls cardiac output by stroke volume and heart rate. The kidney plays a role in the control of volume and the release of renin from the juxtaglomerular cells, leading to vasoconstriction and retention of salt and water. The adrenals control sodium output by aldosterone, and the blood vessels themselves are sensitive to various neurotransmitters and peptides. The degree of hypertrophy caused by constant high pressure in the blood vessels also contributes to the hypertension. Finally, there is the role of the brain in the control of cardiovascular function.

The most apparent controlling system is the baroreceptor reflex, which is activated whenever blood pressure increases, causing it to decrease back toward normal. In an extended state of hypertension, the baroreceptor reflex is impaired or reset to a higher level so that high blood pressure is not compensated for by decreased cardiac output. In addition, the brain controls sympathetic output via the autonomic nervous system, which can directly affect vasoconstriction, and the brain releases hormones that may cause vasoconstriction—e.g., vasopressin, endorphins, and ACTH.

To this list of causative factors in high blood pressure we may now cautiously add that of increased brain angiotensin activity. There is evidence as strong as that for other peptides that angiotensin exists in the brain independently of the peripheral angiotensin levels. This concept has been a little difficult to accept because of the traditional role of the kidneys in producing renin, which acts on angiotensinogen, produced by the liver, to form angiotensin I, which is then converted in the lungs to angiotensin II. It requires a change in thinking to realize that the functions of these large organs might be carried out totally in single cells. Nevertheless, the concept of a brain renin-angiotensin system has gained acceptance after overcoming the hurdles of rigorous testing that have been applied to it. In this chapter, a brief review of the brain renin-angiotensin system is presented.

Renin in the Brain

The first recognition of extra renal renin came with the finding and purification of renin in the salivary glands.[2] If renin could exist outside the kidneys in another organ, then it seemed likely that other tissues would contain it. Renin was first reported in the brains of dogs by Ganten et al.[3] and at the same time Fischer-Ferraro et al.[4] in 1971. A forceful criticism of this finding was made later by Day and Reid,[5] who pointed out that since the renin had been detected at low pH levels, it may well have been confused with cathepsin D, a protease that also has low pH-level optimal activity.

Nevertheless, the appeal of a renin-angiotensin system had been set in motion and was supported by the experiments that were being carried out on the direct effects of angiotensin injections into the brain. In 1969, increased water intake was first reported with injections of angiotensin intravenously. In 1970 the same effects were seen by direct injections into the brain.[6] At the same time, Severs et al.[7] showed that angiotensin directly injected into the cerebral ventricles increased blood pressure. Further studies by Hoffmann and Phillips[8] confirmed these findings and they made an effort to localize the receptor site within the brain for this biological activity. Thus, it seemed that whether angiotensin was formed by renin or formed de novo there was a highly potent effect of the octapeptide in the brain. Direct injection in the cerebral ventricles overcame the blood brain barrier (BBB), which normally excludes peripheral angiotensin from brain tissue. The only exceptions to this were the circumventricular organs, where the BBB is open. In particular, the subfornical organ and organum vasculosum laminae terminalis appeared to contain receptor neurons for angiotensin II.

In 1975, two studies independently demonstrated that blood pressure in spontaneously hypertensive rats (SHR) could be lowered by injections of the angiotensin II antagonist, saralasin, into the brain ventricles but not by intravenous infusion.[9,10] These experiments suggested that there was an overactive angiotensin system in the brains of hypertensive animals, and this brain angiotensin might contribute to the maintenance of the hypertension. These experiments have since been repeated and expanded with the use of both long term infusions of saralasin and other angiotensin inhibitors including converting enzyme inhibitors. In each case, the finding has been consistent.[11–14]

Subsequently, Hirose et al.[15] separated cathepsin D from a brain renin-like substance both on the basis of pH optimum and response to renin antibody. This seemed to settle the confusion over renin and cathepsin D and establish that there was renin in the brain. Nevertheless, the data of Hirose et al. was criticized as representing such a small quantity of renin that it was probably due to plasma renin contamination.[16] Further experiments on human and dog brain in various laboratories established that there is a brain renin distinct from plasma renin or cathepsin D. Its distribution in the brain has been mapped by immunocytochemistry and localized to subcellular fractions (for references, see Table 4-1).

Renin-rich areas in the mouse brain and rat brain were reported by Rix et al.[60] using an antibody against purified submaxillary mouse renin raised in rabbits. The antibody had no cross-reactivity with cathepsin D but fully cross-reacted with mouse kidney renin and rat kidney renin. In both species the most concentrated immunoreactivity was in the supraoptic nucleus and the nuclei of the para- and pariventricularis. Renin-like immunoreactivity was also found in fibers in the dorsal part of the posterior lobe of the pituitary gland. A similar distribution for renin was found by Inagami et al.[49] and Fuxe and his colleagues[21] using the immunofluorescence technique. There appeared to be overlap with the cells staining for renin and those staining for oxytocin in the supraoptic nucleus. The antibody to renin, however, did not cross-react with oxytocin and the results indicate a coexistence of the renin and the peptide in the same cells.

A quantitative study by Schelling et al.[47] using a renin microassay of tissue discretely micropunched from different rat brain areas confirmed that high amounts were in the nuclei described earlier. In addition, a very high concentration was found in the pineal gland.[46,47] Brain renin has similar properties to renal or plasma renin in molecular weight (36,000) and optimal pH of enzyme activity (pH 6.5–7). However, the structure is not identical because the brain renin has lower isoelectric focusing values than plasma or renal renin.[52] Thus, while it may be debated that the original papers claiming to show renin were contaminated with cathepsin D, in the end they stimulated experiments demonstrating the presence of a distinct renin in the brain.

Table 4-1
Evidence for a Brain Renin

1. Presence in brain	Ganten et al., 1971[3]
	Fischer-Ferraro et al., 1971[4]
2. Cathepsin D or renin	Reid and Day, 1976[5]
3. Separation of cathepsin D and renin	Hirose et al., 1978[15]
	Inagami et al., 1978[40]
	Ganten and Speck, 1978[41]
	Osman et al., 1979[42]
4. Measurement and characterization of renin in brain	Haulica et al., 1975[43]
	Dzau et al., 1979[44]
	Hirose et al., 1978[15]
	Speck et al., 1982[45]
5. Distribution in brain	
(Hog)	Hirose et al., 1980[46]
(Rat)	Schelling et al., 1981[47]
6. Immunohistochemical distribution in brain	
(Human)	Slater, 1980[48]
(Mouse)	Inagami, 1980[49]
(Rat)	Fuxe et al., 1982[21]
(Dog)	Smeby et al., 1982[50]
7. Subcellular localization	Smeby et al., 1982[50]
8. Presence in cells (neuroblastoma)	Fishman et al., 1981[51]
	Inagami et al., 1982[52]

Angiotensinogen and Angiotensin in the Brain

If the angiotensin in the brain is formed via a renin-angiotensin cascade, then one would anticipate that the other components of the system would also be present. There was less controversy concerning this part of the story, and angiotensinogen and converting enzyme were found in brain tissue without dispute (Table 4-2). However, there could be contamination of angiotensinogen produced in the brain with that of peripheral origin in the cerebral blood vessels. Printz et al.[17] separated brain angiotensinogen from peripheral angiotensinogen in plasma using ^{3}H-inulin and fully established its quantity and localization within different brain areas. Converting enzyme was found mainly in the choroid plexus within the ventricular system[61] (Table 4-3) and creates a puzzle in that it does not appear to be distributed in the same locations as renin, angiotensinogen or angiotensin II. If it is not in the same place, how can it act in a renin-angiotensin cascade? Fortunately, in cell culture all the components have been found in a

Table 4-2
Evidence for a Brain Angiotensinogen (Renin Substrate)

1.	Renin substrate in brain	Ganten et al., 1971[3]
2.	Quantification in CSF	Reid and Ramsay, 1975[53]
3.	Isoelectric focusing	Printz et al., 1978[54]
4.	Regional distribution	Lewicki et al., 1978[55]
5.	Independent of plasma	Morris and Reid, 1978[56] Printz et al., 1980[57] Eggena et al., 1980[75]
6.	Stimulation by steroids	Printz et al., 1980[57]
7.	Release from hind brain slices	Sernia and Reid, 1980[58]

single cell[41,52] and therefore gross distribution may be a matter of quantity.

Angiotensin II-containing fibers have been localized by immunocytochemistry in several brain regions including the nucleus tractus solitarius, amygdala, and median eminence, but the localization within cell bodies is restricted largely to the supraoptic nucleus and the paraventricular nucleus.[18,19] Other areas such as the hippocampus contain isolated immunoreactive cells, and there are numerous fibers in various localizations. Fibers stained for immunoreactive angiotensin II are frequently found winding around blood vessels (Figure 4-1). This may indicate a role of central angiotensin II in local cerebral blood flow.

Since the supraoptic neurons produce vasopressin, an overlap of vasopressin and angiotensin II is being investigated. Zimmerman et al.[20] claim

Table 4-3
Evidence for Brain Converting Enzyme (CE)

1.	Distribution of CE in neurohypophysis, cerebellum, and lower activities in midbrain, hypothalamus, and choroid plexus	Yang and Neff, 1972[59] Rix et al., 1982[60] Igic et al., 1977[61]
2.	Contained in synaptosomes and membrane bound	Benuck and Marks, 1980[62]
3.	Blockade of CE in SHR lowers blood pressure	Stamler et al., 1980[12] Unger et al., 1981[13]

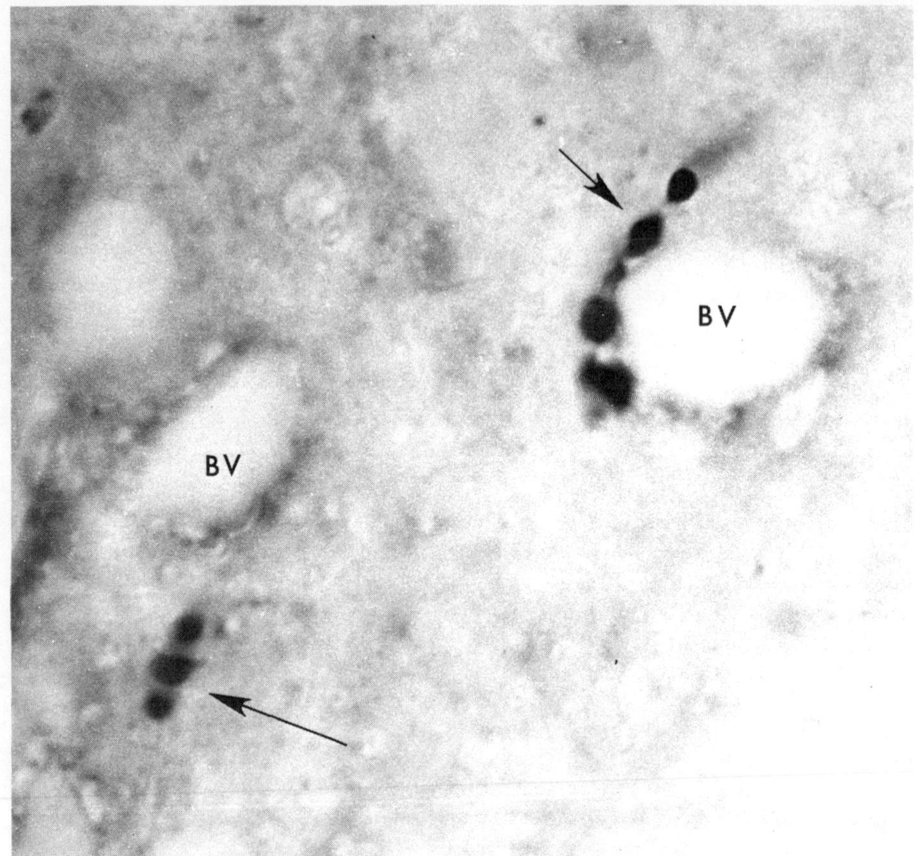

Figure 4-1. Immunoreactive angiotensin II demonstrated by the PAP technique showing fibers (arrow) coursing round a blood vessel (BV). Magnification × 7200. This was from rat; a similar reaction was observed in monkey and human brain.

that angiotensin is localized in the same cells as those containing vasopressin. In thin sections they found both peptides in the same cell. On the other hand, Fuxe et al.[21] claim that angiotensin II is found in cells that contain oxytocin. The significance of this dual packaging is not clear. Vasopressin and angiotensin are not formed from the same prohormone. Further, angiotensin releases vasopressin when injected into the brain.

It appears that angiotensin II can be synthesized in a single cell since ^{3}H-[Ile] and ^{3}H[Val] are incorporated into immunoreactive angiotensin II in primary brain cell cultures.[24] Since the immunoreactive studies show only what the antibody recognizes, our latest approach is to analyze by high pressure liquid chromatography the brain tissue containing immunoreactive angiotensin. To do this we developed a radioimmunoassay for angiotensin II with very high recovery rates (>90%) and assayed the tissue rapidly without freezing and thawing or lyophilizing. We found reasonable amounts of angiotensin II (Ang II) and angiotensin III (Ang III) in the hypothalamus and lower amounts in the cortex of rat brains. Both comigrate with authentic (Ile)[5] angiotensin II and (Ile)[5] angiotensin III on the HPLC. Since the rats were previously nephrectomized and blood levels of Ang II were negligible, the results offer proof of Ang II being endogenously synthesized in the brain.

HPLC assays were run with the hypothalamic tissue, and in each case a clear peak was found in the same fractions that authentic [5](Ile) angiotensin II migrated to (Figure 4-2). Tests with the ^{3}H-Ang II confirmed the position of the peak fraction since it migrated to the same fraction as the hypothalamic Ang II. The results shown in Figures 4-2 and 4-3 demonstrate the presence of a brain peptide that comigrates with the octapeptide an-

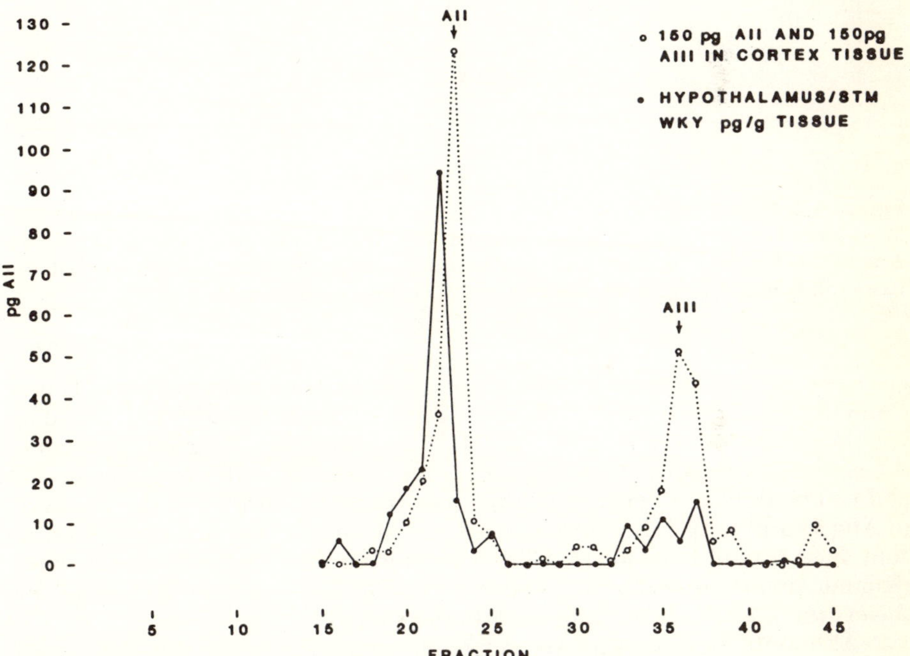

Figure 4-2. Profiles from extracted brain tissue of hypothalamic or cortex origin in a reverse phase HPLC system. Aliquots of each fraction (1 μl) were measured by a high recovery angiotensin II RIA. Prior separation was performed on a Sep-Pac-18 column. UV absorbance was monitored at 210 nm. 90% of the Ang II-like immunoreactivity was recovered from the HPLC column. The result in this profile shows 129 pg/g tissue Ang II and 49 pg/g tissue Ang III, both comigrating with authentic Ang II and III.

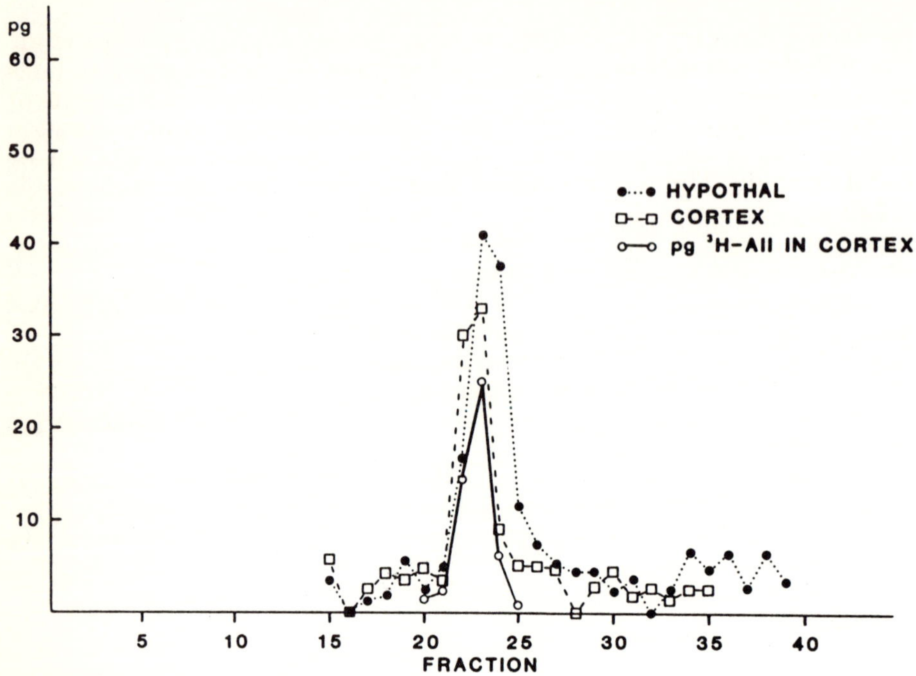

Figure 4-3. Profiles obtained after HPLC using ^{3}H-Ang II added to cortical tissue in order to test precisely to which fraction the Ang II migrated. The peak for ^{3}H-Ang II was fraction 24, and this was also found with both cortical and hypothalamic tissue, showing that these tissues contained endogenous Ang II.

giotensin II. The peptide has the same retention time as angiotensin II and could be measured by radioimmunoassay for Ang II. In addition, the analysis shows that there is angiotensin II$^{2-8}$ heptapeptide (Ang III) present in the brain. This peptide co-migrates with authentic ^{5}(Ile) angiotensin III and can be detected because of the cross-reactivity (100%) of the antibody to Ang II and Ang III. Control tubes tested without the presence of tissue contained no angiotensin II. Cortex treated in the same way as the hypothalamic tissue showed a much reduced amount of angiotensin, but nevertheless there was a detectable peak in the same fractions.

Although the amounts are relatively small (mean = 100–300 pg/g), the results confirm the immunohistochemical studies since the highest concentration of immunoreactive Ang II was in the hypothalamus. We conclude that we were seeing authentic angiotensin II in the supraoptic and paraventricular cells.

Working with cell culture, Raizada et al.[24] have found that radioactive tyrosine can be incorporated into immunoreactive angiotensin. This was done using a tritiated-labelled tyrosine added to brains in cell culture and incubating them for 4–24 hours. In experimental groups, cyclohexamide was added to prevent the protein synthesis and serum-free cultures were grown to avoid uptake of angiotensin from the medium.[24] The results of cultures at 3 days, 5 days, and 7 days revealed a range of incorporation into the angiotensin precipitant, and this incorporation was blocked by cyclohexamide. The results establish that synthesis can occur in the single cell of angiotensin II. In addition to this evidence, angiotensin II has been found in neuroblastoma cells, and all the components of a renin angiotensin system have also been found there.

It still remains to be demonstrated whether angiotensin in the brain is formed by renin angiotensin cascade or by a novel synthetic pathway. Tonin has been proposed as an enzyme that can directly cleave angiotensin II from angiotensinogen.[23] The presence of this type of enzymatic reaction could avoid the necessity of having converting enzyme close to the sites of immunoreactive angiotensin.

In summary, while we may not know yet how angiotensin II is formed in the brain, there does appear to be sufficient evidence for confidence that angiotensin is formed in the brain independently of the peripheral angiotensin system. How it is synthesized, under what conditions, and whether it is identical in all respects to peripheral angiotensin remains to be investigated.

Hypertension and Brain-Renin Angiotensin

How does angiotensin in the brain cause an increase in blood pressure? In the periphery, the major action of angiotensin is direct vasoconstriction. This does not appear to be its main effect in the brain, however, as the pressor action can be reduced or abolished by sympathectomy and hypophysectomy. Sympathectomy induced by injections of 6-hydroxy-dopamine (6-OHDA) centrally abolishes the centrally induced Ang II pressor effect.[25] When given peripherally, 6-OHDA delays the latency of the response to Ang II but does not abolish it.[26] Hypophysectomy reduces the response,[27] and in Brattleboro rats that are genetically incapable of producing vasopressin, the pressor response to central angiotensin II is very small.[28]

These data point to a dual mechanism in the central angiotensin pressor action. Angiotensin stimulates the release of vasopressin into the periphery, which has a direct vasoconstrictive action on blood vessels. Simultaneously, angiotensin triggers activation of sympathetic activity in the periphery, which also increases blood pressure. Removing one or the other does not entirely abolish the pressor action since both mechanisms act in parallel.

It is not yet certain whether angiotensin directly stimulates the supraoptic neurons and causes release of vasopressin or if it does this indirectly. There is evidence for a vasopressin release action on isolated hypothalamic tissue,[29] but the possibility of interneurons being crucial to the release has not been ruled out. The sympathetic activation by central angiotensin appears to involve α-adrenergic receptors since blockade of these by phentolamine reduces the pressor response without altering the drinking response.[30] The actual pathways involved are still unknown.

There is considerable evidence that the starting point for angiotensin activation in the brain is the surface receptor of the organum vasculosum laminae terminalis (OVLT) and subfornical organ (SFO).[31] These are two circumventricular organs set in the anterior wall of the third ventricle. Studies with knife cuts reveal a pathway descending caudally from these sites to the NTS and medulla.[32,33] The present assumption is that angiotensin stimulates the OVLT and triggers neurons in this pathway that activate sympathetic outflow. In models of hypertension such as SHR where the baroreceptor reflex appears to be impaired[34] there is little cardiac compensation for the increased vasoconstriction and hypertension ensues.

In addition, the OVLT and SFO have connections to the supraoptic neurons, and by this route Ang II releases vasopressin which vasoconstricts peripheral vascular beds.[32,34] There are numerous differences in the physiology of spontaneously hypertensive rats (SHR) and their normotensive controls (WKY). No single factor has been isolated (assuming there is one) that could account for the elevated blood pressure. It is hoped that the SHRs offer a model for the most elusive type of hypertension—essential hypertension. In many ways these animals resemble a rat undergoing central angiotensin infusions (see Table 4-4). The rats appear to have higher sympathetic activity and an involvement of vasopressin peripherally.[35,36] They also drink sodium avidly, and it has been observed that rats infused intraventricularly with Ang II will prefer solutions high in sodium (Table 4-5).[64] On the other hand, SH rats do not have increased plasma renin angiotensin levels or overt renal dysfunction, which supports the idea that these effects may be attributed to brain angiotensin.

Table 4-4
Evidence for Involvement of Brain Angiotensin in the
Spontaneously Hypertensive Rats

1. Saralasin lowers blood pressure when injected centrally but not peripherally.[11,39]
2. Captopril lowers blood pressure when injected centrally more than when injected peripherally.[12]
3. MK421 lowers blood pressure centrally (Figure 4-3).
4. More immunoreactive Ang II in the brain is present in SHR than in WKY.[73]
5. Ang II receptor changes in the forebrain are compatible with higher brain Ang II.[38]
6. SHR drink more sodium, which could reflect higher brain Ang II.[74]

Table 4-5
Evidence for a Brain Angiotensin II

1. Biological effects of Ang II	Bickerton and Buckley, 1961[63]
	Fitzsimons, 1972[6]
	Severs and Daniels-Severs, 1973[7]
2. Ang II antagonist lowers blood pressure	Ganten et al., 1975[10]
	Phillips et al., 1975[9]
3. Sodium appetite with Ang II	Buggy and Fisher, 1975[64]
4. Angiotensin receptors in brain	Bennett and Snyder, 1976[65]
	Sirett et al., 1977[66]
5. Immunohistochemical distribution	
(Rat)	Fuxe et al., 1976[18]
	Phillips et al., 1979[19]
	Kilcoyne et al., 1980[67]
(Primate)	Phillips et al., 1980[68]
6. Quantification and characterization	Hutchinson and Csicsman, 1978[69]
	Meyer et al., 1982[22]
	Hermann et al., 1982[70]
7. Angiotensin II in brain cells	
(Receptors)	Raizada et al., 1980[71]
(Immuno-R)	Weyhenmeyer et al., 1980[72]
(Synthesis)	Raizada and Phillips, 1982[24]

Hypertension in spontaneously hypertensive rats can be lowered by the central infusions of angiotensin antagonists[9,10] or converting enzyme inhibitors either acutely or chronically.[12,14] Inhibitors of angiotensin-converting enzyme such as captopril also lower blood pressure peripherally in man and animals with normal or suppressed plasma renin activity. The mechanism of this hypotensive effect is not known, but since it does not appear to depend on peripheral renin levels, the inhibitors may act on the brain. To explore this concept we have studied the central action of converting enzyme inhibition in SHR.[12] Recently, we used the newly developed converting enzyme inhibitor, MK422 (the active diacid form of MK421, made by Merck, Sharpe and Dohme Co.) to interrupt the synthesis of angiotensin II from angiotensin I. MK422 is a potent converting enzyme inhibitor, about 5–7 times more potent than captopril.

In SHR a single injection of 10 μg of MK422 intraventricularly (IVT) produced a biphasic response (Fig. 4-4). For a few minutes there was an increase in blood pressure, which was followed by a prolonged decrease in blood pressure. The pressure was lowered by 25 mm Hg for over 240 minutes. Testing again 24 hours later showed full recovery from the hypoten-

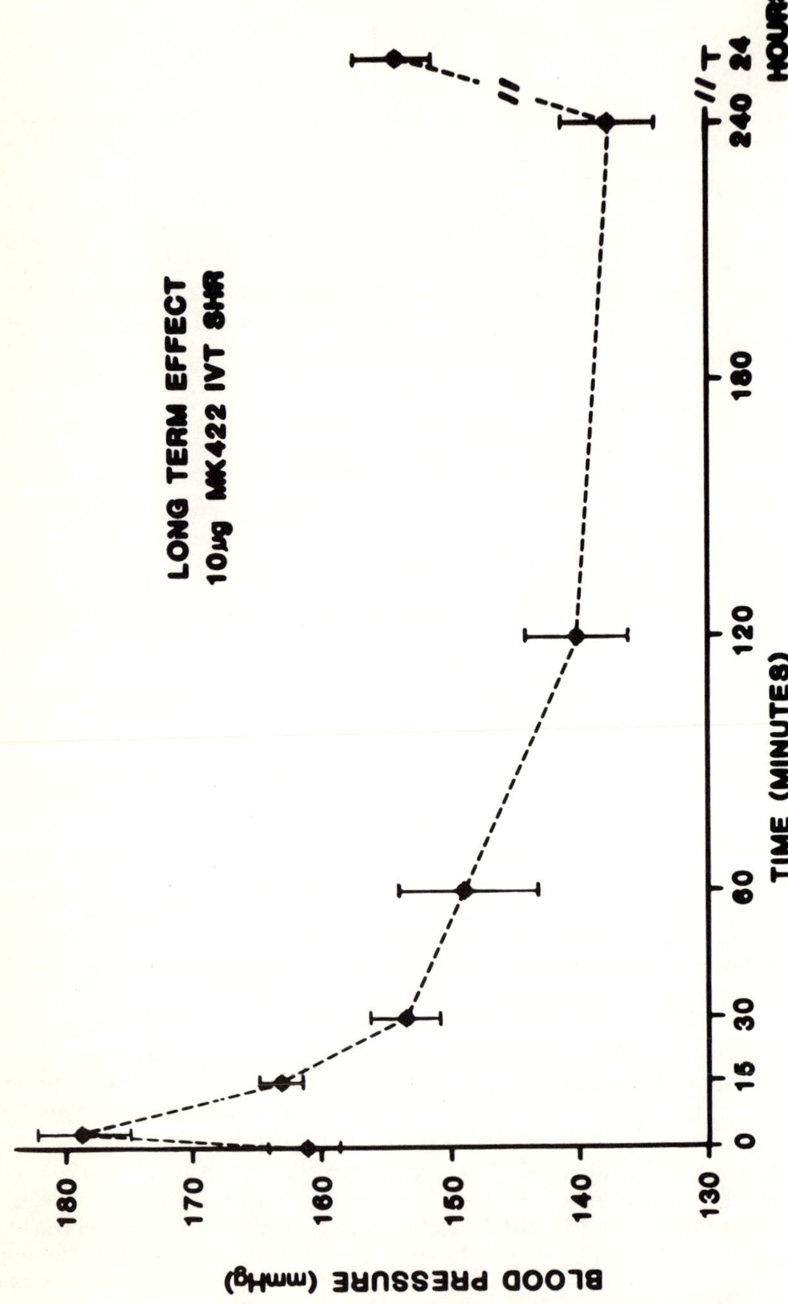

Figure 4-4. The long-term decrease in blood pressure elicited by injecting 10 µg MK422 into the lateral ventricle of spontaneously hypertensive rats. There was no blood-pressure lowering effect on the normotensive Wistar Kyoto control animals. The decrease in blood pressure lasted for at least 10 hours (n = 6).

sive effect. There was no lowering of blood pressure in normotensive rats at this dose level.

A comparison of the different routes of injection revealed that the IVT route was more potent than the intravenous (IV) route. Ten μg of MK422 IVT produced a significant decrease in blood pressure in six SHR (-25 mm Hg $p < .001$). The same dose given IV in these animals produced no significant lowering of blood pressure. Only with the very highest dose tested (2.5 mg IV) was there a significant lowering of blood pressure ($p < 0.001$) with this route of injection.

The results show that MK422 produces a decrease in blood pressure in SHR by a central action on the brain. At 10 μg IVT there was a significant lowering of blood pressure that could not be equalled by the same dose IV, indicating that the effects of the IVT injection were not due to leakage into

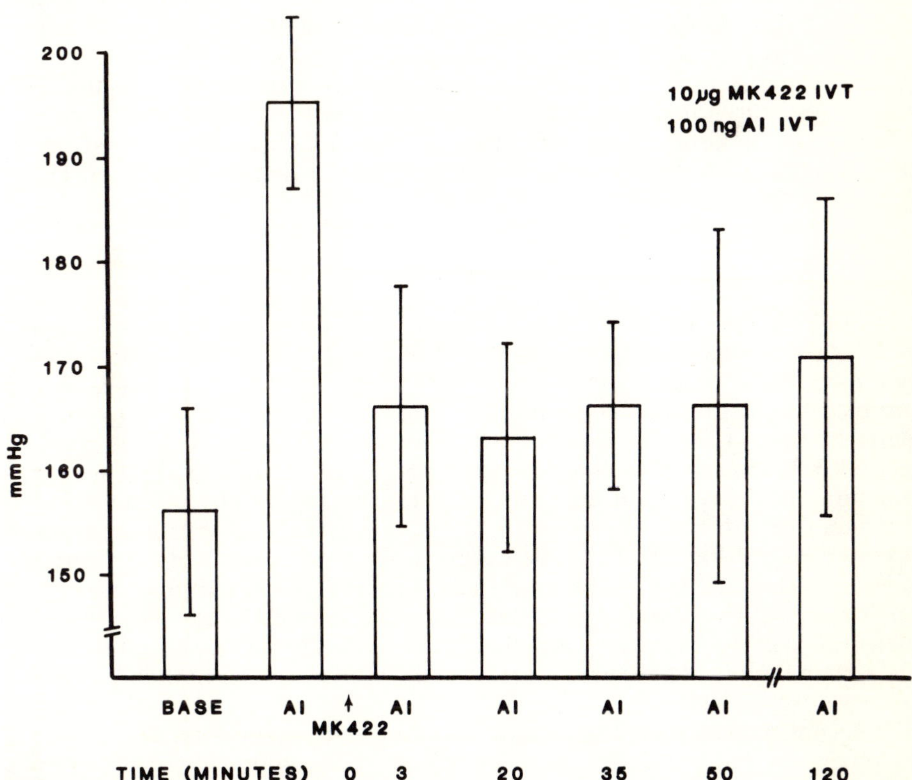

Figure 4-5. Repeated injections of Ang I before and after MK422 was injected IVT reveal that converting enzyme continued to be inhibited during the blood-pressure lowering effect, indicating that the hypotension resulted from the block of Ang II synthesis in the SHR brain.

the periphery. Also, the onset of the depressor effect was rapid (< 30 min.) and long-lasting by both routes when adjusted for the different dose (i.e., higher IV dose). Therefore, the difference in sensitivity between the two routes does not appear to be due to more rapid metabolism in the blood of the IV dose. The lowering of blood pressure with very high doses of MK422 IV may reflect entry into the brain of some portion of the dose from the plasma. Thus, the depressor action of MK422 appears to be on the brain in whole or in part. When angiotensin I was given centrally it was not converted to Ang II, as shown by the reduced pressor response (Figure 4-5). This showed that the MK422 given peripherally or directly into the brain has a central action. Such data as these imply that converting enzyme inhibitors can cross the BBB. Once in the brain they could be effective in lowering blood pressure by preventing the conversion of brain Ang I to Ang II.

In studies on angiotensin receptor binding there are indications that brain receptors may be more sensitive to angiotensin in the hypertensive animals. Microdissection of the circumventricular organs in hypertensive rats revealed that angiotensin II binding was 200% greater in the anterior ventral third ventricle (AV3V) of hypertensive rats than normotensive rats.[37] The initial increase in blood pressure could be explained by an increase in bradykinin. Injections of bradykinin IVT increased blood pressure, in contrast to the depressor effects when the peptide is injected IV.[38]

Summary

The concept of a brain angiotensin system has been established slowly in the face of rigorous questioning. While the amounts of renin and angiotensin in the brain appear to be small, their influence on fluid balance and blood pressure may be profound. The role of multiple organ components of the renin angiotensin cascade in the periphery may be miniaturized in brain tissue to take place in a single cell as indicated in primary neuron cell cultures. In at least one hypertensive model, the spontaneously hypertensive rat, there appears to be an overactivity of the brain renin-angiotensin system, which can be lowered by central angiotensin II antagonists and converting enzyme inhibition. This reveals that angiotensin-converting enzyme inhibitors such as captopril and MK422 may have a therapeutic effect by an action in the brain. Access to the brain could be via the circumventricular organs. This would stimulate sympathetic activity and vasopressin release.

Recently, projections of angiotensin and vasopressin-containing fibers have been found to project to the nucleus tractus solitarius of the brainstem. Here, vasopressin increases the blood pressure when injected directly. Therefore, the triggering action of angiotensin in the brain on vasopressin release may additionally exert an action on the NTS and thus the baroreceptor reflex. These three central actions of angiotensin—increased sympathetic tone, elevated vasopressin release into blood, and vasopressin (or direct angiotensin) mediated alteration of the baroreflex—would produce high blood pressure.

It could be predicted from this that in essential hypertensive patients, elevated levels of angiotensin and/or increased angiotensin receptor binding occurs in the brain. Since angiotensins do not cross the BBB, their presence would be the result of endogenous synthesis of angiotensin in the brain. Ultimately, direct measures in brain tissue or human third ventricle CSF will be required to support this prediction. Based on the studies with the SHR, it would appear that central blockade of brain angiotensin results in a sustained reduction of blood pressure.

References

1. Laragh JH, Buhler FR, Seldin DW: Frontiers in Hypertension Research. New York, Springer Verlag, 1981
2. Cohen S, Taylor JM, Murakami K, Michelakis AM, Inagami T: Isolation and characterization of renin-like enzymes from mouse submaxillary glands. Biochemistry **11:**4286, 1972
3. Ganten D, Minnich JL, Granger P, Hayduk K, Brecht HM, Barbeau A, Boucher R, Genest J: Angiotensin-forming enzyme in brain tissue. Science **173:**64, 1971
4. Fischer-Ferraro C, Nahmod VE, Goldstein DJ, Finkielman S: Angiotensin and renin in rat and dog brain. J Exp Med **133:**353, 1971
5. Day RP, Reid IA: Renin activity in dog brain: enzymological similarity to cathepsin D. Endocrinology **99:**93, 1976
6. Fitzsimons JT: Thirst. Physiol Rev **52:**408, 1972
7. Severs WB, Daniels-Severs AE: Effects of angiotensin on the central nervous system. Pharmacol Rev **25:**415, 1973
8. Hoffman WE, Phillips MI: Regional study of cerebral ventricular sensitive sites to angiotensin II. Brain Res **110:**313, 1976
9. Phillips MI, Phipps J, Hoffman WE, Leavitt M: Reduction of blood pressure by intracranial injection of angiotensin blocker (p113) in spontaneously hypertensive rats (SHR). Physiologist **18**(3):350, 1975 (Abstract)
10. Ganten D, Hutchinson JS, Schelling P: The intrinsic brain iso-renin-angiotensin system in the rat: its possible role in central mechanism of blood pressure regulation. Clin Sci Mol Med **48:**265s, 1975
11. Phillips MI, Mann H, Dietz R, Ganten D: Lowering of hypertension by central saralasin in the absence of plasma renin. Nature **270:**445, 1977
12. Stamler JF, Brody MJ, Phillips MI: The central and peripheral effects of captopril (SQ14225) on the arterial pressure of the spontaneously hypertensive rat. Brain Res **186:**499, 1980
13. Unger T, Kaufman-Buhler I, Scholkens B, Ganten D: Brain-converting enzyme inhibition: a possible mechanism for the antihypertensive action of captopril in spontaneously hypertensive rats. Eur J Pharmacol **70:**467, 1981
14. McDonald W, Wickre C, Aumann S, Ban D, Moffit B: The sustained antihyper-

tensive effect of chronic cerebroventricular infusion of angiotensin antagonist in spontaneously hypertensive rats. Endocrinology **107:**1305, 1980

15. Hirose S, Yokosawa H, Inagami T: Immunochemical identification of renin in rat brain and distinction from acid proteases. Nature **274:**392, 1978
16. Reid IA: Is there a brain renin-angiotensin system? Circ Res **41:**147, 1977
17. Printz MP, Lewicki JA, Wallis CJ: Brain angiotensinogen: origin and evidence for an influence by adrenal corticosteroids. *In* Enzymatic Release of Vasoactive Peptides, edited by Gross F and Vogel G. New York, Raven Press, 1980, p 193
18. Fuxe K, Ganten D, Hokfelt T, Bolme P: Immunohistochemical evidence for the existence of angiotensin II-containing nerve terminals in the brain and spinal cord in the rat. Neurosci Lett **2:**229, 1976
19. Phillips MI, Weyhenmeyer JA, Felix D, Ganten D: Evidence for an endogenous brain renin angiotensin system. Fed Proc **38:**2260, 1979
20. Zimmerman EA, Krupp L, Hoffman DL, Matthew E, Nilaver G: Exploration of peptidergic pathways in brain by immunocytochemistry: a ten year perspective. Peptides **1**(1):3, 1980
21. Fuxe K, Ganten D, Anderson K, Calza L, Agnati LF, Lang RE, Poulsen K, Hokfelt T, Bernardi P: Immunocytochemical demonstration of angiotensin II and renin-like immunoreactive nerve cells in the hypothalamus. Angiotensin peptides as co-modulators in vasopressin and oxytocin neurons and their regulation of various types of central catecholamine nerve terminal systems. *In* The Renin Angiotensin System in the Brain, edited by Ganten D, Printz M, Phillips MI, Scholkens BA. Heidelberg, Springer-Verlag, 1982, p 208
22. Meyer DK, Phillips MI, Eiden L: Studies on the presence of angiotensin II in rat brain. J Neurochem **38:**816, 1982
23. Schiller PW, Demassieux S, Boucher R: Substrate specificity of tonin from rat submaxillary gland. Cir Res **39:**629, 1976
24. Raizada MK, Phillips MI, Gerndt JS: Primary cultures from fetal rat brain incorporate [^{3}H]-isoleucine and [^{3}H]-valine into immunoprecipitable angiotensin II. Neuroendocrinology **36:**64, 1983
25. Gordon FJ, Haywood JR, Brody MJ, Johnson AK: Effect of lesions of the anteroventral third ventricle (AV3V) on the development of hypertension in spontaneously hypertensive rats. Hypertension **4:**387, 1982
26. Falcon JE, Phillips MI, Hoffman WE, Brody MJ: Effects of intraventricular angiotensin II mediated by the sympathetic nervous system. Am J Physiol **235**(4):H392, 1978
27. Severs WB, Summy-Long J, Taylor JS, Connor JD: A central effect of angiotensin: release of pituitary pressor material. J Pharmacol Exp Ther **174:**27, 1970
28. Hutchinson JS, Schelling P, Mohring J, Ganten D: Pressor action of centrally perfused angiotensin II in rats with hereditary hypothalamic diabetes insipidus. Endocrinology **99**(3):819, 1976
29. Sladek CD, Joynt RJ: Characterization of cholinergic control of vasopressin release by the organ-cultured rat hypothalamo-neurohypophyseal system. Endocrinology, **104:**659, 1979
30. Camacho A, Phillips MI: Separation of drinking and pressor responses to central angiotensin by monoamines. Am J Physiol **240:**R106, 1981
31. Phillips MI: Angiotensin in the brain. Neuroendocrinology **25:**354, 1978
32. Phillips MI, Hoffman WE, Bealer SL: Dehydration and fluid balance: central effects of angiotensin. Fed Proc **41:**2520, 1982

33. Hartle DK, Brody MJ: Hypothalamic vasomotor pathways mediating the development of hypertension in the rat. Hypertension **4:**(Supp III)68, 1982
34. Mohring J: Neurohypophyseal vasopressor principle: vasopressor hormone as well as antidiuretic hormone. Klin Wochenschr **56:**71, 1978
35. Schomig A, Dietz R, Rascher W, Luth JB, Mann JFE, Schmidt M, Weber J: Sympathetic vascular tone in spontaneous hypertension of rats. Klin Wochenschr **56:**131, 1978
36. Crofton JT, Share L, Shade RE, Allen C, Tarnowski D: Vasopressin in the rat with spontaneous hypertension. Am Physiol Soc **235:**H361, 1978
37. Stamler JF, Raizada MK, Fellows RE, Phillips MI: Increased specific binding of angiotensin II in the organum vasculosum of the laminae terminalis area of the spontaneously hypertensive rat brain. Neurosci Lett **17:**173, 1980
38. Lewis RE, Hoffman WE and Phillips MI: Angiotensin II and bradykinin: interactions between two centrally active peptides. Am J Physiol **24:**R285, 1983
39. Clough DP, Langmann E, Rettig R, Rockhold R, Unger TH, Ganten D: The effects on blood pressure of central angiotensin blockage in spontaneously hypertensive and sodium depleted rats. Proceedings of the Fourth International Symposium on SHR. Schattauer Verlag, 1982, in press.
40. Inagami T, Yokosawa H, Hirose S: Definitive evidence for renin in rat brain by affinity chromatographic separation from protease. Clin Sci Mol Med **55:**121s, 1978
41. Ganten D, Speck G: The brain renin-angiotensin system: a model for the synthesis of peptides in the brain. Biochem Pharmacol **17:**2379, 1978
42. Osman MY, Smeby BR, Sen S: Separation of dog brain renin-like activity from acid protease activity. Hypertension **1:**53, 1979
43. Haulica I, Branisteanu DD, Bosca V, Stratone A, Berbeleu V, Balan G, Ionescu L: Renin-like activity in pineal gland and hypophysis. Endocrinology **96:**530, 1975
44. Dzau VJ, Slater EE, Haber E: Complete purification of dog renal renin. Biochemistry **18:**5224, 1979
45. Speck GA, Unger T, Lang RE, Ganten D: Isolation and in vivo activity of brain renin for mice and men. *In* The Renin Angiotensin System in the Brain, edited by Ganten D, Pritz M, Phillips MI, Scholkens BA. Heidelberg, Springer-Verlag, 1982, p 76.
46. Hirose S, Yokosawa H, Inagami T, Workman RJ: Renin and prorenin in hog brain: ubiquitous distribution and high concentration in the pituitary and pineal. Brain Res **191:**489, 1980
47. Schelling P, Meyer D, Loos HE, Specle G, Johnson AK, Phillips MI, Ganten D: Renin activity in different brain regions of spontaneously hypertensive rats. *In* Central Nervous System Mechanisms in Hypertension, edited by Buckley JP and Ferrano C, New York, Raven Press, 1981, p 397
48. Slater EE, Defendini R, Zimmerman EA: Wide distribution of immunoreactive renin in nerve cells of human brain. Proc Natl Acad Sci (USA) **77:**5458, 1980
49. Inagami T, Celio MR, Clemens D, Lau D, Takii Y, Kasselberg AG, Hirose S: Renin in rat and mouse brain: immunohistochemical identification and localization. Clin Sci **59**(6):49s, 1980
50. Smeby RR, Husain A, Speth RC: Properties and subcellular localization of brain renin and its substrate. *In* The Renin Angiotensin System in the Brain, edited by Ganten D, Printz M, Phillips MI, Scholkens BA. Heidelberg, Springer-Verlag, 1982, p 118

51. Fishman MC, Zimmerman EA, Slater EE: Renin and angiotensin II: the complete system within the neuroblastoma and glioma. Science **214:**922, 1981
52. Inagami T, Okamura T, Hirose S, Clemens D, Celio MR, Naruse K, Takii Y: Identification, characterization and evidence for interneuronal function of renin in the brain and neuroblastoma cells. *In* The Renin Angiotensin System in the Brain, edited by Ganten D, Printz M, Phillips MI, Scholkens BA. Heidelberg, Springer-Verlag, 1982, p 64
53. Reid IA, Ramsay DJ: The effects of intracerebroventricular administration of renin on drinking and blood pressure. Endocrinology **97:**536, 1975
54. Printz MP, Printz JM, Gregory TJ: Identification of angiotensinogen in animal brain homogenates. Cir Res **43**(1):21, 1978
55. Lewicki JA, Fallon JH, Printz MP: Regional distribution of angiotensinogen in rat brain. Brain Res **158:**359, 1978
56. Morris BJ, Reid IA: The distribution of angiotensinogen in dog brain studied by cell fractionation. Endocrinology **103:**492, 1978
57. Printz MP, Lewicki JA, Wallis CJ: Brain angiotensinogen: origin and evidence for an influence by adrenal corticosteroids. *In* Enzymatic Release of Vasoactive Peptides, edited by Gross F and Vogel G. New York, Raven Press, 1980, p 193
58. Sernia C, Reid IA: Relese of angiotensinogen by rat brain in vitro. Brain Res **192:**217, 1980
59. Yang HYT, Neff NH: Distribution and properties of angiotensin converting enzyme of rat brain. J Neurochem **19:**2243, 1972
60. Rix E, Ganten D, Stock G, Taugner R: Immunocytochemical demonstration of renin and converting enzyme in rat and mouse brain. *In* The Renin Angiotensin System in the Brain, edited by Ganten D, Printz M, Phillips MI, Scholkens BA. Heidelberg, Springer-Verlag, 1982, p 126
61. Igic RP, Robinson CJ, Erdos EG: Angiotensin I converting enzyme activity in the choroid plexus and in the retina. *In* Central Actions of Angiotensin and Related Hormones, edited by Buckley JP and Ferrario C. New York, Pergamon Press, 1977, p 23
62. Benuck M, Marks N: Characterization of a distinct membrane-bound dipeptidylcarboxypeptidase inactivating enkephalin in brain. Biochem Biophys Res Commun **95:**822, 1980
63. Bickerton RK, Buckley JP: Evidence for a central mechanism of angiotensin induced hypertension. Proc Soc Exp Biol Med **106:**834, 1961
64. Buggy J, Fisher AE: Water and sodium intake: evidence for a dual central role for angiotensin: Nature (London) **250:**733, 1975
65. Bennett JP Jr, Snyder SH: Angiotensin II binding to mammalian brain membranes. J Biol Chem **251:**7423, 1976
66. Sirett NE, McLean AS, Bray JJ, Hubbard JI: Distribution of angiotensin II receptors in rat brain. Brain Res **122:**299, 1977
67. Kilcoyne MM, Hoffman DL, Zimmerman EA: Immunocytochemical localization of angiotensin II and vasopressin in rat hypothalamus: evidence for production in the same neuron. Clin Sci **59**(6):57s, 1980
68. Phillips MI, Quinlan JT, and Weyhenmeyer J: An angiotensin-like peptide in the brain. *In* CNS Mechanisms in Hypertension, edited by Buckley JP and Ferrario C. New York, Raven Press, 1981, p 6
69. Hutchinson JS, Csicsmann J: The distribution of immunoreactive angiotensins I and II extracted from rat brain. Acta Med Acad Sci Hung **35:**277, 1978

70. Hermann K, Ganten D, Bayer C, Unger T, Lange RE, Rascher W: Definite evidence for the presence of [Ile^5]-angiotensin I and [Ile^5]-angiotensin II in the brain of rats. *In* The Renin Angiotensin System in the Brain, edited by Ganten D, Printz M, Phillips MI, Scholkens BA. Heidelberg, Springer-Verlag, 1982, p 192

71. Raizada MK, Yang JW, Phillips MI, Fellows RE: Rat brain cells in primary culture: characterization of angiotensin II binding sites. Brain Res **207**(2):343, 1981

72. Weyhenmeyer JA, Raizada MK, Phillips MI, Fellows RE: Presence of angiotensin II in neurons cultured from fetal rat brain. Neurosci Lett **16**:41, 1980

73. Weyhenmeyer JA, Phillips MI: Angiotensin like immunoreactivity in the brain of the spontaneously hypertensive rat. Hypertension **4**:514, 1982

74. Phillips MI: Central effects of angiotensin II on hypertension and sodium intake. *In* Role of Sodium in Cardiovascular Hypertension, edited by Fregly M, Kare M. New York, Academic Press, 1981, p 127

75. Eggena P, Ito T, Barrett JD, Villarreal H, Sambhi MP: A comparison of human renin substrate in plasma and cerebrospinal fluid. *In* The Renin Angiotensin System in the Brain, edited by Ganten D, Printz M, Phillips MI, Scholkens BA. Heidelberg, Springer-Verlag, 1982, p 169

Chapter 5

Central Regulation of Renin Release

K. Bridget Brosnihan and Carlos M. Ferrario

Introduction

The basic structures and physiological factors involved in the release of renin by the kidney are indicated in Figure 5-1. The major factors that regulate renin release are: 1) an intrarenal baroreceptor, 2) the ionic concentration of either sodium (Na^+) and/or chloride (Cl^-) sensed by the macula densa segment in the distal tubule, and 3) the sympathetic nervous system. Early studies showed that the rate of renin secretion is inversely proportional to the pressure in the renal arterioles (intrarenal baroreceptors). This effect may be mediated by a direct inhibitory effect of stretch on the juxtaglomerular cells, a decrease in transmural pressure gradient (i.e., the difference between intraluminal pressure and renal interstitial pressure), or a fall in wall tension at the level of the afferent arteriole. The modulating influence of the sympathetic nervous system on arteriolar smooth muscle tone is also indicated in Figure 5-1.

In addition to these physical factors, circulating hormones or locally generated vasoactive agents may function to change the gain of the intrarenal baroreceptor mechanism. Secretion of renin is also regulated by the macula densa. In this case the rate of secretion is inversely proportional to the amount of Na^+ and/or Cl^- transported across the cells of the macula densa tubular structure. Finally, catecholamines released at the postganglionic sympathetic nerve ending (SN) in the kidney and circulating catecholamines from the adrenal medulla stimulate renin secretion by activation of beta-adrenergic receptors in the juxtaglomerular cells in the kidney. Hormones like angiotensin II, mineralocorticoids, and prostaglandins are other important regulators. These aspects have been recently reviewed in detail[1-5] and will be discussed here only in terms of mechanisms that may be responsible for mediating central release of renin.

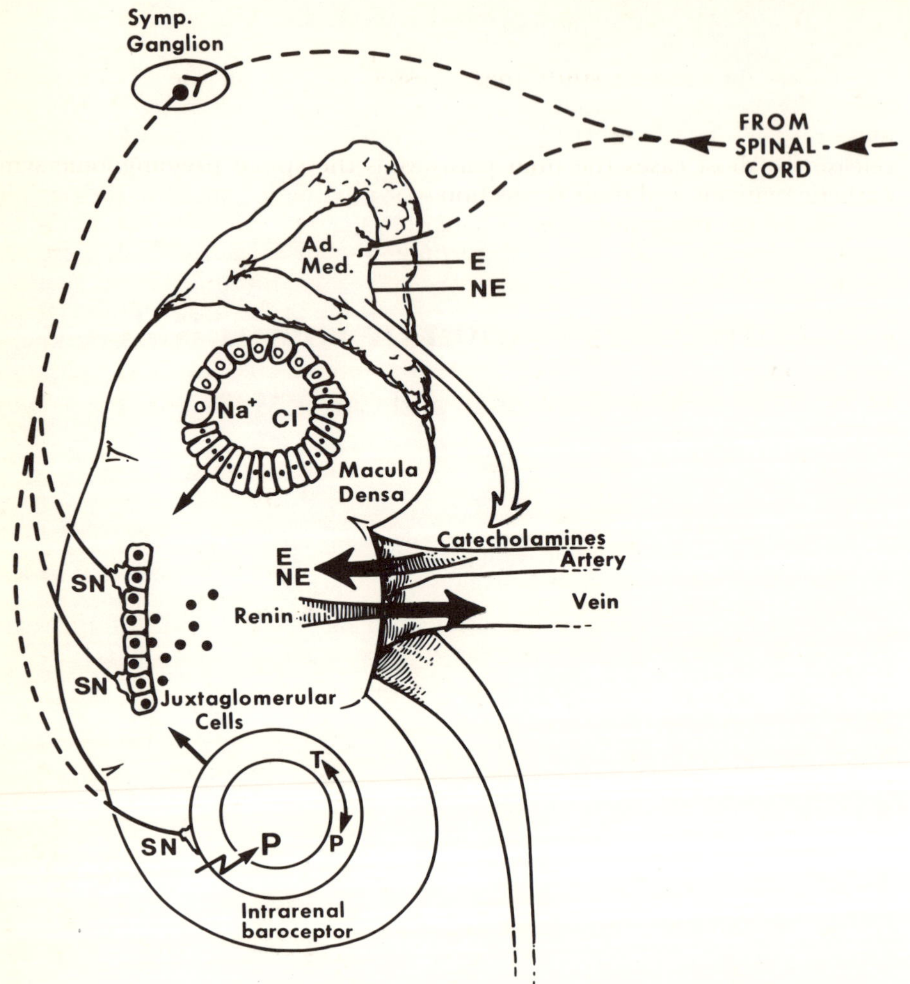

Figure 5-1. Summary of the major modes of control of renin release. See text for explanation. SN = sympathetic nerves; E = epinephrine; NE = norepinephrine; P = pressure; T = tension.

This chapter reviews new information on the central regulation of renin release. Considering the well-known neural aspects of the control of renin release, it is understandable that interest and enthusiasm for clarifying the role of the brain in the regulation of renin release has led to important advances recently. The discovery that neuropeptides in the brain act both independently and in concert with traditional neurotransmitters to influence heart and blood vessel function has also made a mark in elucidating the role of the CNS in the regulation of renin release.

Brain Areas Associated with Renin Secretion

Following the first study that assessed the role of the CNS in renin release by electrical stimulation in 1967,[6] slow but steady progress has permitted mapping the regions of the brain involved in the regulation of renin release. In most cases the final pathway is the spinal preganglionic sympathetic neurons and their projection to sympathetic ganglia in the periphery. However, there are many unanswered questions about the interconnecting networks between the brain and the spinal cord. Both electrical stimulation (Table 5-1) and chemical electrolytic lesion (Table 5-2) studies suffer from the drawback that fibers of passage in the CNS are also stimulated and/or destroyed in the sites studied. A definitive statement of the sites involved cannot always be made. In spite of this drawback, mapping studies have provided us with a basic framework of the pathways effecting changes in the release of renin.

Electrical Stimulation Studies

Electrical stimulation of a wide range of sites within the brain causes changes in renin release. Passo et al.[7,8] stimulated a site in the dorsal medulla (DM) near the obex and observed a 3- to 4-fold increase in plasma renin activity associated with an increase in mean arterial pressure. Both acute and chronic denervation of the kidneys nearly abolished the rise in PRA. Additionally, beta-adrenergic antagonists reduced the response.[8] Since plasma epinephrine levels rose during electrical stimulation of this region, a part of the response may be due to an adrenal medullary component.[7]

Similar results were observed when midbrain regions were electrically stimulated. Ueda et al.[6] stimulated the mesencephalic pressor area around the central gray striatum (periaqueductal gray, PAG) and found that the pressor response was associated with a 5-fold increase in the renal venous arterial difference in renin activity; renal denervation inhibited the neural mediated release of renin.[6]

Comparison of renin release in intact and denervated kidneys enabled Richardson et al.[9,10] to assess the effects of electrical stimulation of the nucleus reticular parvacellularis, a site located near the pontomedullary junction, and to separate the direct effects on renin release from the indirect effects influencing renal vascular resistance. This site is indicated as ventrolateral medulla (VLM) in Figure 5-2. As expected, denervation of the contralateral kidney abolished the increase in renin release following electrical stimulation of the region. Although phenoxybenzamine treatment caused renal vasodilatation, the treatment did not blunt the renin release to stimulation of VLM. Propranolol, on the other hand, abolished the renin release to stimulation of the ventrolateral medulla. The latter finding was consistent with the influence of renal beta-adrenergic receptors on renin

Text continues on page 89

Table 5-1
Summary of Brain Regions that Cause Changes in Renin Release When Electrically Stimulated

Site	Animal	Renin	Blood Pressure	Renal Blood Flow	Femoral Blood Flow	Citation
Posterior hypothalamus (supramammillary nucleus, SMN)	Anesthetized rat	↑ PRA (I) ↔PRA (RD)	NM	NM	NM	Natcheff
SMN	Anesthetized rhesus monkey	↑ PRA (I)	↑	NM	NM	Frankel et al.
Lateral hypothalamus throughout rostral caudal extent (LH)	Conscious dog	↓ PRA (I) ↔PRA (RD)	↓ ↓	↔ ↔	ʾ ↑ ↑	Zehr & Feigl
Lateral hypothalamus (defense area, HDR)	Anesthetized cats	↑ RSR (I) ↔RSR (RD)	↑ ↑	↓ ↔	↑ ↑	Zanchetti et al. Stella et al.
LH	Anesthetized rhesus monkey	↑ PRA (I)	↑	NM	NM	Frankel et al.
Dorsal portion of medulla oblongata (DM)	Anesthetized dogs	↑ PRA (I) ↔PRA (RD)	↑ ↑	NM NM	NM NM	Passo et al. Passo et al.
Nucleus reticularis parvocellularis at the pontomedullary border (ventrolateral medulla, VLM)	Anesthetized cats	↑ RSR (I) ↔RSR (RD)	↑ ↑	↓ ↔	NM	Richardson et al.
Midbrain region—central gray striatum (periaqueductal gray, PAG)	Anesthetized dogs	↑ PRA (I) ↔PRA (RD)	↑ ↑	↓ ↔	NM	Ueda
Fastigial nucleus (FN)	Anesthetized cats	↑ PRA (I)	↑	Constant	NM	Koyama et al.
Cingulate gyrus/corpus callosum (CC)	Anesthetized rhesus monkey	↑ PRA (I)	↓	NM	NM	Frankel et al.
Nucleus septalis medius (NSM)	Anesthetized rhesus monkey	↑ PRA (I)	↑	NM	NM	Frankel et al.
Paracingulate subneocortical white matter (PSWM)	Anesthetized rhesus monkey	↑ PRA (I)	↔	NM	NM	Frankel et al.
Lower medial quadrant of frontal lobe (LMFL)	Anesthetized rhesus monkey	↑ PRA (I)	↑	NM	NM	Frankel et al.

(I) = intact animals; RD = renal denervated animal; NM = not measured; PRA = plasma renin activity; RSR = renin secretion rate.

Table 5-2
Summary of Lesion Sites in the CNS that Were Assessed for an Effect on Renin Release

Site	Animal	Renin	Blood Pressure	RBF	Citation
A. *Electrolytic Lesions*					
Mediobasal hypothalamus sparing median-eminence (MBH-ME)	Anesthetized rat	↔PRA (B)	NM	NM	Karteszi
		↓ PRA (S)	NM	NM	Karteszi
MBH + median eminence (MBH + ME)	Anesthetized rat	↔PRA (B)	NM	NM	Karteszi
		↓ PRA (S)	NM	NM	Karteszi
Anterolateral deafferentation of MBH	Anesthetized rat	↔PRA (B)	NM	NM	Karteszi
		↔PRA (S)	NM	NM	Karteszi
Posterolateral deafferentation of MBH	Anesthetized rat	↔PRA (B)	NM	NM	Karteszi
		↔PRA (S)	NM	NM	Karteszi
Hypophysectomy	Anesthetized rat	↔PRA (B)	NM	NM	Karteszi
		↑ PRA (S)	NM	NM	Karteszi
Anteroventral 3rd ventricle (AV3V)	Anesthetized rat	↑ PRC (B)	NM	NM	Shrager & Johnson
		↑ PRC (S)	NM	NM	Shrager & Johnson
Posterior hypothalamus (supramammillary nuclei, SMN)	Anesthetized rat	↑ PRA (B)	NM	NM	Natcheff et al.
		⇈ PRA (S)	NM	NM	Natcheff et al.
Nucleus tractus solitarius (NTS)	Conscious dog	↑ PRA (B) 1 wk	↑	NM	Ferrario et al.
		↔PRA (B) >2 wk	↑	NM	Ferrario et al.
Area postrema (AP)	Conscious dog	↔PRA (B)	↔/↓	NM	Ferrario et al.
NTS	Anesthetized rat	↑ PRA (Acute)	↑	NM	Zandberg et al.
		↔PRA (>5 wk)	↑	NM	Zandberg et al.
NTS	Conscious dogs	↔PRA (B-chronic)	↑	NM	Carey et al.
B. *Chemical Lesions*					
Dorsal raphe nuclei (DR)	Anesthetized rat	↔PRA (B)	NM	NM	Van de Kar et al.
		↓ PRA (S)	NM	NM	Van de Kar et al.
Median raphe nuclei (MR)	Anesthetized rat	↔PRA (B)	NM	NM	Van de Kar et al.
		↔PRA (S)	NM	NM	Van de Kar et al.

PRA = plasma renin activity; PRC = plasma renin concentration; NM = not measured; (B) = basal, unstimulated conditions; (S) = stimulated conditions.

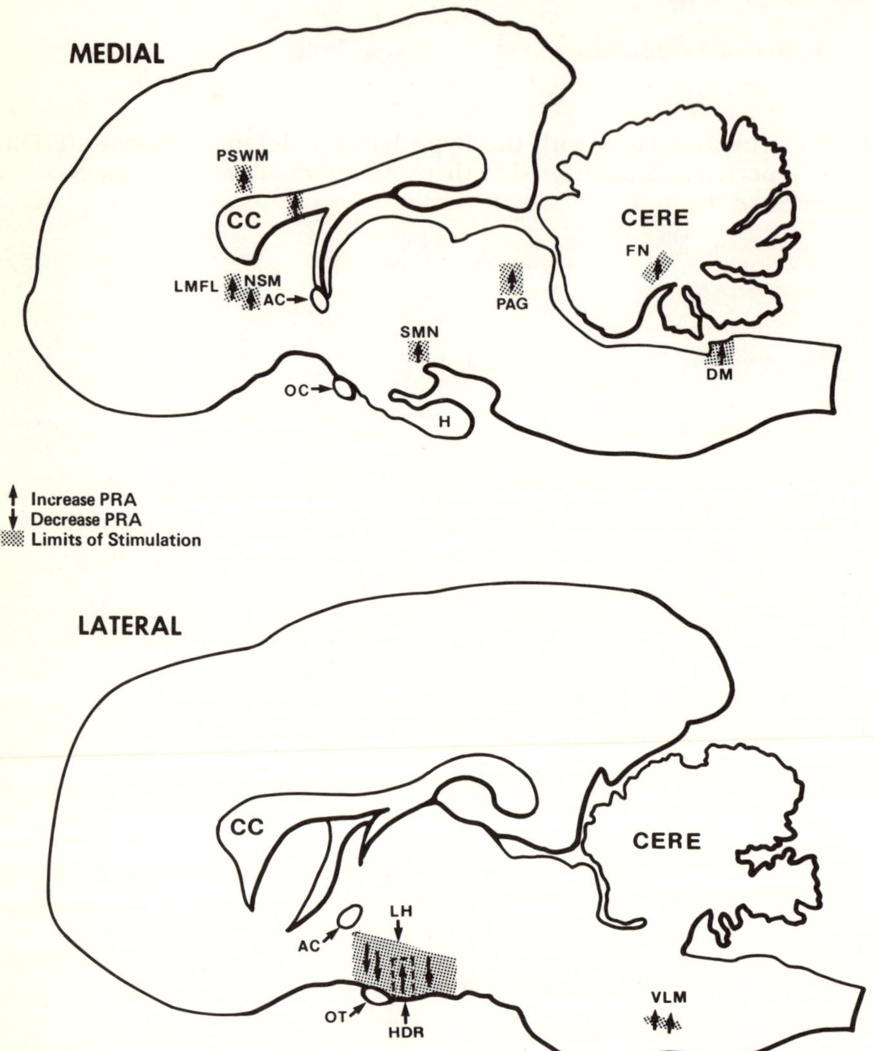

Figure 5-2. Medial and lateral sagittal sections of the brain summarizing regions electrically stimulated in relationship to renin release. *Landmarks:* CC = corpus callosum; AC = anterior commissure; OC = optic chiasm; OT = optic tract; CERE = cerebellum; LH = lateral hypothalamus. *Stimulated sites:* PAG = periaqueductal gray; SMN = supramammillary nucleus; FN = fastigial nucleus; LH = lateral hypothalamus; HDR = hypothalamic defense region within the lateral hypothalamus; VLM = ventral lateral medulla; DM = dorsal medulla at obex; H = hypophysis; PSWM = paracingulate subneocortical white matter; LMFL = lower medial quadrant of frontal lobe; NSM = nucleus septalis medius.

release, although an extrarenal site for the action of propranolol could not be eliminated.

Indicative of the complex functions regulated by the hypothalamus, electrical stimulation at this site causes a variety of cardiovascular and renin release responses. Stimulation of the lateral hypothalamus in anesthetized cats, the area associated with the hypothalamic defense response (HDR), causes hypertension associated with transient renal vasoconstriction.[11–13] The increase in renin release associated with the response was sustained beyond the renal vascular response and could be blocked by transection of the renal nerves. In contrast, Zehr and Feigl[14] showed suppression of plasma renin activity in the conscious dog after stimulation of a sympathoinhibitory site located throughout the anterior-posterior extent of the lateral hypothalamus (LH). At this site, femoral artery flow was increased while renal blood flow did not change. Moreover, mean arterial pressure fell and heart rate (HR) increased. No further lowering of PRA could be elicited by hypothalamic stimulation if propranolol treatment or renal denervation was used. However, the maneuvers lowered renin levels.

These features enabled the authors to consider that the sympathetic nervous system has a "tonic" stimulatory effect on renin release that could be inhibited by increased activity of this hypothalamic area. Additionally, this study suggests that the action of the sympathetic nervous system over the renal release of renin is distinct from the sympathetic vasoconstrictor discharge to the kidney, which has been shown to be low under resting conditions.[15] In anesthetized rhesus monkeys, Frankel et al.[16] stimulated the lateral hypothalamus and found an increase in blood pressure and elevated PRA. Although neither femoral nor renal blood flows were measured, the site of stimulation and responses obtained are more consistent with the results of Zanchetti and coworkers.[11–13] In both anesthetized rats[17] and rhesus monkeys[16] the posterior hypothalamic regions of the supramammillary nucleus (SMN) have been shown to yield similar results—that is, an increase in PRA associated with an increase in mean arterial blood pressure. The dependency of the response on the renal sympathetic nerves was demonstrated in anesthetized rats.[17]

Frankel et al.[16] electrically stimulated various sites within the limbic system and the frontal lobe of the rhesus monkey. They found evidence for increases in PRA during electrical stimulation of certain areas in the cingulate gyrus adjacent to the corpus callosum (CC) and in the paracingulate subneocortical white matter (PSWM). These areas were quite localized since stimulation of other more medial sites was without effect. In most cases there was a tendency for blood pressure to decrease during these stimulations. On the other hand, stimulation of the lower medial quadrant of the frontal lobe (LMFL) and nucleus septalis medius (NSM) resulted in increases in PRA associated with an increase in BP. The pathways for these extrahypothalamic areas connecting to the hypothalamus and brain stem are not known.

The fastigial nucleus (FN) of the cerebellum has been implicated in a variety of autonomic functions associated with sympathoexcitation. In this regard, Koyama et al.[18,19] stimulated the fastigial nucleus of anesthetized cats and found a pressor response associated with a significant increase in PRA and a marked increase in renal vascular resistance. In animals with bilateral lesions of the superior cerebellar peduncle, the pressor response to fastigial stimulation was preserved but the renin release and the renal vascular resistance change were abolished. The lesion itself was without effect on baseline levels of PRA, systemic blood pressure, and renal perfusion pressure assessed at three levels of carotid sinus pressure (Figure 5-3).

Changes in Renin-Releasing Capabilities Following Electrolytic or Chemical Lesions of the CNS

Only a few studies have been completed in which either lesion or knife cuts through the hypothalamus have been done and the effects on renin studied. Bilateral electrocoagulation of the supramammillary nuclei region in the posterior hypothalamus was shown to abolish the increase in PRA following hypoxia but did not interfere with PRA following peritoneal dialysis.[17] Basal levels of PRA were not significantly elevated after destruction of this site.[17]

Electrolytic lesions of the anterior ventral third ventricle (AV3V) in rats, a region shown to be involved in blood pressure regulation and body fluid balance,[20] resulted in sustained elevations of plasma renin concentration (PRC) in animals receiving water ad libitum. Even three months post-surgery, basal PRC levels in AV3V-lesioned rats were still elevated. However, water deprivation causes a similar response in both lesioned and sham lesioned animals. Mediobasal hypothalamic (MBH) lesions either sparing or destroying the median eminence did not influence basal levels of plasma renin activity.[21] Karteszi et al.[21] made a knife cut and deafferented the anterolateral hypothalamus in the rat. In contrast to the results with AV3V lesions, they found no change in basal PRA levels in spite of the presence of polyuria and, presumably, interruption of vasopressin-secreting pathways. The renin response to a serotonin-releasing agent [parachloramphetamine (PCA)] in anterolateral hypothalamic deafferentated animals was increased to a similar level as found in sham-operated controls. Posterolateral lesions, extending from the posterior third of the mammillary bodies up to the level of the aqueduct, but excluding the lateral hypothalamus, did not influence basal levels of plasma renin activity. Renin responses to PCA were attenuated in animals with mediobasal hypothalamic lesions and posterolateral deafferentation.

Chemical lesions of two serotonin-containing midbrain regions, the dorsal (DR) and median (MR) raphe nuclei, were made by local injection of 5,7 dihydroxytryptamine (5,7-DHT) in rats.[22,23] Assessment of post-lesion basal and PCA-stimulated responses was made in these animals with localized serotonin-depleted regions. Basal levels of PRA were not influenced

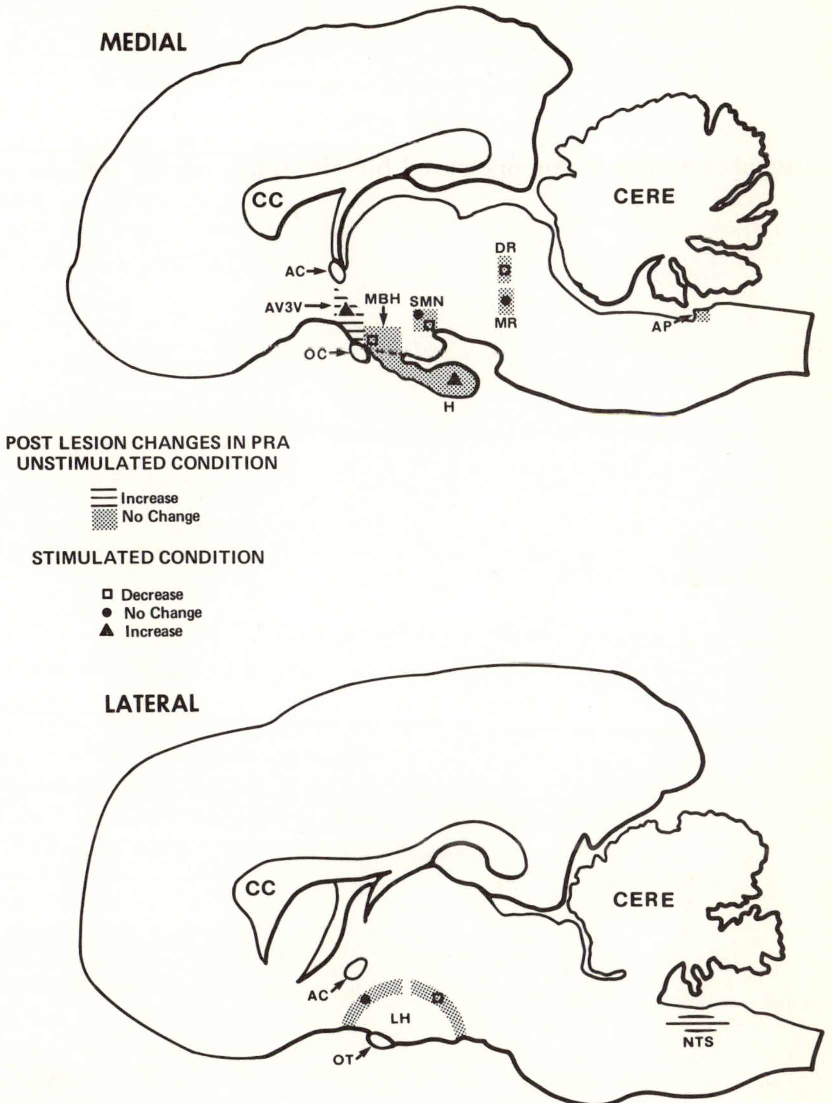

Figure 5-3. Medial and lateral sagittal sections of the brain summarizing lesion sites in the central nervous system in relationship to renin release. *Landmarks:* (same as in Figure 5-2). *Lesion sites:* AV3V = anteroventral III ventricle; MBH = medial basal hypothalamus; SMN = supramammillary nucleus; H = hypophysis; DR = dorsal raphe; MR = medial raphe; AP = area postrema; NTS = nucleus tractus solitarius. In addition, anterolateral deafferentation and posterolateral deafferentation of the mediobasal hypothalamus are illustrated by the two hatched areas around the lateral hypothalamus in the lateral section.

by lesions in the dorsal raphe, median raphe, or combination of both dorsal and median raphe. The effectiveness of the lesion was verified histologically and by a reduction in serotonin levels of these regions. In sham lesioned animals, intraperitoneal injection of PCA caused significant increases in PRA. The effect of PCA on PRA was significantly inhibited by lesions in the dorsal raphe but not by lesions in the median raphe.

The lower medulla may also contain control mechanisms for renin release. The nucleus tractus solitarius (NTS), the primary site of termination of cardiovascular baroreceptors, influences central sympathetic outflow. Lesions of this area have been shown to produce an accelerated form of hypertension in the rat[24] and moderate and labile hypertension in the cat[25] and dog.[26] Ferrario and Barnes[26] demonstrated that lesions of the NTS resulted in an elevation in PRA associated with the elevation in blood pressure in conscious dogs during the first week. After the first week, renin levels returned to normal, while blood pressure was still elevated. Essentially the same results were observed in anesthetized rats with bilateral lesions of the NTS by Zandberg et al.[27] In contrast, NTS lesions in conscious American foxhounds caused mild hypertension and no change in PRA.[28] Chronic lesions of an area immediately adjacent to the NTS, the area postrema, were shown to be without effect on PRA for up to five weeks.[26] The area postrema, a circumventricular organ of the IV ventricle, is known to be sensitive to circulating angiotensin II.

Hypophysectomy has been shown to be without effect on basal circulating levels of PRA.[21,29,30] The PRA response to parachloroamphetamine (PCA), a serotonin-releasing drug, was potentiated in hypophysectomized rats.[21] These findings indicate that the pituitary normally plays an inhibitory role in the response. The potentiated PRA response to PCA after hypophysectomy is probably best explained by the absence of inhibition of renin release by vasopressin. In diabetes insipidus rats, Henderson et al.[31] found that after hypophysectomy, hypotension was associated with reduced basal PRA levels. Subsequent administration of vasopressin in the rats resulted in further lowering of PRA.

In summary, the central regulation of renin originates from regions throughout the rostrocaudal extent of the brainstem and is dependent upon the integrity of the renal sympathetic nerves. Inputs from the lower medulla of the brain to the adrenal medulla also contribute to the regulation of renin release. Some regions, specifically the anterior-lateral hypothalamus, the AV3V region in the upper brainstem, and the NTS in the lower brainstem exert a tonic influence on the levels of circulating renin. Supplemental inputs providing orthostatic and somatosympathetic information feed into the brainstem and interact with the neural regulation of renin. Inputs from and into the pituitary and from higher centers converge upon the brainstem pathways and modulate the final neural outflow to the kidneys.

Central Monoamines in the Regulation of Renin Release

Catecholamines

Alpha Agonists: Clonidine hydrochloride is an alpha$_2$-selective adrenergic agonist that lowers blood pressure in man and experimental animals.[32–35] It is capable of penetrating the blood brain barrier and thus can stimulate both peripheral and central alpha$_2$-adrenergic receptor sites. In animals, clonidine injected intravenously[32,36] produced an initial transient rise in arterial blood pressure, followed by a sustained decrease. When injected into the cisterna magna, a brain ventricle, or the vertebral artery circulation,[36,37] clonidine caused a long-lasting hypotensive effect and bradycardia without the initial transient rise in blood pressure.

Clonidine also acts centrally to suppress renin secretion by a sympathoinhibitory action. Early studies by Onesti et al.,[38] Nolan and Reid,[39] and Ganong[40] demonstrated that either intraventricular or intracisternal administration of clonidine at doses ineffective systemically (1 µg/kg) suppressed renin secretion, lowered blood pressure and plasma ACTH levels, and caused a rise in growth hormone plasma concentration.[41] Clonidine's effect on renin release was observed only when renal perfusion pressure was maintained constant.[39] The central origin and neural mediation of the renin response was confirmed by studies demonstrating that the decrease in renin did not occur if renal nerves were sectioned,[42] autonomic ganglia were blocked,[39] or the spinal cord was sectioned.[43] In animals with spinal cord transected, the ACTH and GH responses to clonidine were still present;[43] the action of clonidine on blood pressure can also be separated from its action on renin by administration of a small dose of the alpha-adrenergic blocking drug phenoxybenzamine into the IV ventricle. Phenoxybenzamine abolished the depressor response to systemic clonidine but the renin-lowering effect persisted.[4] Schultz et al.[44] studied the effects of ventriculocisternal perfusion of clonidine on the renin response to carotid sinus hypotension. Clonidine blocked the increase of renin to carotid sinus hypotension, a finding providing additional support for central alpha-adrenergic receptors modulating baroreceptor input to the CNS. These findings illustrate the multiplicity of sites and mechanisms of clonidine in the brain.

To localize the sites at which clonidine acts, Rudolph et al.[45] injected small doses of the drug into either the carotid or vertebral arteries and also a femoral vein of the dog. Placement of a clip on the basilar artery allowed the forebrain and hindbrain regions to be perfused separately. Before clipping the basilar artery, administration of clonidine into either the vertebral or carotid arteries resulted in a fall in renin secretion. After the basilar artery was clipped, the renin response to clonidine was abolished regardless of route of administration. Although the studies failed to localize a renin-lowering site accessible by one route only, they did demonstrate that after basilar artery clipping, clonidine given via the intracarotid route favored a reduction of ACTH release, while its administration via the intravertebral circulation was more specific for the blood pressure lowering effects. In summary, clonidine acts at a forebrain site to affect the secretion of ACTH and growth hormone, a lower medulla site to influence blood pressure, and a separate site to affect renin secretion.

In order to better understand the nature of the central receptors mediating the renin-lowering action of clonidine, a comparison of the effect of clonidine with other alpha-adrenergic agonists and antagonists was performed.[4,46] Injection of clonidine into the third ventricle or cisterna magna inhibited renin secretion, while injections of epinephrine, norepinephrine, phenylephrine, or methoxyamine stimulated renin secretion. Epinephrine and norepinephrine have approximately equal $alpha_1$ and $alpha_2$ actions, while phenylephrine and methoxyamine have greater $alpha_1$ than $alpha_2$ agonistic actions.[47] These results suggest that central $alpha_2$-adrenergic receptors inhibit the release of renin, while central $alpha_1$-adrenergic receptors stimulate the release of renin. The stimulation of $alpha_1$ receptors to increase renin secretion[46] is associated with little or no effect on blood pressure.

Other comparisons also reveal that ACTH, blood pressure, and growth hormone release are subject to $alpha_2$-adrenergic receptor modulation. In dogs treated with intraventricular 6-hydroxydopamine (6-OHDA) to destroy many of the noradrenergic neurons in the brain, Ganong et al.[46] aimed to separate a pre- and post-synaptic $alpha_2$-adrenergic receptor site of action for clonidine. Such treatment did not alter the fall in blood pressure, ACTH, or renin secretion produced by clonidine but reduced the growth hormone response. Although the data suggest that $alpha_2$-adrenergic receptors are post-synaptic, a pre-synaptic site of action in the medulla could not be ruled out since catecholamine levels in the medulla were not significantly reduced by 6-OHDA treatment.

Antagonism of the renin-lowering response of clonidine with alpha-adrenergic blocking drugs has been difficult to demonstrate. Administration of phentolamine or piperoxane, either intravenously or directly into the III ventricle, failed to prevent the renin-lowing response to clonidine given intravenously. Centrally administered phenoxybenzamine reduced, but did not abolish, the decrease in renin secretion.

The strong evidence supporting a role for central $alpha_2$-adrenergic receptor control in renin release does not necessarily rule out a peripheral $alpha_2$-adrenergic receptor site of action. In the dog, intravenous administration of oxymetazoline, an alpha-agonist similar to clonidine but that does not cross the blood brain barrier, increases PRA.[39] The mechanism for and site of action of this peripheral stimulatory action of this $alpha_2$-adrenergic agonist on plasma renin is unknown. Likely mechanisms and sites of action are a modulatory effect on the intrarenal baroreceptor or macula densa mechanism. Additionally, a direct intrarenal site of action on the juxtaglomerular cells cannot be excluded. These studies in the dog contrast with other findings in rats. Pettinger et al.[48] and others[49,50] have shown that clonidine inhibits renin release by stimulating intrarenal alpha$_2$-adrenergic receptors. Pettinger et al.[48] have suggested that this interaction occurs at the level of the juxtaglomerular apparatus. In studies of sodium-depleted rats, sympathetic inhibition by guanethidine or ganglionic blockade with chlorisoridamine did not abolish the inhibitory effect of clonidine on renin release. However, alpha-adrenergic receptor blockade with phentolamine and phenoxybenzamine abolished the effect of clonidine on renin release.

In summary, clonidine inhibits renin secretion partly by an action on the brain. In dogs the drug acts to decrease ACTH and vasopressin (AVP) release, lower blood pressure, and stimulate growth hormone release. A peripheral site of action is also possible in dogs but the effect appears to be short-lived. In rats, an intrarenal site of action has also been proposed, whereby alpha$_2$-adrenergic agonists directly inhibit the release of renin.

Beta-Adrenergic Agonists: Whereas the involvement of beta-adrenergic-receptor regulation of renin release in the kidney is well established,[1,3,4,29,51] a central role of beta-adrenergic receptors on renin release is still controversial. Intracisternal administration of propranolol decreases PRA by a mechanism mediated by renal sympathetic nerves.[52] Because in this study a large dose of propranolol was given, its passage to the periphery and possible direct action on the kidney could not be excluded. Schultz et al.[44] studied the effects of ventriculocisternal perfusion of propranolol in mediating the renin response to carotid sinus hypotension. Central administration of propranolol did not block the renin response to carotid sinus hypotension[44] under conditions where the passage of propranolol to the periphery was shown to be unlikely. Their studies did not support participation by central beta-receptor mechanisms in the regulation of renin release.

More recently, Privitera et al.[53] studied the effect of intracisternal administration of propranolol at lower doses on plasma renin activity and found dose-dependent decreases in PRA and mean arterial pressure. The same doses given intravenously had no significant effect. Two factors were consistent with a mechanism of reduced sympathetic outflow: intracisternal propranolol reduced plasma norepinephrine levels and renal denervation abolished the reduction in PRA without influencing the hypotensive effect. Administration of both the d- and l-isomers of propranolol lowered plasma renin activity and arterial pressure to a similar extent. Because the two racemic stereoisomers of propranolol gave equivalent results, while lidocaine, which shares the membrane-stabilizing actions of both d- and l-propranolol was without effect, the authors could not attribute the effects of propranolol specifically to either central blockade of beta-adrenergic receptors or a local anesthetic effect.

Serotonin

In order to understand the effects of central serotonergic activity on renin release, knowledge of its biosynthetic pathway is necessary. Since serotonin (5-HT) does not readily cross the blood brain barrier, the brain depends upon "de novo" synthesis of this neurotransmitter within neurons. The precursor, L-tryptophan, is converted to 5-hydroxytryptophan (5-HTP) via a reaction catalyzed by the rate-limiting enzyme, tryptophan hydroxylase. The 5-hydroxytryptophan formed is readily converted to serotonin by the ubiquitous enzyme, L-aromatic amino acid decarboxylase. Brain levels of serotonin can be elevated by systemic injection of tryptophan and reduced by inhibiting tryptophan hydroxylase with para-chlorophenylalanine (PCPA). Interpretation of results following administration of 5-HTP, the immediate precursor of 5-HT, are more complicated, since in addition to the formation of 5-HT at specific serotonin-containing sites, non-5-HT sites possess a similar decarboxylase and can form 5-HT.

In this regard, catecholamine-containing neurons take up 5-HTP and enzymatically form serotonin, which then displaces endogenous catecholamines. This latter effect accounts for some of the different cardiovascular responses observed following administration of L-tryptophan and 5-HTP. It also points out the necessity of confirming results obtained following 5-HTP with more specific antagonists of serotonin. Two analogs of 5-HT—i.e., 5,6- and 5,7-dihydroxytryptamine—are relatively specific cytotoxic agents to the 5-HT system when administered to brain tissue or ventricles. Alterations in either peripheral or central levels of serotonin have been shown to influence renin release. Because serotonin's precursors, tryptophan and 5-hydroxytryptophan, and an antagonist of serotonin, metergoline, penetrate the blood brain barrier and increase serotonin levels or block its actions,[54,55] it has been difficult to separate the peripheral and central effects in some of the early studies.

It is not firmly established whether serotonin has a direct effect on the kidney to alter renin release. Early studies by Bunag et al.[56] showed that serotonin infused into the renal artery was without effect on renin release in anesthetized dogs. While some investigators have confirmed this finding, other studies have not. Meyer et al.[57] showed that intramuscular injections of serotonin resulted in a 5-fold elevation in PRA in ether-anesthetized rats. A peripheral rather than a central site of action was suggested when methysergide, a blocker of the peripheral action of serotonin, was able to prevent the elevated PRA and PRC levels following administration of serotonin. Moreover, beta-receptor blockade with propranolol partially reduced the serotonin-induced elevation in PRA. The precise mechanism for this elevated sympathetic activity was not determined in these studies. A similar 40% reduction in PRA levels after serotonin was found in the presence of camphidonium, a ganglion-blocking agent that does not cross the blood brain barrier. Because serotonin lowers blood pressure in rats, the increase in renin may have been due to hypotension and stimulation of intrarenal baroreceptors or to reflex stimulation of sympathetic outflow.

Because oral intake of tryptophan results in an elevation of PRA that is associated with a delayed rise in aldosterone and cortisol, Modlinger et al.[58] suggested that an elevation in serotonin concentration within the central nervous system may be responsible. More recent studies by Zimmerman and Ganong.[59] have shown that serotonin acts within the central nervous system to influence renin release. Systemic administration of tryptophan and 5-HTP elevated PRA in pentobarbital-anesthetized dogs with renal perfusion pressure maintained at a constant level. Because the effects of these serotonin precursors were prevented by renal denervation,[59] a role for serotonergic neurons in the central nervous system control of renin release was proposed.

By the judicial administration of a series of peripheral and central inhibitors of the enzymatic conversion of these precursors to serotonin, Zimmerman and Ganong[59] uncovered evidence consistent with serotonin having a central site of action in the regulation of renin release. Pretreatment with the peripheral and central aromatic amino acid decarboxylase inhibitor, benserazide, abolished the elevation in PRA following either L-tryptophan or 5-HTP administration. On the other hand, the administration of carbidopa, mainly a peripheral decarboxylase inhibitor, did not reduce the elevated PRA following L-tryptophan or 5-HTP administration. Administration of metergoline, a relatively specific antagonist of peripheral and central serotonin receptors, likewise blocked the response of PRA to L-tryptophan or 5-HTP, consistent with a specific serotonin effect. At the doses of the precursors used there were no changes in blood pressure. These studies indicated that brain serotonin can activate renal sympathetic outflow selectively without a generalized increase in sympathetic outflow to blood vessels, and that the activation of renal sympathetic activity leads to an increase in renin secretion.

Further documentation of the central site of action for serotonin was provided in rats treated with the serotonin-synthesis inhibitor, p-chlorophenylalanine (PCPA), and the neurotoxic agent, 5,7-dihydroxytryptamine (5,7 DHT). PCPA reduced PRA together with brain levels of serotonin.[60] Treatment with 5-HTP, in previously PCPA-treated animals, restored the serotonin levels to normal and elevated PRA. Intraventricular administration of 5,7 DHT produced similar reductions in PRA and brain serotonin levels. In contrast to the results obtained in dogs, L-tryptophan given to rats had no effect on PRA, even though hypothalamic serotonin was elevated in a dose-dependent manner. In rats this may be due to a failure of L-tryptophan to release serotonin.[61] Administration of serotonin agonist, quipizine, and the serotonin-releasing agent, p-chloroamphetamine (PCA), to conscious rats resulted in dose-dependent increases in PRA. Pretreatment with the serotonin-synthesis inhibitor, p-chlorophenylalanine, abolished the effect of PCA.

A definitive study on the contribution of central serotonergic pathways to renin release was completed by Van de Kar et al.[62] Chemical lesions of the dorsal or median raphe nuclei were produced with local microinjection of 5,7-DHT. No alterations in resting plasma renin activity were observed following either lesion. The stimulatory effect of PCA on PRA was significantly inhibited by lesions confined to the dorsal raphe that decreased brain serotonin levels by 60%, but not by lesions confined in the median raphe that similarly reduced brain serotonin levels. Additionally, lesions of the mediobasal hypothalamus were shown to inhibit the renin response to PCA, which implicates this region as part of the pathway by which serotonin release in the brain participates in the regulation of renin.[21,62] Because the serotonergic pathway that orginates in the dorsal raphe has been shown to project to the hypothalamus and other forebrain areas,[63] it is possible that the dorsal raphe stimulates renin release by structures contained within the mediobasal hypothalamic region. Because the PCA response was enhanced by hypophysectomy, the participation of hormones of the pituitary gland was shown not to be necessary for the PCA-stimulatory effect and, if anything, to counteract the response.

To recapitulate, serotonin acts within the brain to influence the level of renin release independently of any hemodynamic alterations. Evidence for an additional peripheral site of action for serotonin on renin release is still controversial.

Hypothalamic-Hypophyseal Factors Involved in Regulation of Renin Release

Evidence has been accruing to support the existence of a separate efferent limb involving components of the pituitary and its releasing factors.

Hypothalamic Factors

Corticotropin-Releasing Factor (CRF): A corticotropin-releasing factor has recently been characterized from extracts of ovine hypothalamus. This 41-amino acid-containing peptide elicits some interesting endocrine, physiological, and behavioral changes, in addition to its potent action of stimulating the pituitary release of ACTH.[64,65] Pertinent to this review is the property of centrally administered CRF to cause a prompt and long-lasting elevation of plasma epinephrine and norepinephrine in conscious rats and dogs associated with an increase in mean arterial pressure and heart rate.[64–66] Others have reported that intraventricular (IVT) administration of CRF causes a slight increase in BP and no change in HR in conscious monkeys.[67] The CRF-induced cardiovascular changes were not dependent on the release of a pituitary hormone or adrenomedullary epinephrine, since similar responses were found in hypophysectomized rats, animals treated with dexamethasone, or adrenalectomized rats. Blockade of circulating levels of vasopressin and/or angiotensin II (Ang II) formation were also without effect on the cardiovascular response to IVT CRF administration.[65] Although the pressor responses were not dependent upon elevation of circulating Ang II, in the study no measurement of Ang II (or PRA) was made.[65] An action of CRF on renin release independent from the elevation of circulating catecholamines or of blood pressure has not yet been studied.

Intravenous (IV) administration of CRF has been reported to decrease blood pressure in dog,[66] rat,[65,66] and monkey[67] but not in sheep.[68] The mechanisms of this decrease are thought to be due solely to increased blood flow in the mesenteric circulation.[69] Whether this decrease in blood pressure is associated with stimulation of renin release by way of an intrarenal baroreceptor mechanism has not yet been assessed. No evidence for a direct action of CRF or juxtaglomerular cells has been presented.

In dogs, IV or IVT CRF was shown to be accompanied by a marked increase in plasma vasopressin,[66] whereas in sheep CRF does not influence plasma vasopressin.[68] In conscious sheep, circulating Ang II (presumably PRA although it was not measured) did not change[68] after intravenous CRF administration.

Somatostatin: Since somatostatin, a tetradecapeptide, was first isolated from ovine hypothalamus as a growth hormone-release inhibitory factor by Brazeau et al.,[70] it has been shown to inhibit the secretion of insulin, glucagon, gastrin, TSH, and ACTH.[71,75] It is present in many different parts of the peripheral and central nervous system, the pancreas, and the gastrointestinal tract.[76] Circulating levels of somatostatin have been reported, and the gastrointestinal tract is considered to be the major source of circulating somatostatin.[77] Its widespread influence and distribution suggest an action directed to common secretory mechanisms of these endocrine and exocrine systems. Consistent with this it has been demonstrated that somatostatin impairs cyclic adenosine-monophosphate production by the pituitary gland[78] and blocks calcium influx, a necessary step in many secretory processes.[79] In regard to renin release, however, the exact mechanism is not known.

Somatostatin is without effect on resting levels of PRA, but inhibits the rise in PRA produced by a number of maneuvers. In normal man, Gomez-Pan et al.[80] showed that furosemide-induced elevations in PRA are inhibited by somatostatin without affecting plasma aldosterone levels. Although pretreatment with somatostatin was without effect on BP, HR, or PRA of normal male volunteers, such pretreatment markedly attenuated the increase in blood pressure, heart rate, and PRA elicited by infusion of orciprenaline, a beta-agonist.[81] Because intraventricular administration of somatostatin and its analogs has been shown to act within the CNS to suppress the rise in plasma catecholamines associated with a variety of neurally elicited stimuli,[82] it is anticipated that somatostatin may interfere with neurally elicited release of renin.

In addition, evidence for a direct effect of somatostatin on the dog kidney and dog renal cortical cell suspensions has been obtained by Izumi et al.[83] Intrarenal infusions of low, but not high, doses of somatostatin were effective in reducing furosemide-elevated PRA levels 50 to 70%. Confirmation of a direct site of action was obtained in studies using dog renal cortical cell suspensions where somatostatin-reduced renin released into the medium.[83]

Thyrotropin-Releasing Hormone (TRH): TRH, a tripeptide hormone, was first identified in 1970[70,84] in pigs and cows. In addition to its potent stimulatory effects on thyroid-stimulating hormone (TSH) secretion and prolactin,[85] TRH has been shown to possess a number of unusual biological actions as a physiological opioid antagonist in shock.[86] TRH-induced release of prolactin and TSH were not accompanied by any change in PRA in normal male volunteers.[87] Brown and Tache[88] have shown that TRH acts on the CNS to increase heart rate and blood pressure, as well as to increase transiently the secretion of adrenal catecholamines. Additionally, IVT but not IV administration of TRH has been shown to increase vasopressin release.[89] No measurements of PRA were made in any of these studies. Although an effect on renin release seems likely, it may be difficult to find since both arginine vasopressin and catecholamines modulate the release of renin in opposite directions.

Vasoactive Intestinal Peptide (VIP): Vasoactive intestinal peptide, a 28 amino acid peptide, was originally isolated from porcine duodenum by Said and Mutt,[90,91] but subsequently has been found in neurons of the central and peripheral nervous system,[92] in autonomic ganglia,[92] and in hypophyseal portal blood.[93] Its localization has led to the suggestion that VIP may be a neurotransmitter or a neuromodulator of hormone secretion.[4,94] It exhibits a wide range of biological actions (for example, relaxation of smooth muscle, stimulation of intestinal water and electrolyte secretion, and release of insulin, glucagon, and several anterior pituitary hormones[95-97]).

VIP infused directly into the renal artery of anesthetized dogs causes a fourfold elevation of renin secretion reflected in a concomitant elevation of PRA.[94,98] These changes occurred without any change in sodium excretion or plasma potassium concentration. The response was found whether or not renal perfusion pressure was maintained at a constant level, suggesting a role independent of the intrarenal baroreceptor. The effect appeared to be directly on the kidney since the same dose given intravenously was without effect.

Definitive evidence for a direct action of the peptide on renin release was obtained by Porter et al.[99] using an isolated superfused rat glomerular preparation. At doses of 10^{-9}M to 10^{-7}M, VIP was shown to be effective in stimulating renin release within five minutes. At a lower dose (10^{-10}M), VIP was ineffective. The mechanism of action on VIP on the juxtaglomerular cell is still under investigation.

The report by Hokfelt et al.[92] that VIP-immunoreactivity is present in nerve fibers in the renal cortex makes it likely that VIP-containing nerves could be involved in the regulation of renin secretion. Other reports, however, have been unable to document its presence in the renal nerves.[100,101] The question of a central role for VIP in the regulation of renin has not yet been addressed.

Neurotensin: Neurotensin, the hypothalamic tridecapeptide, causes hypotension after its IV administration[102] and hypertension after its IVT administration.[103,104] Since its isolation from the hypothalamus it has been found to have a widespread distribution within the CNS and in selected areas of the gastrointestinal tract. Indirect evidence that inhibition of the renin-angiotensin system may participate in the hypotensive response to neurotensin was reported by Kcrouac et al.[104] Bilateral nephrectomy or pretreatment of rats with captopril or with saralasin was found to inhibit the hypotensive response of neurotensin. The central pressor response to neurotensin was blocked by centrally administered alpha-adrenergic antagonists;[103] this finding suggests an involvement of the sympathetic nervous system in the response. A central role for neurotensin in augmenting renin release as a component of the enhanced sympathetic outflow seems likely, but studies measuring PRA have not been reported.

Posterior Pituitary Factors

Vasopressin: The oligopeptide hormone arginine vasopressin (AVP), together with its carrier neurophysin, is synthesized in the supraoptic and paraventricular nuclei of the hypothalamus and subsequently released from the posterior pituitary. The first demonstration of an effect of vasopressin on renin release was conducted by Bunag et al.[105] In anesthetized dogs with maintained renal artery constriction and elevated PRA levels, vasopressin infused intravenously or intrarenally produced inhibition of renin release in 17 of 21 dogs (IV) and two of two dogs in which the peptide was injected into the renal artery. Hemodynamic results were variable, with no effect or a slight increase in brachial pressure being associated with no change in renal blood flow in most animals. Oxytocin given at comparable doses produced no significant effects on renin release.

In conscious sodium depleted dogs, Tagawa et al.[106] showed that intravenous infusion of vasopressin reduced plasma renin activity in a dose-dependent manner. These changes in renin were not accompanied by a change in plasma osmolality, electrolytes, mean arterial pressure, or heart rate. Because the vasopressin infusion was shown to elevate plasma vasopressin levels in small physiological increments, a physiological role of AVP as an inhibitor for renin release acting directly on the kidney was proposed. A similar dose response curve for intravenous vasopressin decreasing PRA was found by Malayan et al.[107] in normal conscious dogs. A linear relationship was found between plasma and infused vasopressin levels. Only at the higher rates of infusion were significant changes in blood pressure and heart rate observed. Similar findings have been reported for AVP infusion into normal, healthy male volunteers.[108] Liard et al.,[109] however, found no change in PRA after a one-hour vasopressin infusion in conscious dogs. In their study, plasma AVP was elevated 11 pg/ml, a value shown by Malayan et al.[107] to be sufficient to reduce PRA. The difference between the two results may reflect a difficulty in demonstrating a further lowering of PRA in unanesthetized trained dogs.

The chronic inhibitory influence of vasopressin in renin release has been confirmed in the Brattleboro rat strain, a genetic model lacking the synthetic and releasing capabilities for AVP.[31,110,111] Such homozygous Brattleboro rats develop the condition of diabetes insipidus (DI). In the anesthetized DI male rat, basal PRC is elevated twofold compared with the heterogeneous Brattleboro rat,[110] Sabra control rats,[110] or Long-Evans control rats.[31] Renin content of the kidney was chronically elevated. Gutman and Benzakein[111] showed that exogenous AVP administration reduced PRA and PRC.

In normal subjects and patients maintained on diuretic treatment, a 60-minute infusion of AVP at a low rate resulted in a gradual reduction in PRA.[112] On the other hand, in patients with the syndrome of inappropriate secretion of antidiuretic hormone (SIADH), Fichman et al.[113] have demonstrated that the elevated AVP found in these patients is associated with PRA values that are low to undetectable. Stimuli such as change of posture or salt restriction that normally result in elevation of PRA provoked little or no response in these patients.

Because vasopressin induces natriuresis in water-loaded dogs and rats, a change in the macula densa sodium concentration might be considered as a mechanism to explain the reduction in PRA. Shade et al.[114] eliminated this possibility by preventing the filtering function of the kidney in anesthetized dogs and showed that the inhibitory action of AVP administered into the renal artery on PRA was still present. With this route of administration, neither renal blood flow nor mean arterial pressure was affected, eliminating an intrarenal baroreceptor participation.

During mild hemorrhage a role for vasopressin in blood pressure regulation and modulation of renin release was demonstrated by Schwartz and Reid.[115] In conscious dogs, mild hemorrhage (15 ml/kg) was associated with no change in blood pressure, heart rate, and a slight increase in PRA of 7 ng/ml/hr. Administration of vasopressin antagonist during mild hemorrhage decreased mean arterial pressure by 32 mm Hg, increased heart rate by 59 beats/min, and resulted in a further elevation of PRA to 23 ng/ml/hr. During mild hemorrhage, AVP tonically exerts an inhibitory effect on renin secretion.

Anterior Pituitary Factors

Adrenocorticotrophic Hormone (ACTH): The anterior pituitary hormone ACTH is well known and characterized as the primary regulator of adrenal steroid secretion. A role for ACTH in the regulation of renin release has been sought for a number of years. Haynes et al.[116] first reported that administration of ACTH results in a transitory increase in PRA in anesthetized dogs. In rats, Hauger-Klevene et al.[117] reported that ACTH injection increases PRA. Part of the problem in assessing the role of ACTH on renin release is the inhibitory action of glucocorticoids on renin release.[117] In adrenalectomized animals, ACTH administration results in a potentiation of renin release. Another complicating factor is the ability of glucocorticoids to augment the synthesis of renin substrate by the liver.[5]

Chronic infusion of ACTH for 10 days resulted in no significant change in mean arterial pressure but substantial natriuresis, kaliuresis, diuresis, hypernatremia, and hypokalemia.[118] These changes were associated with a significant suppression of PRA to nearly undetectable levels, which were maintained for the 10 days of ACTH infusion. The changes in PRA resembled those of excess mineralocorticoids. However, in this study, plasma aldosterone was only transiently elevated. Similar findings were reported by McCaa[119] in regard to the PRA levels. Chronic infusion of ACTH for seven days in conscious dogs resulted in suppression of PRA levels and hypertension. Because chronic ACTH infusion reduced PRA whether or not an increase of blood pressure was found, it does seem unlikely that a baroreceptor mechanism is importantly involved in this response.

The ability of ACTH to suppress PRA is consistent with the findings in other species and also in humans.[120–123] The precise mechanism by which ACTH inhibits renin secretion has not been established. In the chronic studies the effect appears to be secondary to an expansion of extracellular fluid volume. In patients treated with dexamethasone to suppress endogenous ACTH levels, infusion of ACTH did not alter PRA.[124] In sodium deficient subjects either in an upright or recumbent position, ACTH infusion was able to reduce PRA.[120] Chronic infusion of cortisol, on the other hand, resulted in significant hypotension and no significant influence on PRA or plasma aldosterone.[118]

The effects of hypophysectomy with or without supplemental ACTH on renal renin release and content, as well as circulating levels, are controversial. Hypophysectomized rats maintained on either normal or sodium-deficient diets had similar levels of PRA when compared with intact animals on the same diet.[125] Long-term treatment of hypophysectomized rats with ACTH or a combination of ACTH and GH for three weeks did not alter PRA levels.[125] Bozovic et al.[126] observed that the rate of release of renin from kidney slices of rats pretreated with ACTH was greater than those of control rats.

Growth Hormone: Growth hormone (GH), a polypeptide of 191 amino acids, originates from the anterior pituitary and is the most abundant of all active substances studied to date in the gland. Growth hormone primarily influences the growth in all tissues of the body. GH appears to play a minor role, if any, in renin release in intact subjects. Intravenous administration of human GH in two doses (4 or 12 IU) did not elevate PRA in human subjects.[127] Hypophysectomized rats on sodium deficient or normal diets treated chronically with growth hormone had unaltered plasma renin levels.[125] Similarly, Honeyman et al.[128] showed that the PRA and the kidney renin content were not altered in control rats, hypophysectomized rats, or hypophysectomized rats treated with growth hormone. When renin release was assessed using the perfused kidney, hypophysectomized rats had markedly lower secretion rates than normal rats at two levels of perfusion pressure. Kidneys from hypophysectomized rats treated with growth hormone had a much higher rate of renin secretion in spite of similar renin kidney content.[128] Although these effects of GH were observed only in hypophysectomized animals, they point out the modulatory influence of growth hormone on renin release in the absence of other pituitary influences.

Prolactin: The anterior pituitary hormone prolactin has been reported to influence water balance and body fluid homeostasis. In rats and man, prolactin causes dipsogenesis and antidiuresis.[129] A role for prolactin in the regulation of renin and aldosterone secretion has been suggested. Such a role seems unlikely in regard to renin release since plasma prolactin levels do not correlate with plasma renin activity in normal individuals.[130] In normal males, Epstein et al.[127] injected TRH to induce changes in TSH and prolactin. The changes in prolactin were not associated with changes in urinary Na^+ and K^+ excretion, free water clearance, or PRA.

Conclusions

In summary, although a number of pituitary hormones have a direct action on renin release, other factors influence the level of renin indirectly by altering extracellular fluid volume, stimulating the intrarenal baroreceptor and altering electrolyte excretion. Recent characterizations of the releasing hormones, CRF and somatostatin, have shown that in addition to their "primary" function of releasing or inhibiting the release of pituitary hormones, they can activate or depress sympathetic outflow and thus have the potential for eliciting neural release of many peripheral hormones, including renin. The latter action can occur independently of pituitary function.

Acknowledgment: The authors would like to acknowledge Amy W. Lammert and Cheryl L. Chernicky for their assistance.

References

1. Keeton TK, Campbell WB: The pharmacologic alterations of renin release. Pharmacol Rev **31**:81, 1981
2. Davis JO, Freeman RH: Mechanisms regulating renin release. Physiol Rev **56**:1, 1976

3. Donald DE: Studies on the release of renin by direct and reflex activation of renal sympathetic nerves. Physiologist **22**:39, 1979

4. Ganong WF, Barbieri C: Neuroendocrine components in the regulation of renin secretion. *In* Frontiers in Neuroendocrinology, Vol. 7, edited by Ganong WF, Martini LF. New York, Raven Press, 1982, p 231

5. Reid IA, Morris BJ, Ganong WF: The renin-angiotensin system. Ann Rev Physiol **40**:377, 1978

6. Ueda H, Yasuda H, Takabatake Y, Iizuka M, Iizuka T, Ihori M, Yamamoto M, Sakamoto Y: Increased renin release evoked by mesencephalic stimulation in the dog. Jap Heart J **8**:498, 1967

7. Passo SS, Assaykeen TA, Otsuka K, Wise BL, Goldfien A, Ganong WF: Effect of stimulation of the medulla oblongata on renin secretion in dogs. Neuroendocrinology **7**:1, 1971

8. Passo SS, Assaykeen TA, Goldfien A, Ganong WF: Effect of alpha- and beta-adrenergic blocking agents on the increase in renin secretion produced by stimulation of the medulla oblongata in dogs. Neuroendocrinology **7**:97, 1971

9. Richardson D, Stella A, Leonetti G, Bartorelli A, Zanchetti A: Renin release and renal vasomotor changes during stimulation of the brain stem in the cat. Clin Sci Mol Med **45**:243s, 1973

10. Richardson D, Stella A, Leonetti G, Bartorelli A, Zanchetti A: Mechanisms of renal release of renin by electrical stimulation of the brainstem in the cat. Circ Res **34**:425, 1974

11. Zanchetti A, Stella A: Neural control of renin release. Clin Sci Mol Med **48**:215s, 1975

12. Zanchetti A: Hypothalamic control of circulation. A Review. *In* The Nervous System in Arterial Hypertension, edited by Julius S, Esler MO. Springfield, CC Thomas, 1976, p 397

13. Zanchetti A, Stella A, Dampney R: Central and reflex control of renin release. *In* Hypertension and Brain Mechanisms, edited by DeJong W, Provoost AP, Shapiro AP. Amsterdam, Elsevier, 1977, p 397

14. Zehr JE, Feigl EO: Suppression of renin activity by hypothalamic stimulation. Circ Res **32 & 33**:1–17, 1973

15. Folkow B, Neil E: Circulation. New York, Oxford University Press, 1971, p 511

16. Frankel RJ, Jenkins JS, Wright JJ, Khan MUA: Effect of brain stimulation on aldosterone secretion in the rhesus monkey (Macaca Mulatta). J Endocrin **71**:383, 1976

17. Natcheff N, Logofeton A, Tzaneva N: Hypothalamic control of plasma renin activity. Pflugers Archiv **371**:279, 1977

18. Koyama S, Ammons WS, Manning JW: Altered renal vascular tone and plasma renin activity due to fastigial and baroreceptor activation. Am J Physiol **239**:H232, 1980

19. Koyama S, Ammons WS, Manning JW: Visceral afferents and the fastigial nucleus in vascular and plasma renin adjustments to head-up tilting. J Autonom Nerv Sys **4**:381, 1981

20. Shrager EE, Johnson AK: Anteroventral third ventricle (AV3V) region ablation: chronic elevations of plasma renin concentration. Brain Res **190**:554, 1980

21. Karteszi M, Van de Kar LD, Makara GB, Stark E, Ganong WF: Evidence that the mediobasal hypothalamus is involved in serotonergic stimulation of renin secretion. Neuroendocrinology **34**:323, 1982

22. Van de Kar LD, Wilkinson CW, Ganong WF: Pharmacological evidence for a role of brain serotonin in the maintenance of plasma renin activity in unanesthetized rats. J Pharmacol Exp Ther **219:**85, 1981
23. Van de Kar LD, Wilkinson CW, Skrobik Y, Brownfield MS, Ganong WF: Evidence that serotonergic neurons in the dorsal raphe nucleus exert a stimulatory effect on the secretion of renin but not of corticosterone. Brain Res **235:**233, 1982
24. Doba N, Reis DJ: Acute fulminating neurogenic hypertension produced by brainstem lesions in the rat. Circ Res **32:**584, 1973
25. Nathan MA, Reis DJ: Chronic labile hypertension produced by lesions of the nucleus tractus solitarii in the cat. Circ Res **40:**72, 1977
26. Ferrario CM, Barnes KL: Inactivation of either the area postrema or the nucleus tractus solitarii produces opposite changes in the hemodynamic characteristics of conscious trained dogs. *In* Central Nervous System Mechanisms in Hypertension, edited by Buckley JP, Ferrario CM. New York, Raven Press, 1981, p 61
27. Zandberg P, Palkovits M, De Jong W: Effect of various lesions in the nucleus tractus solitarii of the rat on blood pressure, heart rate and cardiovascular reflex response. Clin Exp Hyperten **1:**355, 1978
28. Carey RM, Dacey RG, Jane JA, Winn HR, Ayers CR, Tyson GW: Production of sustained hypertension by lesions in the nucleus tractus solitarii of the American foxhound. Hypertension **1:**246, 1979
29. Ganong WF, Reid IA: Role of the sympathetic nervous system and central alpha- and beta-adrenergic receptors in regulation of renin secretion. *In* Regulation of Blood Pressure by the Central Nervous System, edited by Onesti G, Fernandes M, Kim KE, New York, Grune & Stratton, 1976, p 261
30. Palkovits M, DeJong W, Van Der Wal B, De Wied D: Effect of adrenocorticotrophic and growth hormones on aldosterone production and plasma renin activity in chronically hypophysectomized sodium-deficient rats. J Endocrin **47:**243, 1970
31. Henderson IW, Balment RJ, Oliver JA: Vasopressin effects on plasma renin activity in male and female rats. Clin Sci Mol Med **55:**301, 1978
32. Kobinger W, Walland A: Investigations into the mechanism of the hypotensive effect of 2-(2,-6-dichlorophenylamino)-2-imidazoline-HCl. Eur J Pharmacol **2:**155, 1967
33. Laubie M, Delbarre B, Bogaeievsky D, Bogaeievsky Y, Tsoucaris-Kupfer D, Senon D, Schmitt H, Schmitt H: Pharmacologic evidence for a central alpha-sympathomimetic mechanism controlling blood pressure and heart rate. Circ Res **38** (Suppl II):35, 1976
34. Reid JL: Central action of antihypertensive drugs. *In* Drug Therapeutics. Concepts for Physicians, edited by Melmon K. New York, Elsevier, 1979, p 135
35. Isaac L: Clonidine in the central nervous system: site and mechanism of hypertensive action. Cardiovascular Pharmacol **2**(Suppl 1): S5, 1980
36. Reid IA, MacDonald DM, Pachnis B, Ganong WF: Studies concerning the mechanism of suppression of renin secretion by clonidine. J Pharmacol Exp Ther **192:**713, 1975
37. Itskovitz, HD: Clonidine and the kidney. J Cardiovasc Pharmacol **2**(Suppl 1): S47, 1980

38. Onesti G, Schwartz AB, Kim KE, Paz Martinez V, Schwartz C: Antihypertensive effect of clonidine. Circ Res **28–29**(Suppl II): 53, 1971
39. Nolan PL, Reid IA: Mechanism of suppression of renin secretion by clonidine in the dog. Circ Res **42**:206, 1978
40. Ganong WF: The renin-angiotensin system and the central nervous system. Fed Proc 36:1771, 1977
41. Ganong WF, Kramer N, Salmon J, Reid IA, Lovinger R, Scapagnini U, Boryczka AT, Shackelford R: Pharmacological evidence for inhibition of ACTH secretion by a central noradrenergic system in the dog. Neuroscience **1**:167, 1976
42. Reid IA, MacDonald DM, Pachnis B, Ganong WF: Studies concerning the mechanism of suppression of renin secretion by clonidine. J Pharmacol Exp Ther **192**:713, 1975
43. Ganong WF, Reid IA, Holland J, Kaplan S, Shackelford R, Boryczka AT: Effect of spinal cord transection on the endocrine and blood pressure responses to intravenous clonidine. Neuroendocrinology **25**:105, 1978
44. Schultz HD, Zehr JE, Livnat A: Central and peripheral adrenergic modulation of carotid sinus-induced renin release. Am J Physiol **242**:R318, 1982
45. Rudolph CD, Kaplan SL, Ganong WF: Sites at which clonidine acts to affect blood pressure and the secretion of renin, growth hormone, and ACTH. Neuroendocrinology **31**:121, 1980
46. Ganong WF, Chalett J, Jones JH, Kaplan SL, Karteszi M, Stith RD, Van de Kar LD: Further characterization of putative alpha-adrenergic receptors in brain that affect blood pressure and the secretion of ACTH, GH, and renin in the dog. Endocrinol Exper **16**:191, 1982
47. Langer SZ: Presynaptic regulation of the release of catecholamines. Pharmacol Rev **32**:337, 1981
48. Pettinger WA, Keeton TK, Campbell WB, Harper DC: Evidence for a renal alpha-adrenergic receptor inhibiting renin release. Circ Res **38**:338, 1976
49. Kirchertz EJ, Peters G: The effect of clonidine (catapres) and other hypotensive agents on plasma renin activity (PRA) in rats. Experientia (Basel) **29**:764, 1973
50. Vandongen R, Greenwood DM: The inhibition of renin secretion in the isolated rat kidney by clonidine hydrochloride (catapres). Clin Exp Pharmacol Physiol **2**:583, 1975
51. Ganong WF: Effects of sympathetic activity and ACTH on renin and aldosterone secretion. *In* Hypertension, edited by Genest J, Koiw E. New York, Springer-Verlag, 1972, p 4
52. Privitera PJ, Walle T, Knapp DR, Gaffney TE: Central renin suppressing action of propranolol. *In* Regulation of Blood Pressure by the Central Nervous System, edited by Onesti G, Fernandes M, Kim KE. New York, Grune & Stratton, 1976, p 443
53. Privitera PJ, Webb JG, Walle T: Effects of centrally administered propranolol on plasma renin activity, plasma norepinephrine and arterial pressure. Eur J Pharmacol **54**:51, 1979
54. Kuhn DM, Wolf WA, Lovenberg W: Review of the role of the central serotonergic neuronal system in blood pressure regulation. Hypertension **2**:243, 1980

55. Sanders-Bush E, Massari VJ: Actions of drugs that deplete serotonin. Fed Proc **36:**2149, 1977
56. Bunag RD, Page IH, McCubbin JW: Neural stimulation of release of renin. Circ Res **19:**851, 1966
57. Meyer D, Abele M, Hertting G: Influence of serotonin on water intake and the renin-angiotensin system in the rat. Arch Int Pharmacodyn **212:**130, 1974
58. Modlinger RS, Schonmuller JM, Arora SP: Stimulation of aldosterone, renin, and cortisol by tryptophan. J Clin Endocrinol Metab **48:**599, 1979
59. Zimmerman H, Ganong WF: Pharmacological evidence that stimulation of central serotonergic pathways increases renin secretion. Neuroendocrinology **30:**101, 1980
60. Van de Kar LD, Wilkinson CW, Ganong WF: Pharmacological evidence for a role of brain serotonin in the maintenance of plasma renin activity in unanesthetized rats. J Pharmacol Exp Ther **219:**85, 1981
61. Marsden CA, Conti J, Strope E, Curzon G, Adams RN: Monitoring 5-hydroxytryptoamine release in the brain of the freely moving unanesthetized rat using in vivo voltametry. Brain Res **171:**85, 1979
62. Van de Kar LD, Wilkinson CW, Skrobik Y, Brownfield MS, Ganong WF: Evidence that serotonergic neurons in the dorsal raphe nucleus exert a stimulatory effect on the secretion of renin but not of corticosterone. Brain Res **235:**233, 1982
63. Steinbusch HW: Distribution of serotonin-immunoreactivity in the central nervous system of the rat-cell bodies and terminals. Neuroscience **6:**557, 1981
64. Brown MR, Fisher LA, Rivier J, Spiess J, Rivier C, Vale W: Corticotropin-releasing factor: effects on the sympathetic nervous system and oxygen consumption. Life Sci **30:**207, 1982
65. Fisher LA, Jessen G, Brown MR: Corticotropin-releasing factor (CRF): mechanism to elevate mean arterial pressure and heart rate. Regulatory Peptides **5:**153, 1983
66. Brown M, Fisher L, Spiess J, Rivier J, Rivier C, Vale W: Corticotropin-releasing factor (CRF): effects on the sympathetic nervous system (SNS), vasopressin release and cardiovascular function. Program of the 64 Annual Meeting of the Endocrine Society, 1982, p 212
67. Kalin NH, Shelton SE, Kraemer GW, McKinney WJ: Corticotropin-releasing factor administered intraventricularly to rhesus monkey. Peptides **4:**217, 1983
68. Donald RA, Redekopp C, Cameron V, Nicholls MG, Bolton J, Livesey J, Espiner EA, Rivier J, Vale W: Hormonal actions of corticotropin-releasing factor in sheep: effect of intravenous and intracerebroventricular injection. Endocrinology **113:**866, 1983
69. Brown MR, Fisher LA, Spiess J, Rivier J, Rivier C, Vale W: Comparison of the biologic actions of corticotropin-releasing factor and sauvagine. Regulatory Peptides **4:**107, 1982
70. Brazeau P, Vale W, Burgus R, Ling N, Butcher M, Rivier J, Guillemin R: Hypothalamic polypeptide that inhibits the secretion of immunoreactive pituitary growth hormone. Science **179:**77, 1973
71. Bloom SR, Mortimer CH, Thorner MO, Besser GM, Hall R, Gomez-Pan A, Roy VM, Russell RCG, Coy DH, Kastin AJ, Schally AV: Inhibition of gastrin and gastric acid secretion by growth hormone-release inhibiting hormone. Lancet **2:**1106, 1974

72. Alberti KGMM, Christensen SE, Iversen J, Seyer-Hansen K, Christensen NJ, Prange Hansen A, Lundbaek K, Orskov H: Inhibition of insulin secretion by somatostatin. Lancet **2**:1299, 1973

73. Mortimer CH, Carr D, Lind T, Bloom SR, Mallinson CN, Schally AV, Tunbridge WMG, Yeomans L, Coy DH, Kastin A, Besser GM, Hall R: Effects of growth-hormone release-inhibiting hormone on circulating glucagon, insulin, and growth hormone in normal, diabetic, acromegalic, and hypopituitary patients. Lancet **1**: 697, 1974

74. Siler TM, Yen SSC, Vale W, Guillemin R: Inhibition by somatostatin on the release of TSH induced in man by thyrotropin-releasing factor. J Clin Endocrinol Metab **38**:742, 1974

75. Fehm HL, Voight KH, Lang R, Beinert KE, Raptis S, Pfeiffer EF: Somatostatin: a potent inhibitor of ACTH hypersecretion in adrenal insufficiency. Klin Wschr **54**:173, 1976

76. Vale WC, Rivier C, Brown M: Regulatory peptides of the hypothalamus. Ann Rev Physiol **29**:473, 1977

77. Schusdziarra V, Zyznar E, Rouiller D, Boden G, Brown JC, Arimura A, Unger RH: Splanchnic somatostatin: a hormonal regulator of nutrient homeostasis. Science **207**:530, 1980

78. Labrie F, Borgeat P, Ferland L, Dupont A, Lemaire S, Pelletier G, Barden N, Drouin J, DeLean A, Belanger A, Jolicoeur P: Hypophysiotropic hormones. *In* Hypothalamic Hormones, edited by Motta M, Crosignani PG, Martini L. New York, Academic Press, 1975, p 109

79. Taminato T, Seino N, Coto Y, Imura H: Interaction of somatostatin and calcium in regulating insulin release from isolated pancreatic islets of rats. Biochem Biophys Res Comm **66**:928, 1975

80. Gomez-Pan A, Snow MH, Piercy DA, Robson V, Wilkinson R, Hall R, Evered DC: Actions of growth hormone-release inhibiting hormone (somatostatin) on the renin aldosterone system. J Clin Endocrinol Metab **43**:240, 1976

81. Rosenthal J, Escobar-Jimenez F, Raptis S: Prevention by somatostatin of rise in blood pressure and plasma renin mediated by beta-receptor stimulation. Clinical Endocrinol **6**:455, 1977

82. Fisher DA, Brown MR: Somatostatin analog: plasma catecholamine suppression mediated by the central nervous system. Endocrinology **107**:714, 1980

83. Izumi Y, Honda M, Hatano M: Effect of somatostatin on plasma renin activity. Endocrinol Japon **26**:389, 1979

84. Boller J, Enzmann F, Folkers K, Bowers Cy, Schally AV: The identity of chemical and hormonal properties of the thyrotropin-releasing hormone and pyroglutamyl-histidyl-proline amide. Biochem Biophys Res Comm **37**:705, 1969

85. Bowers CY, Friesen HG, Hwang P, Guyda HJ, Folkers K: Prolactin and thyrotropin release in man by synthetic pyroglutamylhistidyl-prolinamide. Biochem Biophys Res Comm **45**:1033, 1971

86. Holaday JW, D'Amato RJ, Ruvio BA, Faden AI: Action of naloxone and TRH on the autonomic regulation of the circulation. *In* Regulatory Peptides: From Molecular Biology to Function, edited by Costa E, Trabucchi M. New York, Raven Press, 1982, p 353

87. Epstein S, Van Zyl-Smit R, LeRoith D, Vinik A, Pimstone B: The effects of

TRH on prolactin, plasma renin activity, water, and electrolyte excretion in normal males. Hormone Metab Res **9:**495, 1977

88. Brown M, Tache Y: Hypothalamic peptides: central nervous system control of visceral function. Fed Proc **40:**2565, 1981

89. Weitzman RE, Firemark HM, Glatz TH, Fisher DA: Thyrotropin-releasing hormone stimulates release of arginine vasopressin and oxytocin in vivo. Endocrinology **104:**904, 1979

90. Said SI, Mutt V: Polypeptide with broad biological activity: isolation from small intestine. Science **169:**1217, 1970

91. Said SI, Mutt V: Isolation from porcine-intestinal wall of a vasoactive octacosapeptide related to secretion and to glucagon. Eur J Biochem **28:**199, 1972

92. Hokfelt T, Schultzberg M, Elde R, Nilsson G, Terenius L, Said S, Goldstein M: Peptide neurons in peripheral tissues including the urinary tract: immunohistochemical studies. Acta Pharmacol Toxicol **43** (Suppl II): 79, 1978

93. Said SI, Porter JC: Vasoactive intestinal polypeptide: release into hypophyseal blood. Life Sci **24:**227, 1979

94. Porter JP, Reid IA, Said SI, Ganong WF: Stimulation of renin secretion by vasoactive intestinal peptide. Am J Physiol **234:**F306, 1982

95. Besson J, Rotsztejn WH, Bataille D: Involvement of VIP in neuroendocrine function. *In* Vasoactive Intestinal Peptide, edited by Said SI. New York, Raven Press, 1982, p 253

96. Said SI: Vasodilator action of VIP: Introduction and general consideration. *In* Vasoactive Intestinal Peptide, edited by Said SI. New York, Raven Press, 1982, p 145

97. Krep GJ: Effect of VIP infusion on water and electrolyte transport in the human intestine. *In* Vasoactive Intestinal Peptide, edited by Said SI. New York, Raven Press, 1982, p 193

98. Porter JP, Ganong WF: Relation of vasoactive intestinal polypeptide to renin secretion. *In:* Vasoactive Intestinal Peptide, edited by Said SI. New York, Raven Press, 1982, p 285

99. Porter JP, Said SI, Ganong WF: Vasoactive intestinal peptide stimulates renin secretion in vivo: evidence for a direct action of the peptide on the renal juxtaglomerular cells. Neuroendocrinology **36:**404, 1983

100. Alm P, Alumets J, Hakason R, Owman C, Sjoberg NO, Sundler P, Wallen B: Origin and distribution of VIP (vasoactive intestinal peptide) nerve in the genitourinary tract. Cell Tissue Res **205:**337, 1980

101. Larsson LI, Fahrenkrug J, Schaffalitzky de Muckadell OB: Vasoactive intestinal polypeptide occurs in nerves of the female genito-urinary tract. Science **197:**1374, 1977

102. Carraway RF, Leeman SE: The isolation of a new hypotensive peptide, neurotensin, from bovine hypothalamus. J Biol Chem **284:**6854, 1973

103. Sumners C, Phillips MI, Richards EM: Central pressor actions of neurotensin in conscious rats. Hypertension **4:**888, 1982

104. Kerouac R, St-Pierre S, Manning M, Rioux F: Partial blockade of neurotensin-induced hypotension in rats by nephrectomy, captopril and saralasin: possible mechanisms. Neuropeptides **3:**295, 1983

105. Bunag RD, Page IH, McCubbin JW: Inhibition of renin release by vasopressin and angiotensin. Cardiovasc Res **1:**67, 1967

106. Tagawa H, Vander AJ, Bonjour J, Malvin L: Inhibition of renin secretion by vasopressin in unanesthetized sodium-deprived dogs. Am J Physiol **220:**949, 1971

107. Malayan SA, Ramsay DJ, Keil LC, Reid IA: Effects of increases in plasma vasopressin concentration in plasma renin activity, blood pressure, heart rate, and plasma corticosteroid concentration in conscious dogs. Endocrinology **107:**1899, 1980

108. Khokhar AM, Slater JDH, Forsling ML, Payne NN: Effect of vasopressin on plasma volume and renin release in man. Clin Sci Mol Med **50:**415, 1976

109. Liard JF, Deriaz O, Schelling P, Thibonnier M: Cardiac output distribution during vasopressin infusion or dehydration in conscious dogs. Am J Physiol **243:**H663, 1982

110. Gutman Y, Benzakein F: Antidiuretic hormone and renin in rats with diabetes insipidus. Eur J Pharmacol **2:**114, 1974

111. Gutman Y, Benzakein F: Effects of an increase and lack of antidiuretic hormone on plasma renin activity in the rat. Life Sci **10:**1081, 1971

112. Hesse B, Nielsen I: Suppression of plasma renin activity by intravenous infusion of antidiuretic hormone in man. Clin Sci Mol Med **52:**357, 1977

113. Fichman MP, Michelakis AM, Horton R: Regulation of aldosterone in the syndrome of inappropriate antidiuretic hormone secretion (SIADH). J Clin Endocrinol Metab **39:**136, 1974

114. Shade RE, Davis JO, Johnson JA, Gotshall RW, Spielman WS: Mechanism of action of angiotensin II and antidiuretic hormone on renin secretion. Am J Physiol **224:**926, 1973

115. Schwartz J, Reid IA: Effect of vasopressin blockade on blood pressure regulation during hemorrhage in conscious dogs. Endocrinology **109:**1778, 1981

116. Haynes FW, Forsham PH, Hume DM: Effects of ACTH, cortisone, desoxycorticosterone, and epinephrine on the plasma hypertensinogen and renin concentration of dogs. Am J Physiol **172:**265, 1953

117. Hauger-Klevene JH, Brown H, Fleischer N: ACTH stimulation and glucocorticoid inhibition of renin release in the rat. Proc Soc Exp Biol Med **131:**539, 1964

118. Lohmeier T, Kastner PR: Chronic effects of ACTH and cortisol excess on arterial pressure in normotensive and hypertensive dogs. Hypertension **4:**652, 1982

119. McCaa RE: Aldosterone fluid balance. *In* Angiotensin Converting Enzyme Inhibitors: Mechanisms of Action and Clinical Complications, edited by Horovitz ZP. Baltimore, Urban & Schwarzenberg, 1981, p 199

120. Benraad TJ, Kloppenborg PWC: Plasma renin activity and aldosterone secretion rate in man during chronic ACTH administration. J Clin Endocrinol Metab **31:**581, 1970

121. Freeman RH, Davis JO, Fullerton D: Chronic ACTH administration and the development of hypertension in rats. Proc Soc Exp Biol Med **163:**473, 1980

122. Rauh W, Levine LS, Gottesdiener K, Chow D, Oberfield SE, Gunczler P, Pareira J, New MI: Adrenocortical function, electrolyte metabolism, and blood pressure during prolonged adrenocorticotropin infusion in juvenile hypertension. J Clin Endocrinol Metab **49:**52, 1979

123. Stewart KW, Coghlan JP, Denton DA, Fei DT, Mason RT, Scoggins BA, Whitworth JA: Effect of angiotensin converting enzyme inhibition with SQ 14225 on blood pressure in sheep. Clin Exp Hyperten **3:**159, 1981

124. Kem DC, Gomez-Sanchez C, Kramer NJ, Holland OB, Higgins JR: Plasma aldosterone and renin activity response to ACTH infusion in dexamethasone-suppressed normal and sodium-depleted man. J Clin Endocrinol Metab **40:**116, 1975

125. Palkovits M, deJong W, Van der Wal B, de Wied D: Effect of adrenocorticotrophic and growth hormone on aldosterone production and plasma renin activity in chronically hypophysectomized sodium-deficient rats. J Endocrinol **47:**243, 1970
126. Bozovic L, Efendic S, Rosenquist U: The effect of ACTH on plasma renin activity. Acta Endocrinol **138:**123, 1969
127. Epstein S, LeRoith D, Rabkin R: The effect of different preparations of human growth hormone on plasma renin activity in normal males. J Clin Endocrinol Metab **42:**390, 1976
128. Honeyman TW, Goodman HM, Fray JCS: The effects of growth hormone on blood pressure and renin secretion in hypophysectomized rats. Endocrinology **112:**1613, 1983
129. Bern MA, Nicoll CS: The comparative endocrinology of prolactin. Recent Prog Horm Res **24:**681, 1968
130. Meier A, Weidmann P, Hennes U, Ziegler WH: Plasma prolactin in normal and hypertensive subjects: relationship with age, posture, blood pressure, catecholamines, and renin. J Clin Endocrinol Metab **50:**304, 1980

Chapter 6

Neural Regulation of Renal Function: Sodium Excretion and Renin Release

Ulla C. Kopp, Hallvard Holdaas,
and Gerald F. DiBona

The structure and function of the intrinsic innervation of the kidney has been studied for over 100 years. It was initially observed that nerve fibers entered the kidney along the main renal artery and ran along it to its finest branches. However, most previous studies concerning the functional importance of the renal nerves in the control of kidney function involved stressful anesthesia and surgery, which caused Homer Smith[1] to conclude:

"For the moment it may be said that substantial evidence of the neural control of either the tubular excretion or reabsorption of any urinary constituent is lacking."

However, recent advances in our anatomical knowledge of distribution of nerve endings in the kidney requires a revision of this view.

Renal Neuroanatomy

Electron microscopic and histochemical fluorescence methods have demonstrated a rich innervation of the kidney.[2] This renal innervation is predominantly adrenergic, as both morphological and functional studies exclude a role for cholinergic innervation. Adrenergic innervation has been demonstrated along the vascular tree including the interlobar, arcuate, and interlobular arteries and the afferent and efferent arterioles. The proximal and distal convoluted tubules, the thick ascending limb of Henle's loop, and the juxtaglomerular granular cells also receive adrenergic innervation. The renal innervation consists mainly of efferent unmyelinated fibers with fewer afferent myelinated fibers. Radioligand binding studies have demonstrated that both the renal vasculature and the tubules possess alpha and beta adrenoceptors as well as dopaminergic receptors.

Neural Regulation of Renal Sodium Excretion

The role of the renal nerves in the control of renal sodium and water excretion has been extensively studied since Claude Bernard[3] demonstrated an ipsilateral diuresis and natriuresis following section of the greater splanchnic nerve. Research on the neural control of water and solute excretion has employed two different approaches. If the renal nerves are involved in renal tubular sodium and water reabsorption, it has been reasoned that renal denervation should result in a diuresis and natriuresis, whereas stimulation of the renal nerves, directly or indirectly by reflex stimulation, should result in a decreased water and sodium excretion.

In the past it has been argued that denervation diuresis and natriuresis were consequences of altered renal hemodynamic factors such as changes in renal blood flow and/or glomerular filtration rate. However, Bencsath et al.,[4] using micropuncture technique in rats, demonstrated that acute renal denervation decreased proximal tubular reabsorption of sodium and water without changing single nephron glomerular filtration rate. Bello-Reuss et al.[5,6] demonstrated that the tubular fluid-to-plasma concentration ratio of inulin decreased in samples of tubular fluid collected from late proximal tubules and from early and late distal convolutions following acute renal denervation. There were no changes in hydrostatic pressures measured in renal cortical microvascular structures. The effect of renal denervation is not a transient effect that is only observed immediately after denervation since denervation diuresis and natriuresis are also observed 2–3 weeks after renal denervation.[7] Rogenes and Gottschalk[8] have demonstrated that chronic renal denervation in rats results in a diuresis and natriuresis not only in anesthetized rats but also in conscious rats.

Pharmacological renal denervation has also been employed to demonstrate the role of the renal nerves in the control of renal tubular sodium and water reabsorption. Renal alpha-adrenoceptor blockade with phenoxybenzamine increased urinary flow rate and urinary sodium excretion in anesthetized[9] but not in conscious normal dogs.[10] Studies in conscious dogs,[11] rabbits,[12] and rats[13] (Figure 6-1) demonstrate that during dietary sodium deprivation chronic renal denervation impairs the ability of the kidney to reduce urinary sodium excretion sufficiently in order to avoid negative external sodium balance. In agreement with these studies in animals there are several studies in man demonstrating the inability of either normal subjects treated with guanethidine[14] or patients with idiopathic autonomic insufficiency[15] to avoid negative sodium balance during dietary sodium deprivation.

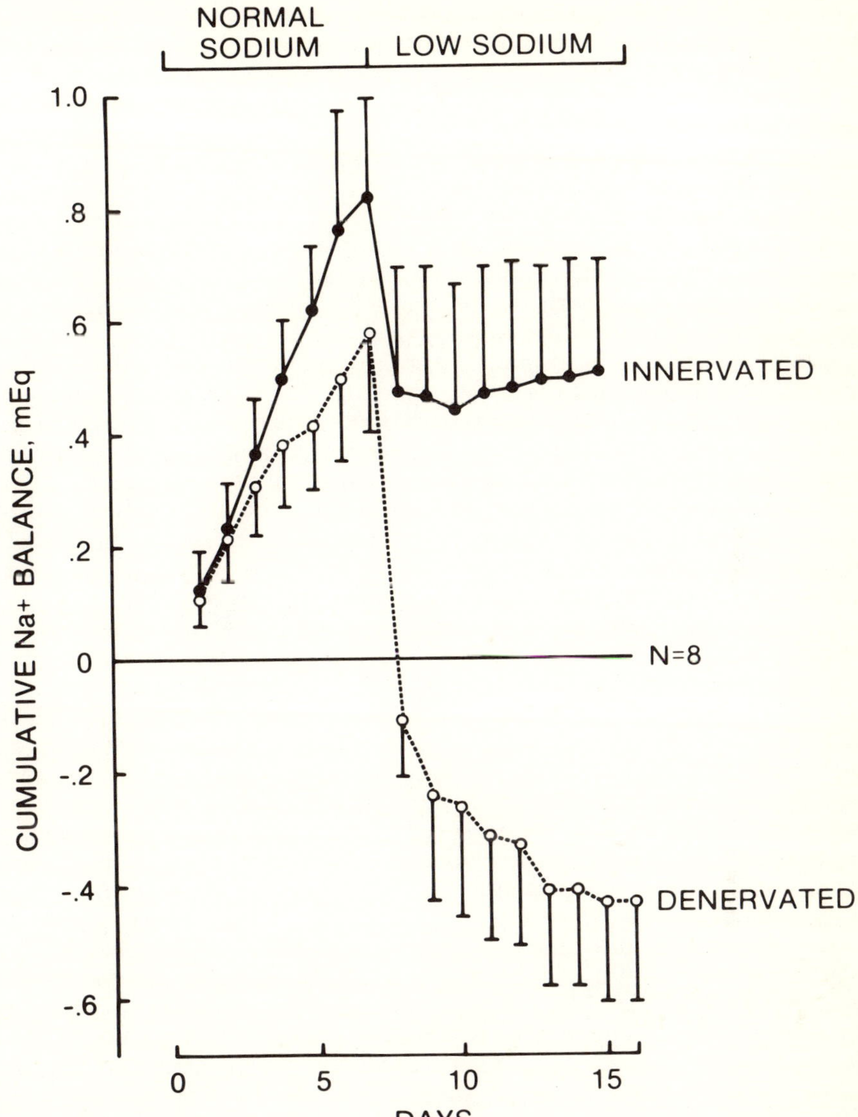

Figure 6-1. The effect of chronic bilateral renal denervation on the renal adaptation to dietary sodium deprivation.

Thus, the renal nerves are an important component of the efferent mechanisms involved in the normal regulation of renal tubular sodium transport and the maintenance of external sodium balance.

In previous studies the effect of electrical renal nerve stimulation on urinary water and sodium excretion was confounded by the high nerve-stimulation frequency used, which caused a decrease in urinary sodium excretion associated with marked reductions in renal blood flow and glomerular filtration rate. It was thus difficult to differentiate between a direct effect on renal tubular sodium transport and an indirect effect mediated by alterations in renal hemodynamics.

In conscious dogs with congestive heart failure, unilateral renal arterial administration of the alpha-adrenoceptor antagonist, phenoxybenzamine, produced an ipsilateral diuresis and natriuresis without changing renal blood flow or glomerular filtration rate.[10] In anesthetized dogs with thoracic inferior vena cava constriction, renal denervation, surgical or pharmacological, partially restored the natriuretic and diuretic response to saline volume expansion without changes in renal hemodynamics; the diuretic and natriuretic responses were associated with an inhibition of proximal tubular sodium reabsorption.[16] These studies demonstrated a role for efferent renal sympathetic nerves in the renal sodium retention of edema-forming states and suggested that there was a level of efferent renal nerve activity that directly affects renal tubular sodium reabsorption without concomitant changes in renal blood flow or glomerular filtration rate.

Using direct electrical stimulation of the severed peripheral renal nerves, La Grange et al.[17] demonstrated that, indeed, there is such a level. They showed that electrical renal nerve stimulation in a frequency range of 0.3–1.0 Hz reduced urinary sodium excretion without affecting renal blood flow or glomerular filtration rate. Slick[16] et. al., using a renal nerve stimulation frequency just subthreshold for a reduction in renal blood flow, demonstrated an ipsilateral reversible decrease in urinary sodium excretion without changes in renal blood flow, glomerular filtration rate, or intrarenal distribution of blood flow. There was no change in urinary sodium excretion from the contralateral unstimulated kidney. The ipsilateral decrease in urinary sodium excretion was abolished by renal alpha adrenoceptor blockade with phenoxybenzamine[2] or renal adrenergic blockade with guanethidine.[2] The antidiuretic and antinatriuretic responses to low-level renal nerve stimulation were not mediated by the intrarenal action of circulating angiotensin II or prostaglandins as inhibition of either hormonal system with saralasin[2] and indomethacin,[2] respectively, did not influence the antidiuretic or antinatriuretic responses.

Using micropuncture techniques in rats, Bello-Reuss et al.[18] demonstrated that similar low-frequency renal nerve stimulation increased proximal tubular fractional and absolute sodium and water reabsorption without changes in single nephron or whole kidney glomerular filtration rate or renal plasma flow; urinary sodium excretion decreased 25%. A recent study by DiBona and Sawin[19] showed that low-level renal nerve stimulation also results in an increase in sodium chloride but not water reabsorption in the loop of Henle, presumably in the thick ascending portion.

The effects on renal tubular sodium reabsorption of renal adrenergic stimulation with pharmacological agents have also been examined. In conscious dogs, intrarenal administration of norepinephrine at doses that do not change renal blood flow or glomerular filtration rate results in a decrease in urinary sodium excretion that is abolished by phenoxybenzamine.[10] However, recent studies[20] show that the antinatriuretic response to physiological doses of norepinephrine is modest. Rat renal microperfusion studies show that adding norepinephrine to the peritubular capillary perfusate results in increased fluid reabsorption, while adding norepinephrine to the lumen of the proximal convoluted tubules has no effect.[21] These results indicate that the receptors mediating the antinatriuretic response to norepinephrine are situated on the basolateral aspect of the proximal tubule.

The effects of reflex alterations of efferent renal nerve activity on renal function have been examined. Lowering carotid sinus pressure results in an increase in peripheral sympathetic activity. Gross et al.[22] demonstrated a 62% increase in efferent renal sympathetic nerve activity in response to bilateral carotid occlusion in conscious dogs. With renal perfusion pressure held constant, lowering carotid sinus pressure in an isolated carotid sinus perfusion preparation reduces urinary sodium excretion without changing renal hemodynamics. This reflex reduction in urinary sodium excretion is abolished by either phenoxybenzamine or guanethidine.[2]

Carotid baroreceptor reflex activation of efferent renal sympathetic nerve activity by a 60° head-up tilt in anesthetized dogs did not change renal hemodynamics but decreased urinary sodium excretion at unchanged renal perfusion pressure. The antidiuretic and antinatriuretic responses were abolished by surgical or pharmacological renal denervation and by bilateral carotid sinus denervation but not by cervical vagotomy.[2] Hypercapnic acidosis has also been observed to produce an antinatriuresis without accompanying changes in renal hemodynamics; the antinatriuresis was significantly reversed by renal denervation.[23]

Thus, increased efferent renal sympathetic nerve activity produced by either direct electrical or indirect reflex renal nerve stimulation causes increased renal tubular sodium reabsorption without concomitant changes in renal hemodynamics.

Several studies have examined whether decreased efferent renal nerve activity results in diuresis and natriuresis. Inflation of a balloon placed in the left atrium to increase left atrial pressure activates cardiopulmonary baroreceptors, increases afferent vagal firing, and decreases efferent renal sympathetic nerve activity[2,24] and plasma antidiuretic hormone concentration.[25] Prosnitz and DiBona[2] showed that left atrial ballon inflation produced a reversible decrease in efferent renal sympathetic nerve activity that was associated with an increase in urinary water and sodium excretion in the absence of renal hemodynamic changes. Bilateral cervical vagotomy abolished the responses in efferent renal sympathetic nerve activity and urinary water and sodium excretion. Exogenous antidiuretic hormone abolished the diuretic response but did not affect the decrease in efferent renal sympathetic nerve activity or the natriuretic response. These findings suggested that stimulation of cardiopulmonary receptors by increasing left atrial pressures produces a reflex response via afferent vagal fibers whose efferent limb consists of suppression of both antidiuretic hormone release and efferent renal sympathetic nerve activity.

Using simultaneous proximal tubular and peritubular capillary micro-perfusion techniques in the rat, it was shown that net proximal tubular fluid absorption was increased by norepinephrine and decreased by the alpha-adrenoceptor antagonists, phentolamine or phenoxybenzamine, when added to the peritubular capillary perfusate. Perfusion of the proximal tubular lumen with norepinephrine or either antagonist was without effect.[21] These results suggest that proximal tubular fluid absorption is regulated by stimulation of alpha-adrenoceptors located on the antiluminal aspect of the tubule. In agreement with these findings are the results from a study in anesthetized dogs in which methoxamine, infused intrarenally at a dose that did not reduce renal blood flow or glomerular filtration rate, resulted in a reduction in urinary flow rate and sodium excretion.[26]

Studies by DiBona and Osborn[27] (Figure 6-2) examining the adrenoceptors involved in mediating the antinatriuretic response to low-frequency renal nerve stimulation demonstrate that neither renal beta-1 adrenoceptors (atenolol) nor beta-1,2 adrenoceptor (propranolol) blockade affects the antinatriuretic response. However, renal alpha-adrenoceptor blockade with either prazosin (alpha-1) phentolamine or phenoxybenzamine (alpha-1,2) markedly inhibits this response. Furthermore, the antinatriuretic response to reflex renal nerve stimulation (lowering carotid sinus pressure) is blocked by phenoxybenzamine but not affected by beta-1 adrenoceptor blockade with metoprolol.[2,28]

In summary, bidirectional alterations in efferent renal sympathetic nerve activity, produced either directly (renal nerve stimulation, renal denervation) or by activation of physiological reflexes (carotid sinus baroreceptors, left atrial mechanoreceptors) cause parallel changes in renal tubular sodium and water reabsorption that are directly mediated by adrenergic nerve terminals in contact with the peritubular basement membrane of renal tubular epithelial cells. Renal hemodynamic factors, peritubular physical forces, and circulating humoral substances are not involved. The proximal tubule and thick ascending limb of Henle's loop have been identified as sites of action for this neural control mechanism of sodium and water transport.

The efferent renal sympathetic nerves are participants in the efferent

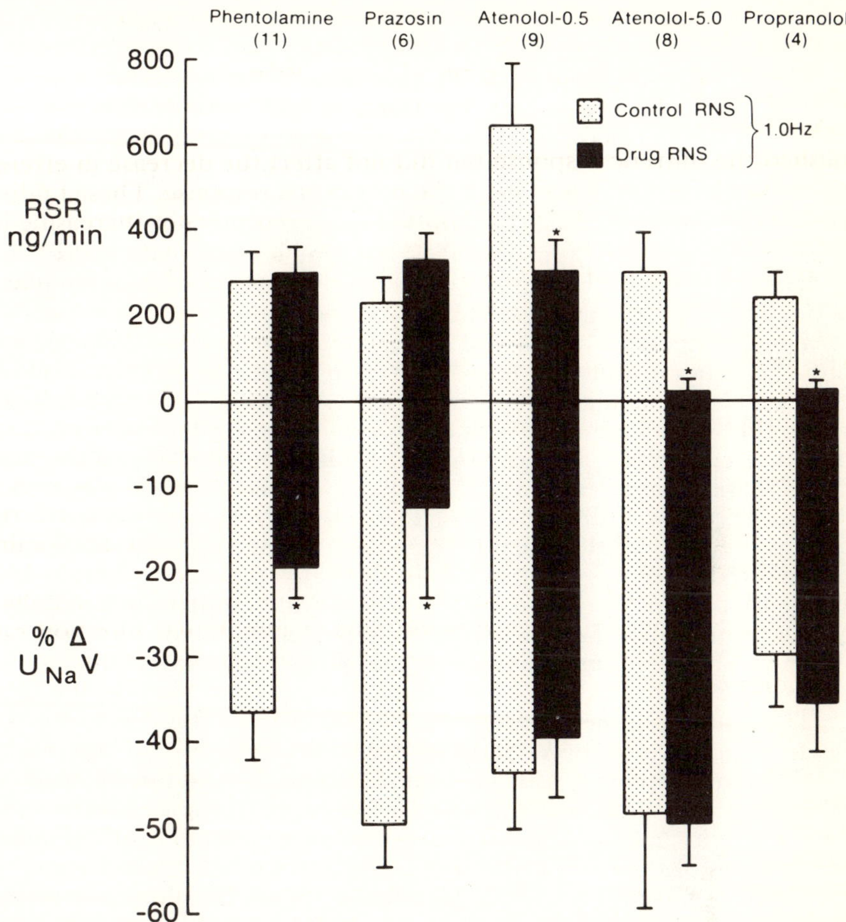

Figure 6-2. The effect of various adrenoceptor antagonists (administered into the renal artery) on the antinatriuretic and renin secretion rate response to 1.0 Hz renal nerve stimulation in anesthetized dogs.

limb(s) of the mechanism(s) involved in the avid renal sodium retention of certain edema-forming conditions as well as in the normal physiological response to dietary sodium deprivation. This neural control mechanism is operative in the conscious unanesthetized animal. Current evidence favors the view that the mechanism operates via renal tubular alpha-1 adrenoceptors, although improved ability to characterize renal tubular epithelial cell membrane catecholamine receptor anatomy will provide further information on this issue.

Neural Regulation of Renal Renin Release

There is considerable evidence that three primary mechanisms regulate renin release by the kidney: the renal vascular baroreceptor, the renal tubular macula densa receptor, and the renal sympathetic nerves.[29]

Increases in efferent renal sympathetic nerve activity, produced either directly or by reflex, are known to increase renin release.[30] However, increases in efferent renal sympathetic nerve activity are also capable of producing changes in the input stimuli to both the baroreceptor and the macula densa receptor mechanisms, which confounds a precise definition of the mechanism of the renin release.

The endogenous release of norepinephrine during efferent renal sympathetic nerve stimulation may increase renin release by activation of either alpha or beta adrenoceptors, or both. Activation of alpha adrenoceptors on the renal vasculature results in renal vasoconstriction with reductions in renal blood flow and glomerular filtration rate. These alterations may increase renin release by a hemodynamic stimulus to the baroreceptor or by reduced distal tubular sodium chloride delivery stimulus to the macula densa receptor. Additionally, activation of alpha adrenoceptors on the proximal renal tubules results in increased renal proximal tubular sodium reabsorption, contributing to the decreased distal tubular sodium chloride delivery stimulus to the macula densa receptor. Activation of beta adrenoceptors on the juxtaglomerular granular cells directly increases renin release.

Thus, multiple mechanisms are capable of contributing to the renin release response to efferent renal sympathetic nerve stimulation. Further investigations employing various levels of intensity of efferent renal sympathetic nerve stimulation and specific adrenoceptor stimulatory and inhibitory agents have permitted a more precise definition of the relative contributions of the various mechanisms.

Low-frequency renal nerve stimulation (0.25 Hz) does not produce any change in renal blood flow, glomerular filtration rate, or urinary sodium excretion, and is without effect on renin release in a filtering kidney at control renal arterial pressure. However, this low-frequency renal nerve stimulation significantly augments the renin release response to reduction in renal arterial pressure to 50 mm Hg—i.e., below the range of renal blood flow autoregulation.[31]

Reduction of renal arterial pressure below the range of renal blood flow autoregulation stimulates the baroreceptor by afferent arteriolar dilatation. Therefore, low-frequency (0.25 Hz) renal nerve stimulation enhances the renin release response to baroreceptor activation, a non-neural stimulus to renin release. Similarly, increasing ureteral pressure at control renal arterial pressure produces afferent arteriolar dilatation and baroreceptor stimulation; in this setting, low-frequency (0.25 Hz) renal nerve stimulation increases renin release.[32]

The augmentation of renin release by low-frequency (0.25 Hz) renal nerve stimulation is dependent on a functionally operative macula densa receptor mechanism.[32,33] The neural augmentation of renin release is mediated by renal beta-1 adrenoceptors located on the juxtaglomerular granular cells.[32] In agreement with these findings of an augmentation of non-neural stimulus-mediated renin release by subthreshold neural stimuli, it has been shown that the renin release response to baroreceptor activation is augmented by renal arterial administration of humoral adrenergic agonists.[34] Slightly higher levels (i.e., > 0.25 Hz) of efferent renal sympathetic activity, such as those prevailing in the innervated kidney, enhance the renin release response to reduction in renal arterial pressure within[35] or below[36] the range of renal blood flow autoregulation, compared with the denervated kidney.

In light of these observations it is clear that levels of efferent renal sympathetic nerve activity that do not affect renal hemodynamics, urinary sodium excretion, or renin release can significantly augment the renin release response to non-neural stimuli such as reductions in renal arterial pressure or increases in ureteral pressure. The clinical correlates of this experimental finding might include renal artery stenosis, systemic hypotension, or ureteral obstruction.

Renal nerve stimulation at a frequency of 0.5 Hz increases renin release without changing renal blood flow, glomerular filtration rate, or urinary sodium excretion.[37] In the absence of changes in the input stimuli to the baroreceptor and macula densa receptor mechanisms for renin release, the renin release occurring during 0.5 Hz renal nerve stimulation may be considered to be derived from direct neural activation of juxtaglomerular granular cells.

This renin release response was abolished by renal beta-1 adrenoceptor blockade with atenolol but was unaffected by renal beta-2 adrenoceptor blockade with butoxamine, renal alpha-1,2 adrenoceptor blockade with phentolamine, or renal alpha-1 adrenoceptor blockade with prazosin.[26,37] Thus, renin release elicited solely by neural stimulation of juxtaglomerular granular cells is mediated by renal beta-1 adrenoceptors. Neither renal beta-2, alpha-1, or alpha-2 adrenoceptors are involved.

Further evidence that stimulation of renal alpha-1 adrenoceptors does not affect renin release in the absence of changes in input stimuli to the baroreceptor and macula densa receptor derives from studies using the selective alpha-1 adrenoceptor agonist, methoxamine. When infused into the renal artery at doses that did not change renal blood flow or glomerular filtration rate, and either did not affect, or decreased, urinary sodium excretion, renin release was not increased. However, when infused at higher doses that resulted in decreases in renal blood flow, glomerular filtration rate, and urinary sodium excretion, there was an increase in renin release.[26]

Renal nerve stimulation at a frequency of about 1.0 Hz increases renin release with no change in glomerular filtration rate, a small decrease or no change in renal blood flow, and a 30–40% reduction in urinary sodium excretion.[27,38] The renin release response is abolished by renal beta-1,2 adrenoceptor blockade with propranolol and renal beta-1 adrenoceptor blockade with metoprolol or atenolol, but is not affected by renal alpha-1,2 adrenoceptor blockade with phentolamine or renal alpha-1 adrenoceptor blockade with prazosin (Figure 6-2). Renal beta adrenoceptor blockade abolished the renin release response without affecting the antinatriuretic response, while renal alpha adrenoceptor blockade abolished the anti-natriuretic response without affecting the renin release response.

Therefore, these studies indicate that neurally stimulated increases in renin release are mediated by renal beta-1 adrenoceptors, and neurally stimulated increases in renal tubular sodium reabsorption are mediated by renal alpha-1 adrenoceptors. These studies also indicate that the decrease in urinary sodium excretion and sodium chloride delivery to the macula densa receptor does not contribute to the renin release observed at this level of renal nerve stimulation.

Renal nerve stimulation at frequencies in excess of 1.0 Hz increases renin release in association with decreases in renal blood flow, glomerular filtration rate, and urinary sodium excretion. The renin release results from a complex interaction of mechanisms[39]—renal vasoconstriction and hemodynamic alterations (baroreceptor), reduction in glomerular filtration rate and increase in renal tubular sodium reabsorption with decreased sodium chloride delivery to the macula densa receptor, and direct neuroadrenergic stimulation of juxtaglomerular granular cells.

Renal alpha adrenoceptor blockade with phenoxybenzamine abolishes the renal vasoconstriction and significantly reduces the renin release response. Renal beta-1 adrenoceptor blockade with metoprolol also significantly reduces the renin release response. The combination of renal alpha and beta-1 adrenoceptor blockade with phenoxybenzamine and metoprolol totally abolishes the renin release response. Since the antinatriuretic response is relatively unaffected by these adrenoceptor blocking agents compared with their effect on the renin release response, there is little evidence for a substantial role of the macula densa receptor mechanism in the renin release response.

These studies indicate a major role for the vascular baroreceptor mechanism in the renin release response to renal vasoconstrictor intensities of renal nerve stimulation. It has been hypothesized[40] that such renal nerve stimulation exerts a preferential vasoconstrictor effect on the renal vasculature proximal to the afferent arterioles, resulting in a decrease in afferent arteriolar pressure, which elicits afferent arteriolar vasodilatation and activation of the baroreceptor mechanism. However, there are no direct measurements indicating that during intense renal vasoconstriction with marked reductions in total renal blood flow and increases in total renal vascular resistance there is a selective afferent arteriolar vasodilatation.

Thus, graded intensities of renal nerve stimulation influence renin release through a complex interaction of neural and non-neural mechanisms (Figure 6-3). At increasing intensities, there is progressive recruitment of the various mechanisms that are additive in their contribution to the observed renin release.

INFLUENCE OF RENAL NERVES ON RENIN SECRETION

RENAL NERVE STIMULATION	EFFECT ON RENIN SECRETION RATE
0.25 Hz	Modulation of non-neural mechanisms
0.50 Hz	Direct neural release from juxtaglomerular granular cells without alterations in stimuli to macula densa or baroreceptor
1.00 Hz	Alteration in stimulus to macula densa receptor
2.00 - 2.50 Hz	Alteration in stimulus to vascular baroreceptor

Effects become additive as frequency of renal nerve stimulation increases.

Figure 6-3. The influence of renal nerves on renin secretion.

Efferent renal sympathetic nerve traffic can be modulated by activation of several important cardiovascular and somatic reflexes. The high-pressure aortic and carotid baroreceptors and low-pressure cardiopulmonary baroreceptors can interact to produce alterations in efferent renal sympathetic nerve activity that represent the sum of the two reflex inputs. Activation of somatic sensory receptors in muscles can produce profound changes in efferent renal sympathetic nerve traffic. Such reflex activation results in alterations in renin release that are dependent on intact renal innervation and may be considered to be dependent on intrarenal mechanisms similar to those outlined for direct renal nerve stimulation.

Hypertension

In both human and experimental hypertension, there is abundant evidence for an important contribution of sodium, the sympathetic nervous system, and the renin-angiotensin system to the raised arterial pressure. The ability of heightened activity of the renal sympathetic nerves to produce selective increases in both renin release and renal tubular sodium and water reabsorption without alterations in renal hemodynamics allows the possibility that a small increase in activity of the sympathetic nervous system can contribute to the hypertensive process in the absence of detectable changes in systemic and regional cardiovascular hemodynamics. In this regard it is noteworthy that renal denervation[41] or destruction of the antero-ventral portion of the third ventricle of the hypothalamus,[42] which receives afferent renal neural projections, delays the onset or prevents the development of some but not all forms of experimental renal hypertension.

Acknowledgments: The research performed in the author's laboratory was supported by USPHS-NIH Research Grants AM 15843, HL 23898 and HL 14388 and by research grants from the American Heart Association—Iowa Affiliate and the Veterans Administration. Dr. Kopp was supported by a postdoctoral research fellowship from the National Kidney Foundation—Iowa Affiliate. Dr. Holdaas was supported by a Fogarty International Center Senior International Fellowship (TW 03120) from the NIH.

References

1. Smith, HW: The Kidney: Structure and Function in Health and Disease, New York, Oxford University Press, 1937
2. DiBona, GF: The functions of the renal nerves. Rev Physiol Biochem Pharmacol **94:**75, 1982
3. Bernard, C: Leçons sur les proprietes physiologiques des liquides de l'organisme, Paris, Bailliere, 1859
4. Bencsath P, Bonvalet J-P, De Rouffigmac C: Tubular factors in denervation diuresis and natriuresis. *In* Recent Advances in Renal Physiology, edited by Wirz H, Spinelli F, Basel, Karger, 1972, p 96
5. Bello-Reuss, E, Colindres RE, Pastoriza-Munoz E, Mueller, RA, Gottschalk CW: Effects of acute unilateral denervation in the rat. J Clin Invest **56:**208, 1975
6. Bello-Reuss E, Pastoriza-Munoz E, Colindres RE: Acute unilateral renal denervation in rats with extracellular volume expansion. Am J Physiol **232:**F26, 1977
7. Benscath P, Asztalos B, Szalay L, Takacs L: Renal handling of sodium after chronic renal sympathectomy in the anesthetized rat. Am J Physiol **236:**F513, 1979
8. Rogenes PR, Gottschalk CW: Renal function in conscious rats with chronic unilateral renal denervation. Am J Physiol **242:**F140, 1982
9. Strandhoy JW, Schneider EG, Willis, LR, Knox FG: Intrarenal effects of phenoxybenzamine on sodium reabsorption. J Lab Clin Med **83:**263, 1974
10. Barger AC, Muldowney FP, Liebowitz MR: Role of the kidney in the pathogenesis of congestive heart failure. Circulation **20:**273, 1959
11. Schneider EG, McLane-Vega L, Hanson R, Childers J, Gleason S: Effect of chronic bilateral renal denervation on daily sodium excretion in the conscious dog. Fed Proc **37:**645, 1978
12. Gordon D, Peart WS, Wilcox CS: Requirement of the adrenergic nervous system for conservation of sodium by the rabbit kidney. J Physiol **293:**24P, 1979.
13. DiBona GF, Sawin LL: Role of renal nerves in renal adaptation to dietary sodium restriction. Am J Physiol **245:**F322, 1983
14. Gill JR, Bartter FC: Adrenergic nervous system in sodium metabolism. II. Effects of guanethidine on the renal response to sodium deprivation in normal man. New Engl J Med **275:**1466, 1966
15. Wilcox, CS, Aminoff MJ, Slater JDH: Sodium homeostasis in patients with autonomic failure. Clin Sci **53:**321, 1977
16. Slick GL, DiBona GF, Kaloyanides GJ: Renal sympathetic nerve activity in sodium retention of acute caval constriction. Am J Physiol **226:**925, 1974.

17. LaGrange RG, Sloop CH, Schmid HE: Selective stimulation of renal nerves in the anesthetized dog. Circ Res **33:**704, 1973
18. Bello-Reuss E, Trevino DL, Gottschalk CW: Effect of renal sympathetic nerve stimulation on proximal water and sodium reabsorption. J Clin Invest **57:**1104, 1976
19. DiBona GF, Sawin LL: Effect of renal nerve stimulation on NaCl and H_2O transport in Henle's loop of the rat. Am J Physiol **243:**576, 1982
20. Johnson MD. Barger AC: Circulating catecholamines in control of renal electrolyte and water excretion. Am J Physiol **240:**F192, 1981
21. Chan YL: The role of norepinephrine in the regulation of fluid absorption in the rat proximal tubule. J Pharmacol Exp Ther **215:**65, 1980
22. Gross R, Kirchheim H: Effects of bilateral carotid occlusion and auditory stimulation on renal blood flow and sympathetic nerve activity in the conscious dog. Pfluegers Arch **383:**233, 1980
23. Anderson RJ, Henrich WL, Gross RA, Dillingham MA: Role of renal nerves, angiotensin II and prostaglandins in the antinatriuretic response to acute hypercapnic acidosis in the dog. Circ Res **50:**294, 1982
24. Karim F, Kidd C, Malpus CM, Penna PE: Effects of stimulation of the left atrial receptors on sympathetic efferent nerve activity. J Physiol **227:**243, 1972
25. DeTorrente A, Robertson GL, McDonald KM, Schrier RW: Mechanism of the diuretic response to increased left atrial pressure in the anesthetized dog. Kidney Int **8:**355, 1975
26. Osborn JL, DiBona GF, Thames MD: Role of renal alpha adrenoceptors mediating renin secretion. Am J Physiol **242:**F620, 1982
27. Osborn JL, Holdaas H: Renal adrenoceptor mediation of antinatriuretic and renin secretion responses to low frequency renal nerve stimulation in the dog. Circ Res **53:**298, 1983
28. Kopp UC, DiBona GF: Interaction of renal beta-1 adrenoceptors and prostaglandins in reflex renin release. Am J Physiol **244:**F418, 1983
29. Reid IA, Morris BJ, Ganong WF: The renin-angiotensin system. Ann Rev Physiol **40:**377, 1978.
30. Torretti J: Sympathetic control of renin release. Ann Rev Pharmacol Toxicol **22:**167, 1982
31. Thames MD, DiBona GF: Renal nerves modulate the secretion of renin mediated by non-neural mechanisms. Circ Res **44:**645, 1979
32. Holdaas H, DiBona GF, Kiil F: Effect of low-level renal nerve stimulation on renin release from nonfiltering kidneys. Am J Physiol **241:**F156, 1981
33. Osborn JL, Thames MD, DiBona GF: Role of macula densa in renal nerve modulation of renin secretion. Am J Physiol **242:**R367, 1982
34. Langard O, Holdaas H, Eide I, Kiil F: Conditions for humoral alpha adrenoceptor stimulation of renin release in anesthetized dogs. Scand J Clin Lab Invest **41:**527, 1981
35. Osborn JL, Thames MD, DiBona GF: Renal nerves modulate renin secretion during autoregulation. Proc Soc Exp Biol Med **169:**432, 1982
36. Stella A, Calaresu F, Zanchetti A: Neural factors contributing to renin release during reduction in renal perfusion pressure and blood flow in cats. Clin Sci Mol Med **51:**453, 1976
37. Osborn JL, DiBona GF, Thames MD: Beta-1 receptor mediation of renin secretion elicited by low-frequency renal nerve stimulation. J Pharmacol Exp Ther **216:**265, 1981

38. Kopp, U, Aurell M, Nilsson IM, Ablad B: The role of beta-1 adrenoceptors in the renin release response to graded renal sympathetic nerve stimulation. Pfluegers Arch **387**:107, 1980
39. Kopp U, Aurell M, Sjolander M, Ablad B: The role of prostaglandins in the alpha and beta adrenoceptor mediated renin release response to graded renal nerve stimulation. Pfluegers Arch **391**:1, 1981
40. Holdaas, H, Langard O, Eide I, Kiil F: Mechanism of renin release during renal nerve stimulation in dogs. Scand J Clin Lab Invest **41**:617, 1981
41. Winternitz SR, Oparil S: Importance of renal nerves in the pathogenesis of experimental hypertension. Hypertension **4**:III-108, 1982
42. Brody MJ, Johnson AK: Role of the anteroventral third ventricle region in fluid and electrolyte balance, arterial pressure regulation and hypertension. *In* Frontiers in Neuroendocrinology, edited by Martini L, Ganong WF, New York, Raven, 1980, p 249

Chapter 7

Endogenous Opioid Peptides in the Regulation of Arterial Blood Pressure

Glen R. Van Loon

Effects of opiates on arterial blood pressure and other cardiovascular parameters have been known for a long time.[1] In the course of studies designed to elucidate the mechanism of action of morphine and attempts to develop a nonaddictive analgesic, it became clear that opiates must bind stereospecifically to sites on brain cells in order to trigger their many effects. Evidence for the existence of specific opiate-binding sites in brain was presented by a number of laboratories in 1973,[2] and this led to an active search for endogenous ligands. The first characterization of endogenous opioid peptides was provided in 1973,[3] and this isolation of the enkephalins was followed by an explosion of knowledge on the chemistry, pharmacology, physiology, and anatomy of opioid peptides. The distribution of opioids in brain areas known to be important for the regulation of cardiovascular function, and the known effects of morphine and other opiate drugs on blood pressure and heart rate, has led to a considerable number of studies on the effects of endogenous opioid peptides on cardiovascular parameters.

Classes and Distribution of Endogenous Opioid Peptides

Much of the confusion that exists regarding the effects of endogenous opioid peptides on a wide number of parameters relates to the complexity of families of endogenous opioids and their receptors. In 1975, two pentapeptides, Tyr-Gly-Gly-Phe-Met and Tyr-Gly-Gly-Phe-Leu were identified in pig brain and named met- and leu-enkephalin.[3] It was also noted that the sequence of met-enkephalin was uniquely present as the 61–65 amino acid residues of β-lipotropin, a 91 amino acid peptide hormone that had been characterized in 1965,[4] although its function remained unknown. Shortly after, a number of peptides were extracted from pituitary glands and hypothalami and found to represent sequences of β-lipotropin.[5,6] These included the 61–76, 61–77, and 61–91 sequences, which were named α, γ, and β respectively. β-endorphin was the most potent and most widely distributed of these peptides. Subsequently, it has become clear that β-endorphin is derived from β-lipotropin, which is in turn derived from a 31,000-Dalton precursor molecule termed proopiomelanocortin.[7]

Although the met-enkephalin structure represents a sequence of β-endorphin, it has also become clear that it is not derived from the same precursor molecule. Rather, studies of the adrenal have provided strong evidence that met-enkephalin is derived from a different gene product than β-endorphin.[8,9] This precursor molecule is also large (about 30,000 Daltons) and contains six met-enkephalin sequences and one leu-enkephalin sequence. Leu-enkephalin represents the N-terminus of both a 17 amino acid opioid peptide named dynorphin[10] and another opioid named β-neo-endorphin.[11] The precursor relationships of these peptides remain unclear, but they are genetically distinct from the precursors of β-endorphin and met-enkephalin. These opioid peptide-precursor relationships are outlined in Figure 7-1.

The endogenous opioid peptides are widely distributed in brain and in peripheral tissues including pituitary, adrenal medulla, sympathetic nerve endings and ganglia, pancreas, and gastrointestinal tract. The distribution of the various opioid peptides in brain and peripheral tissues has been studied primarily with immunochemical methods, and marked differences in distribution patterns have been demonstrated.[12–14]

Another perplexing aspect of the opiate field relates to the number of different opiate receptors and the variable affinities of the endogenous ligands for these receptors.[15,16] The most simplistic concept of opioid ligand-receptor interactions at present suggests that β-endorphin is an endogenous μ-receptor ligand, met- and leu-enkephalin are δ-receptor ligands, and dynorphin is a κ-receptor ligand. However, β-endorphin does bind to δ-receptors also. The opioid antagonist, naloxone, is a μ-receptor antagonist, which in high concentrations binds also to δ receptors.

In addition to the different opioids and opioid systems in brain and peripheral nerves that may function to regulate arterial blood pressure, opioids from a number of peripheral tissues are humoral substances circulating in plasma, and these may also function in blood pressure regulation. They include not only β-endorphin from the pituitary,[17] but enkephalins[18,19] presumably from adrenal medulla and peripheral sympathetic nerves, and other forms of opioid peptides.[20] The co-localization of enkephalins with catecholamines in chromaffin cells and their co-secretion[21] suggests further a homeostatic role for these substances in cardiovascular as well as metabolic regulation. Enkephalins are degraded rapidly in plasma,[22] and changes in circulating levels in response to stimuli have been

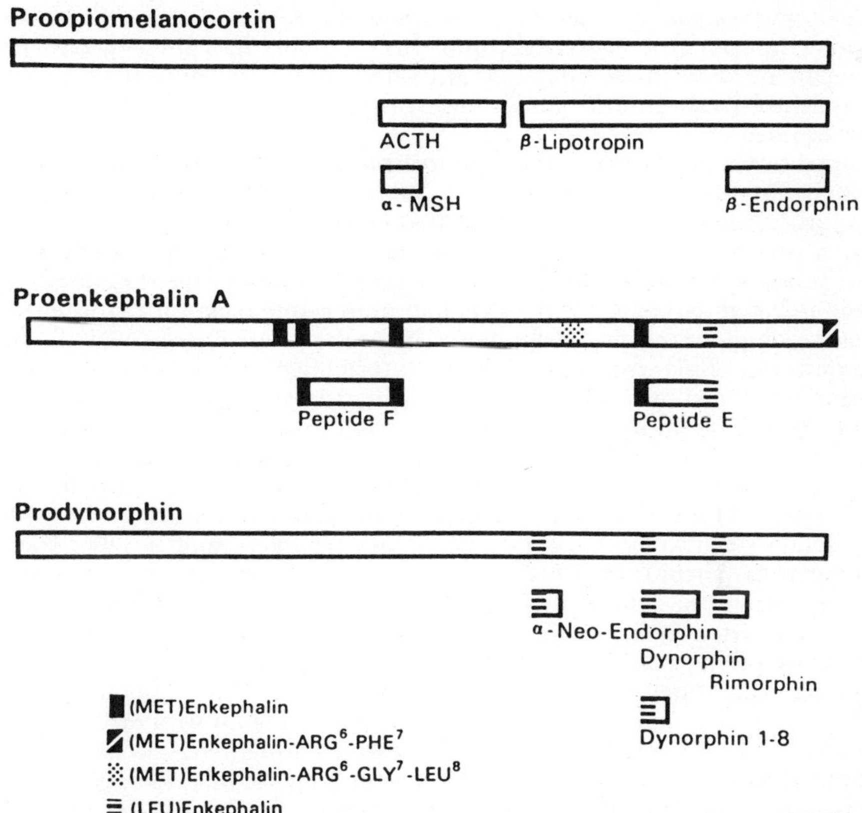

Figure 7-1. Relationships of the opioid peptides to their precursors. Three families of opioid peptides are depicted with their precursor molecules. A number of other opioid peptides representing fragments of these precursors have been isolated but are not shown.

difficult to document.[19] It remains unclear whether enkephalins are secreted into the circulation as pentapeptides or in a larger protected form.

Effects of Morphine on Arterial Blood Pressure

Morphine and opiate-like drugs have complex effects on the circulation[23,24] and species differences are apparent. Intravenous injection of morphine in rats produces a precipitous but transient fall in blood pressure and heart rate.[25,26] The bradycardia appears to be vagally mediated since it is blocked by transection of the vagus nerves. The depressor effect of morphine is also blocked by vagotomy and may result from a combination of vagal bradycardia and decreased sympathetic vasomotor tone.[25] In other studies in spontaneously breathing rats, systemic morphine produced a brief increase in blood pressure after a period of bradycardia and transient, mild hypotension; all of these responses were blocked by bilateral cervical vagotomy.[27]

Systemic administration of morphine in cats produces decreases in both blood pressure and heart rate that are not affected by cutting the vagi; thus, these effects seem to be mediated by changes in sympathetic tone of blood vessels and heart.[24] Intravenous naloxone in chloralose-anesthetized cats produced a pressor response only if morphine or opioid peptides had been injected earlier, or if the cats had undergone bilateral vagotomy and stellate ganglion removal.[28] Similarly, in awake squirrel monkeys, naloxone was without effect unless morphine was also injected.[29] In this study, morphine produced an initial increase followed by a decrease in blood pressure. Pretreatment with naloxone resulted in a prolonged increase in blood pressure after administration of morphine. In man, morphine frequently produces orthostatic hypotension,[30] but has little effect on supine blood pressure.[31] These effects of morphine in man appear to result from central inhibition of sympathetic tone,[32] but it seems likely that in most species some direct peripheral effects occur to alter cardiovascular parameters.

Intracerebral administration of morphine in cats produces varied effects, dependent on its site of action.[24,33] By acting on structures adjacent to the obex of the medulla and causing reduced sympathetic tone and increased vagal tone, morphine produced bradycardia and hypotension following intracisternal injection. In contrast, by acting on structures adjacent to the third ventricle and causing increased sympathetic discharge, morphine produced tachycardia and a transient increase in blood pressure following injection into the third or lateral ventricles. In rats, intracisternal administration of morphine produced pressor and tachycardic responses,[34] probably by increasing sympathetic tone. In dogs, morphine and morphine-like drugs appear to decrease blood pressure and heart rate by an action in the medulla oblongata to decrease sympathetic tone and increase vagal tone.[35–37] The vagal bradycardia seems to result from an action in the nucleus ambiguous rather than in the nucleus tractus solitarius.[38]

Effects of Opioid Peptide Administration
on Arterial Blood Pressure

Responses to Enkephalins

Variable blood pressure responses have been demonstrated following administration of a number of synthetic opioid peptides. This variability relates to the specific peptide, dosage, route of administration, time after administration, state of consciousness of the animal, and species of animal, and probably depends largely on the anatomical site of action and type of opiate receptor involved.

Leu-enkephalin increased blood pressure after administration into the lateral brain ventricle, the cisterna magna, or intravenously in conscious unrestrained cats and rats.[39,40] In contrast, in anesthetized cats, D-ala[2]-D-leu-enkephalin[41] or leu-enkephalin[42] decreased blood pressure,[41,42] after a transient increase with the latter.[42] Naloxone inhibited both the hypertensive and hypotensive responses in this study.

Met-enkephalin is almost inactive in vivo because of its rapid rate of enzymic degradation. Thus, it is not surprising that met-enkephalin did not alter blood pressure after intraventricular or intracisternal administration unless administered intracisternally in very high dosages.[24,39] High doses intraventricularly increased blood pressure in awake rats[39] and high doses intracisternally transiently lowered blood pressure in anesthetized cats.[41] In pentobarbital-anesthetized cats, intravenous administration of met-enkephalin caused a decline in blood pressure.[42]

D-ala[2]-met-enkephalinamide or D-ala[2]-met-enkephalin in low dosages increased blood pressure after intracisternal injection in conscious spontaneously breathing or artificially ventilated rats[43,44] or after intraventricular injection in cats.[45] In contrast, high dosages produced a biphasic effect, with an initial pressor effect and a delayed, more prolonged depressor effect.[40,46] Since both respiratory depression and hypotension have been described following application of met-enkephalin to the ventral surface of the brain stem,[47] it has been suggested that the hypotension produced by high dosages may be secondary to hypoxemia.[43,44] Others have emphasized the state of consciousness as a variable affecting responses to opioids.

Although D-ala[2]-met-enkephalin produced dose-dependent increases in blood pressure after intraventricular injection in awake rats, the same doses produced decreases in blood pressure in chloralose-anesthetized rats.[48] Also, the pressor responses in awake rats were blocked by the opiate receptor antagonists, diprenorphine and naloxone, whereas the depressor effects under anesthesia were blocked by diprenorphine but not naloxone. Systemic administration of D-ala[2]-MePhe[4]-Met(O)[5]-ol-enkephalin in urethane-anesthetized rats decreased blood pressure and heart rate.[49]

Since the increases in blood pressure just noted after central injections of enkephalins were not followed by a reflex bradycardia, it appears that the enkephalins may not only activate the sympathetic nervous system but also inhibit the vagal component of the baroreceptor reflex.[40,45] A descarboxy analog of leu-enkephalin (RX783016; Reckitt and Colman), a relatively specific μ-receptor agonist, decreased baroreflex sensitivity at low doses that alone did not affect blood pressure and heart rate.[50] On the other hand, an α-receptor agonist, BW180C (Wellcome) and a κ-receptor agonist, ketocyclazocine, increased baroreflex sensitivity.

The multiplicity of opioid receptors may account for some of the variability in the effects of opioids on blood pressure. It has been suggested [51] that anterior third ventricle receptors are of the α-type and respond to intraventricular injections of opioids with increases in blood pressure. In contrast, the receptors of the medulla oblongata and peripheral receptors, responding to intracisternal and systemic opioid administration, respectively, with decreases in blood pressure may be of the α-type and more sensitive to naloxone. However, these conclusions have been questioned[52,53] in view of the fact that intraventricular and intracisternal injections spread to multiple sites along the ventricular system.

Systemic administration of enkephalins has been reported by some investigators to produce decreases in blood pressure,[42,49,54] although others[39,40] have reported no change or hypertensive responses. In humans, systemic administration of D-ala^2-MePhe^4-Met(O)^5-ol-enkephalin produced no change in blood pressure.[55]

The carboxy terminus of proenkephalin A in the adrenal medulla contains the heptapeptide sequences Tyr-Gly-Gly-Phe-Met-Arg-Phe-OH.[8] The rodent brain contains a neuronal system[56] that is specifically labeled by antibodies raised to the shorter peptide sequence, Phe-Met-Arg-Phe-amide, a cardioexcitatory peptide first identified in the invertebrate nervous system.[57] Systemic administration of these peptides in anesthetized rats produced marked increases in systolic and diastolic blood pressure and heart rate.[58] The effects were dependent on the carboxyterminal Arg-Phe configuration and were stereospecific for these two amino acids.

Responses to β-endorphin

β-endorphin injected intracisternally in dogs produced a small transient increase and prolonged decrease in arterial blood pressure.[46] In chloralose-anesthetized cats, intracisternal β-endorphin was 10–20 times more potent than morphine in producing sustained hypotension.[41] In our own studies in awake rats, intracisternal β-endorphin produced variable blood pressure responses; decreased blood pressure and heart rate were seen in some animals; and increased blood pressure and heart rate were seen in other animals after β-endorphin, but overall no significant mean changes were noted.[59]

The intravenous administration of similar doses of β-endorphin, which crosses the blood brain barrier only poorly, produced in urethane-anesthetized rats a transient fall followed by a small increase in blood pressure and finally prolonged hypotension.[60,61] These effects were completely blocked by naloxone. Adrenalectomy blunted the first depressor response and potentiated the later hypotension; dexamethasone blocked the adrenalectomy-induced potentiation of the hypotensive effect of intravenous endorphin. Adrenal demedullation also greatly reduced the initial depressor response. In humans, intravenous β-endorphin[62] in the dosages (1–10 mg) examined produced no change in blood pressure.

Response to Naloxone

Intravenous naloxone increased systolic blood pressure in normotensive humans when doses greater than 1 mg/kg were given.[63] Others have reported that intravenous naloxone does not alter mean arterial pressure in normotensive or hypertensive subjects, either awake or anesthetized,[64] but these authors gave less than 1 mg/kg.

Peripheral Effects

In addition to local release of enkephalins from peripheral nerve terminals, opioid peptides from pituitary, adrenal, and perhaps other organs such as the gut and its derivatives are released into the peripheral circulation. It remains unknown which of these may be involved in mediating peripheral cardiovascular responses and at what sites, especially in view of the indirect effects brain opioid peptides appear to have on peripheral autonomic function. In any case, some direct peripheral effects of opioids have been described.

Both leu- and met-enkephalin decreased perfusion pressure when injected intra-arterially in isolated perfused femoral artery preparations in pentobarbital anesthetized cats.[65] These effects were antagonized by naloxone, suggesting a specific opioid-receptor mediated vasodilatory effect in skeletal muscle. Although the effect on perfusion occurred within 20 to 30 seconds after drug administration, intravenous enkephalin also decreased the animals' mean arterial pressure, and the effect on isolated femoral vasculature may have been indirectly mediated by the effect on the general circulation or on sympathetic nervous system activity. Others have noted vasodilatory effects of intra-arterial met-enkephalin to increase blood flow in the gastric mucosa.[66,67]

Localization of Opioid Peptide Effects on Arterial Blood Pressure

The nucleus tractus solitarius (NTS), a hindbrain region known to mediate cardiovascular activity,[68] contains β-endorphin nerve terminals[69] and opiate binding sites.[70–72] Thus, a number of investigators have examined the effects of opioids injected specifically into this brain nucleus. Fentanyl, a μ-receptor agonist, did not alter blood pressure or heart rate when microinjected into the NTS of chloralose-anesthetized dogs.[38] In contrast, unilateral injection of β-endorphin into the NTS of urethane-anesthetized, normotensive male rats resulted in a U-shaped dose-response relationship, with decreases in mean arterial pressure and heart rate occurring at doses < 5 ng and increases in mean arterial pressure occurring at doses > 10 ng.[73–75] Decreases in blood pressure resulted after doses as low as 10–100 pg injected unilaterally into the NTS or the caudally adjacent nucleus commissuralis, but not after injections dorsal, lateral, ventral or rostral to the NTS.

Naloxone administered into the NTS did not alter blood pressure or heart rate of control rats, but naloxone injected into the NTS or subcutaneously prevented the hypotensive effect of β-endorphin injected subsequently into the NTS. In addition, the injection of antiserum to β-endorphin directly into the NTS produced a delayed increase in blood pressure and prevented the hypotensive effect of β-endorphin injected into the NTS. This β-endorphin antiserum did not cross-react with the enkephalins, and an antiserum to met-enkephalin did not prevent the β-endorphin effect.

In contrast to the hypotensive effects of low doses of β-endorphin but similar to the high doses of β-endorphin, unilateral injections of Des-tyr-β-endorphin or D-ala^2-met-enkephalin into the NTS produced increases in blood pressure.[73] Thus, two separate opioid systems with different receptors may exist in the brain stem to regulate cardiovascular function. One may involve β-endorphin or μ-receptors and be depressor in nature; the other may involve met-enkephalin or δ-receptors and be pressor in nature. Such an inverse relationship between two opioid systems may explain the failure of naloxone to clearly affect blood pressure in normotensive animals.[73]

Other data are not consistent with this hypothesis.[76] These authors found that in chloralose/urethane-anesthetized cats, injection into the NTS of the μ-receptor agonists, morphine, morphiceptin, or D-ala^2-MePhe^4-Gly^5-ol-enkephalin, or the κ-receptor agonist, dynorphin, failed to alter blood pressure, whereas the δ-receptor agonist, D-ala^2-D-leu-enkephalin, produced a dose-dependent naloxone-reversible decrease in mean arterial pressure.

The nucleus ambiguus of the medulla oblongata is richly innervated by enkephalin-positive nerve terminals,[77] and electrical stimulation of this nucleus produced a frequency-dependent bradycardia.[38] Although fentanyl did not alter blood pressure when injected into the NTS, it produced a striking decrease in heart rate and a small decrease in blood pressure when injected into the nucleus ambiguus.[38] Injection of met-enkephalinamide into the nucleus ambiguus produced bradycardia without a change in blood pressure. Microinjection into the nucleus ambiguus of chloralose-anesthetized dogs of a number of substances including veratridine, L-Tyr-D-Arg, and physostigmine, which are thought to release enkephalins from nerve endings, and D-phenylalanine, puromycin, captopril, and Gly-Gly-Phe-Met, which are known to decrease enkephalin degradation, resulted in naloxone-reversible bradycardia but no changes in blood pressure.[78]

Recently, the effects of administration of opioid agonists of different receptor subtypes directly into the hypothalamus have been examined.[51,52] In preliminary studies, these authors found that a highly (200 to 400-fold) selective μ-receptor agonist, D-ala^2-MePhe^4-Gly^5-ol-enkephalin, was 10-fold more potent than the less (2 to 10-fold) selective δ-receptor agonist, D-ala^2-leu-enkephalin, in increasing blood pressure and heart rate after injection into the anterior hypothalamus of awake rats.[51] They suggested that these findings, which were naloxone-reversible, were consistent with an action of both enkephalins as μ-opiate receptors. The κ-receptor agonist, MR 2034 (Boehringer-Ingelheim), had no effect on blood pressure or heart rate.

These authors suggested further that activation of the sympathetic nervous system balances the cardiodepressant action of the opioid, with the adrenal medulla maintaining heart rate and the sympathetic nerves maintaining blood pressure in the normal range despite marked respiratory depression and vagal activation.[51] The highly specific μ-receptor agonist produced a decrease in heart rate with no change in blood pressure in adrenal-demedullated rats, and decreases in both heart rate and blood pressure in adrenal-demedullated rats in which sympathetic outflow was blocked by bretylium tosylate.

Subsequently, these authors have injected a number of opiate receptor agonists into two hypothalamic nuclei of pentobarbital-anesthetized rats.[52] In contrast to their data in awake rats, in anesthetized rats D-ala^2-MePhe^4-Gly^5-ol enkephalin produced a marked decrease in blood pressure after injection into the medial preoptic nucleus. Morphine, a μ-receptor agonist, and D-ala^2-leu^5-enkephalin produced mild pressor responses after injection into the medial preoptic nucleus and more marked depressor responses after injection into the periventricular hypothalamic nucleus. Although dynorphin decreased blood pressure after injection into the periventricular hypothalamic nucleus, this hypotension was probably secondary to marked respiratory depression.

Interactions with Other Drugs and Neurotransmitters in Blood Pressure Modulation

Interactions between brain opioids and α-adrenergic systems have been suggested.[79–82] Both clonidine, an antihypertensive drug that stimulates adrenergic α-receptors, and morphine, which also decreases blood pressure and heart rate, appear to produce these effects in part by decreasing central sympathetic outflow. Clonidine has a number of other effects similar to morphine.[80] It can produce analgesia; its withdrawal elicits symptoms similar to those of morphine withdrawal; it reverses symptoms of opiate withdrawal, whereas adrenergic α-receptor antagonists elicit symptoms of opiate withdrawal. The hypotension produced by clonidine in awake or anesthetized normotensive rats is not reversed by naloxone.[79] In contrast, in spontaneously hypertensive rats naloxone reversed the decrease in blood pressure produced by clonidine. These data are discussed more extensively next.

Interaction between β-adrenergic receptors and endogenous opioids in brain has also been suggested.[39] Intraventricular administration of propranolol in normotensive awake rats inhibited the pressor responses to intraventricular but not to intravenous met- and leu-enkephalin. However, propranolol did not alter the hypotensive responses to met- or leu-enkephalin in cats.[42]

Angiotensin II increases blood pressure when injected into brain.[83] Recently, it has been suggested that an endogenous opioid system is involved in mediating the central nervous system cardiovascular effects of angiotensin II, perhaps at the area postrema.[84] Naloxone blunted the pressor response of angiotensin II administered into the vertebral arteries of chloralose-anesthetized dogs without affecting the pressor responses to intravenous angiotensin II. Morphine potentiated the pressor response to intravertebral angiotensin II, and naloxone completely reversed this effect.

Other investigators have suggested that endogenous opioid peptides may inhibit the central pressor actions of angiotensin II by acting at a number of brain sites to decrease the angiotensin II-induced increases in sympathetic outflow, in vasopressin secretion, and in sensitivity to vasopressin.[85] Met-enkephalin, leu-enkephalin, β-endorphin, or morphine administered into a lateral cerebral ventricle inhibited the pressor response to intraventricular angiotensin II in conscious rats.[85] Naloxone blocked the effects of all these opioids. Also, all of these opioids inhibited the angiotensin II-induced increases in plasma vasopressin without affecting the basal concentration.

Involvement of a serotonergic pathway in the action of β-endorphin on arterial blood pressure has been suggested.[60] Depletion of serotonin stores with p-chlorophenylalanine or blockade of serotonin receptors with cyproheptadine, mianserin, or metergoline prevented the initial depressor effect of intravenous β-endorphin in anesthetized rats. Also, fluoxetine, a serotonin uptake inhibitor, potentiated the initial depressor effect of intravenous β-endorphin in these studies.

A possible effect of histamine in mediating the hypotensive effects of morphine in humans has been suggested. The combination of the H_1 receptor antagonist, diphenhydramine, and the H_2 receptor antagonist, cimetidine, blunted minimally the decreases in mean blood pressure and systemic vascular resistance produced by intravenous morphine.[86] Diphenhydramine antagonized the hypertensive and hypotensive responses to intravenous leu-enkephalin in cats, but did not affect the hypotensive response to met-enkephalin.[42]

Endogenous Opioid Peptides in Animal Models of Hypertension

Blood Pressure Responses to Opioid Peptides and Antagonists in Genetic Spontaneously Hypertensive Rats

A number of biogenic amines and neuropeptides appear to be primarily or secondarily involved in the central regulation of blood pressure in the genetic spontaneously hypertensive rat (SHR).[87] Thus, it would be expected that investigators would examine a possible role of endogenous opioid peptides in these hypertensive rats, especially in view of the effects of opioid peptides in normotensive animals already discussed. Intraventricular injections of either D-ala^2-met-enkephalin[48] or leu-enkephalin[40] produced greater pressor responses in SHR rats than in normotensive WKY control rats. Intravenous leu-enkephalin also produced greater pressor responses in SHR than in WKY rats.[40] Intravenous but not intraventricular naloxone blunted these pressor responses of leu-enkephalin. In contrast, in this study intracisternal leu-enkephalin did not produce greater pressor responses in spontaneously hypertensive rats than in WKY rats, but naloxone blunted these pressor responses in both groups.

The apparent importance of central sympathetic tone in the physiologic regulation of arterial blood pressure and the similarities between some effects of clonidine and opioids led to investigation of the interactions between some effects of clonidine and opioids led to investigation of the interactions between central opiate and alpha adrenergic systems in the control of cardiovascular function not only in normotensive rats but also in SHR. In unanesthetized SHR, naloxone or naltrexone inhibited the hypotension and bradycardia produced by either the acute or chronic systemic administration of clonidine.[79] Naloxone also reversed the hypotension produced by systemic α-methyldopa. The authors suggested that the cardiovascular effects of central α-adrenoceptor stimulation in SHR are mediated by the release of an endogenous opioid.[79]

The hypotension and bradycardia produced by clonidine were also inhibited by naloxone in pentobarbital-anesthetized rats. Furthermore, the reductions in heart rate and blood pressure produced in normotensive control rats by clonidine or α-methyldopa were smaller than in SHR, and these effects were not influenced by naloxone. Naloxone also reduced the pressor effects of morphine in SHR. In contrast, the α-adrenoceptor antagonist, yohimbine, blocked the pressor effect of clonidine but not of morphine. These latter data are in agreement with earlier findings.[35] The authors believe that in the sequence of clonidine-induced hypotension and bradycardia in SHR, activation of opiate receptors occurs distal to the activation of α-receptors—that is, an opioid system is present somewhere in the descending sympathetic outflow tract.[79] This suggestion is in keeping with our own hypothesis,[82] which will be discussed in more detail later.

Following sudden cessation of treatment with clonidine, there is a period of tachycardia and swings of increased blood pressure. Intraventricular morphine suppresses the upswings of blood pressure following withdrawal of clonidine in SHR without affecting the tachycardia, and naloxone abolished the inhibitory effect of morphine.[88] Subcutaneous morphine was much less effective in antagonizing the blood pressure lability during clonidine withdrawal. In a subsequent study these authors demonstrated that intraventricular morphine suppressed the labile hypertensive overshoot following cessation of treatment of SHR with a selective α$_2$-adrenoceptor agonist, azepexole.[89]

The centrally mediated hypotensive effect of propranolol may be sim-

ilar to that of clonidine. Naltrexone inhibited the hypotension and bradycardia produced by either acute intracisternal or chronic oral propranolol in anesthetized SHR.[90]

Prolonged low-frequency stimulation of the sciatic nerve elicits a post-
stimulatory long-lasting decrease in arterial blood pressure secondary to
inhibition of central sympathetic activity in awake SHR. This depressor
effect is suppressed by naloxone but not by dexamethasone, suggesting a
role of brain opioids but not of pituitary β-endorphin in this depressor
response.[91] The time course of the depressor response was much different
from that of the increase in pain threshold produced by sciatic nerve stimulation, and the dose of naloxone required to attenuate the depressor response was much greater, suggesting that the brain site of action and opiate
receptor type may be different for the two responses. Administration of
the serotonin synthesis inhibitor, p-chlorophenylalanine, abolished the depressor response, and administration of the serotonin precursor, 5-hy-
droxytryptophan, or the serotonin uptake inhibitor, zimelidine, enhanced
the depressor response, suggesting that a serotonergic system is involved in
this opioid-mediated depressor response in SHR rats.[91]

Brain serotonin systems appear to be involved in some pathophysiologic aspects of the regulation of blood pressure[92] and other cardiovascular
parameters.[93,94] Also, the effects of opioids on brain serotonin metabolism[95,96] and the effects of serotonin depletion on the depressor response to
β-endorphin[60] provide further basis for interactions between serotonin
and opioid systems that are consistent with these findings in SHR. Of some
interest also is the finding of these authors that diazepam abolished the
depressor response following sciatic nerve stimulation.[91]

Although plasma and pituitary concentrations of arginine vasopressin
are elevated in SHR, and enkephalins can increase vasopressin secretion,
the cardiovascular effects of brain enkephalins do not seem to be due to
vasopressin.[97,98] Plasma vasopressin was unchanged two minutes after administration of intraventricular D-ala^2-met-enkephalin as blood pressure is
first increased, and plasma vasopressin was decreased 25 minutes after enkephalin administration during the later prolonged pressor response. Intravenous injection of a vasopressin pressor antagonist inhibited the
pressor response to intravenous vasopressin in normotensive rats and in
SHR. However, this vasopressin antagonist did not block the pressor response to intraventricular D-ala^2-met-enkephalin.[98] Thus, the depressor
response to intraventricular leu-enkephalin in Brattleboro rats with hereditary hypothalamic diabetes insipidus—which contrasts with the pressor response in control WKY or Long Evans rats[40]—may not relate simply to the
lack of vasopressin in these rats.

*Measurements of Endogenous Opioids in Genetic Spontaneously
Hypertensive Rats*

Activation of α$_2$-receptors in brain stem of SHR results in the release
of a substance with β-endorphin immunoreactivity.[80] Clonidine and L-α-

methylnoradrenaline but not D-α-methylnoradrenaline increase the release of β-endorphin immunoreactivity from brain stem slices from SHR but not from normotensive WKY rats. Yohimbine reduced the basal release and prevented the clonidine-induced increase in release of β-endorphin from these SHR brain stem slices. Activation of α_2-receptors in brain, then, results in the release of β-endorphin, which inhibits sympathetic outflow and decreases blood pressure.

Since naloxone did not alter either the basal release or the clonidine-stimulated release of β-endorphin in these studies, it appears that naloxone antagonizes the clonidine effect by preventing the action rather than the release of the endogenous opiate,[80] although inhibition by naloxone of the morphine-induced increase in opiate activity of cerebrospinal fluid has been reported.[99] The specific brain site of release and action of this endogenous opioid mediating the depressor effect of clonidine in SHR is not known, but the nucleus tractus solitarius or a related neuronal pathway seem likely. Also, it is not known whether this opioid mechanism is limited to SHR or has implications for hypertension generally.

These findings raised the possibility that some brain opioid neurons are altered in SHR. Met-enkephalin immunoreactivity and met-enkephalin binding have been measured in a large number of brain areas of SHR and compared with data of normotensive WKY rats.[100] Met-enkephalin concentration and binding were higher in young SHR than young WKY rats in some brain nuclei such as the dorsal nucleus of the vagus, and lower in others such as the arcuate nucleus. However, these differences did not persist in adult rats in which differences were noted in nuclei that had not shown these variations in young rats. It remains entirely unknown whether activation of some met-enkephalin neurons such as those in the dorsal nucleus of the vagus or the amygdala or suppression of other met-enkephalin neurons may be causally related to the development of hypertension in SHR.

In a number of peripheral tissues of SHR rats including the coeliac and superior cervical ganglia, salivary gland, and adrenal gland, met- and leu-enkephalin immunoreactivity are reduced when compared with normotensive WKY controls.[101] A chromatographic profile of immunoreactive met-enkephalin-like peptides in the coeliac gland disclosed that SHR contain less of the low molecular weight peptides but an equal amount of the high molecular weight peptides. These authors[101] and others[102] have found no differences in met-enkephalin contents of hypothalamus or striatum between SHR and WKY rats. Others have reported increases in total posterior pituitary enkephalin immunoreactivity in SHR compared with WKY controls, but no increases in rats with DOCA/salt hypertension compared with their normotensive controls.[102]

β-endorphin immunoreactivity is also higher in neurointermediate lobe of pituitary in SHR, and plasma levels of β-endorphin are lower than in normotensive WKY controls.[103] The dopamine agonist, bromocriptine, decreased not only blood pressure but also neurointermediate lobe β-endorphin concentration in SHR, further supporting the hypothesis of a dopaminergic defect in this model of hypertension.[103] In a subsequent study these authors compared β-endorphin levels in neurointermediate lobe of pituitary and plasma in the Japanese and New Zealand strains of genetically hypertensive rats.[104] The hypertensive rats of the New Zealand strain did not show the differences in β-endorphin levels seen in the SHR of the Okamoto strain, suggesting that the differences noted in the Japanese strain may reflect a genetic difference not necessarily related to elevated blood pressure.[104]

Opioid Peptides in Other Animal Models of Hypertension

Endogenous opioids also appear to be involved in the regulation of blood pressure in some other animal models of hypertension. Intraventricular β-endorphin produced a greater fall in arterial blood pressure in urethane-anesthetized renal hypertensive rats of the two-kidney, one-clip Goldblatt model than in controls.[75] Naloxone attenuated the α-methyldopa-induced depressor response in conscious renal hypertensive rats of this model.[81]

Pain Threshold in Hypertension

Several lines of evidence suggest an interaction between blood pressure and pain regulatory mechanisms. Experimentally induced and genetically hypertensive rats are less sensitive to painful stimuli than normal controls,[87,105,106] and this decrease in pain sensitivity is naloxone-reversible.[87] Also, an acute increase in blood pressure in rats reduces reactivity to noxious stimuli.[107] Furthermore, humans with essential hypertension have a higher threshold for pain in response to tooth pulp stimulation than normotensive controls.[108] Possible involvement of an opioid mechanism in this correlation remains to be clearly established.

Role of Endogenous Opioid Peptides in Hypotension

Treatment of Hypotension With Opioid Antagonists in Animal Models of Shock

Since exogenous and endogenous opioids produce hypotension at doses even lower than required for analgesia, it was considered that endogenous opioids might contribute to the hypotension of experimental or clinical shock. This hypothesis has been tested by evaluating the therapeutic effects of the opiate antagonist in animal models of shock.[109–118] In endotoxin shock produced in rats by the intravenous administration of purified lipopolysaccharide of *Escherichia coli*, intravenous naloxone attenuated the decrease in blood pressure.[109] This naloxone effect was dose-dependent and stereospecific. Although naloxone consistently improved blood pressure in these studies, the 24-hour survival rate was not significantly improved. However, naloxone-treated animals were significantly hypertensive at the time of death in contrast with the hypotensive controls, suggesting that noncardiovascular factors may critically affect survival in rat endotoxin shock.[109]

In endotoxin shock in pentobarbital-anesthetized dogs, naloxone attenuated the decreases in mean arterial blood pressure, left ventricular contractility, and cardiac output without affecting pulmonary wedge pressure, heart rate, or total peripheral vascular resistance.[110] In view of the dramatic effect of naloxone on left ventricular contractility, it is possible that the primary therapeutic effect of naloxone in canine endotoxin shock is to reverse the depression of myocardial contractility, and the naloxone-induced increase in arterial pressure may be secondary to its inotropic effects.[110] Furthermore, the survival rate was significantly improved by naloxone when used in high doses in this shock model.

The beneficial effects of naloxone in canine endotoxin shock appear to be mediated in brain since ventriculocisternal administration of naloxone increased blood pressure to normal in endotoxin shock.[111] The timing of administration of naloxone after the onset of shock may be important since, in a porcine model of endotoxin shock, blood pressure was increased only transiently when naloxone was given late in the development of the shock state.[112] These authors also demonstrated that morphine injected after the onset of endotoxin shock produced a further decrease in blood pressure.

Naloxone increased arterial pressure and 24-hour survival rate in hypovolemic shock produced by withdrawing blood from awake rats[113,114] and these findings have been confirmed in pentobarbital-anesthetized dogs.[115] It has been suggested that enhancement of survival by naloxone in hemorrhagic shock may result from nonopiate effects, since morphine did not adversely influence survival.[113]

The effect of naloxone has been examined in yet another animal model of shock. Transection of the spinal cord at C_7 in rats[116] or cats[117] produced a fall in blood pressure, and intravenous naloxone increased arterial blood pressure in both of these shock models. Furthermore, a systemically ineffective dose of naloxone injected intraventricularly increased blood pressure in spinally transected rats. Bilateral cervical vagotomy blocked the pressor effect of naloxone in spinally transected rats or cats.[117] In these "spinal" rats and cats, vagotomy produced an increase in blood pressure similar to that produced by naloxone. Methylatropine, which is relatively impermeable to the blood brain barrier, produced an increase in blood pressure in spinally transected rats, and blocked the effect of intraventricular naloxone on blood pressure.[117] Atropine blocked the effect of naloxone in "spinal" cats, but had little effect alone on the hypotension of these animals.[117]

These studies suggest that the effects of naloxone on blood pressure after spinal transection result from an action on parasympathetic efferent pathways in brain. Similar to the data in the canine endotoxin shock model,[110] in "spinal" cats naloxone produced greater improvement in left ventricular contractility than in mean arterial pressure. These findings again suggest that the primary effect of naloxone in shock may be to antagonize the negative inotropic effects, and that the effects of naloxone on blood pressure may be secondary.

It has been suggested that β-endorphin released from the pituitary may potentiate the hypotension of these shock models by acting at brain opiate receptors after penetrating brain through circumventricular areas such as the area postrema.[118] This hypothesis is based on the failure of naloxone to increase blood pressure in hypovolemic shock in hypophysectomized rats. However, the authors have not adequately considered the possibility that lack of adrenal glucocorticoid or pituitary antidiuretic hormone may be responsible for this failure of naloxone to increase blood pressure in hypophysectomized animals made acutely hypovolemic.

Hemorrhagic shock in pentobarbital-anesthetized dogs was associated with increases in plasma concentrations of β-endorphin, met-enkephalin, and leu-enkephalin immunoreactivities, and volume repletion decreased the plasma levels of these opioid peptides.[119]

Administration of endotoxin in awake sheep produced an initial transient increase in blood pressure, followed by a period of hypotension, then return to a level slightly above baseline. Plasma β-endorphin immunoreactivity increased during the initial period of hypertension, fell almost to normal as blood pressure fell, then rose to a peak concentration late in the period of hypotension and remained elevated for a few hours.[120] In the first phase of secretion, more β-endorphin was released than β-lipotropin, whereas in the second phase the proportion of β-lipotropin was greater than β-endorphin. This pattern of secretion is similar to the pattern we found in rats in response to multiple stresses.[121]

Following an initial restraint stress, equal amounts of β-lipotropin and β-endorphin were secreted, whereas following a second restraint stress five minutes later, the ratio of β-lipotropin to β-endorphin increased markedly. The significance of this change in secretion pattern remains unknown, but β-lipotropin does not have opioid activity; thus β-endorphin immunoreactivity does not always reflect opioid bioactivity. The initial release of β-endorphin and β-lipotropin occurred before, hence not in response to, endotoxin-induced hypotension or hyperthermia, but the transient hypertension could have resulted from β-endorphin.[120] Also, it appears unlikely that the second phase of β-endorphin secretion was secondary to hypotension since this occurred during the recovery from hypotension.

Naloxone given together with endotoxin resulted in a potentiation of the initial pressor response to endotoxin and had little effect on the hypotension. Naloxone potentiated both early and late phases of endorphin secretion into plasma. Cerebrospinal fluid levels of β-endorphin increased during the second increase in plasma β-endorphin and were not affected by naloxone.

Clinical Effects of Opioids in Shock

The effect of naloxone to increase blood pressure in animal models of shock has stimulated a number of studies of the effects of naloxone on shock in humans. Intravenous naloxone increased systolic blood pressure within minutes in 8 of 13 patients with septic shock.[122] Many of these patients were receiving dopamine concurrently. Of the four patients who failed to respond to naloxone, three were receiving high doses of corticosteroids and one had secondary adrenocortical insufficiency. Promising results have been obtained by others treating individual patients with septic[123–125] or cardiogenic[124,126] shock with naloxone.

Naloxone may also have therapeutic benefit in treating cerebral ischemia. Naloxone was infused (in a double-blind study with saline) in two patients with cerebral ischemia and one with cerebral infarction.[127] Naloxone produced considerable reversal of the neurological deficits in the patients with ischemia, without altering systemic arterial blood pressure.

Role of Endogenous Opioids in Other Forms of Hypotension

Blood pressure normally decreases during sleep, reaching its nadir during stages 3–4 of slow-wave or nonrapid eye movement sleep. This decrease in blood pressure seems to result from a fall in peripheral vascular resistance since cardiac output is normal in early sleep when blood pressure is falling. In addition, baroreflex sensitivity increases during sleep. Recently, it has been found that naloxone did not affect the very early decrease in systolic blood pressure after the onset of sleep, but did prevent the later decrease during the second sleep cycle.[81] These data suggest that endogenous opioids may be involved in the fall in blood pressure seen during sleep.

The hypotensive effect of fasting or caloric restriction is greater in hypertensive than normotensive humans[129] and rats.[130] In normotensive rats the small decrease in blood pressure induced by fasting may be secondary to suppression of cardiac sympathetic nervous system activity, whereas in SHR the larger decrease appears to be secondary to decreased sympathetic nervous system activity plus an opiate-mediated vasodepressor mechanism.[131] In food-deprived SHR but not in WKY control rats, naltrexone produced an increase in systolic blood pressure.

A number of visceroautonomic reflexes are associated with alterations in blood pressure. Distension of the renal pelvis results in a fall in mean arterial blood pressure, which is abolished by morphine or the decapeptide, caerulein.[132] Naloxone prevented the effect of morphine without altering the effect of caerulein.

Regulation of Catecholamine Secretion by Endogenous Opioid Peptides

Although it is controversial whether plasma catecholamine measurements provide an index of sympathetic tone in the resting state, it does appear that plasma catecholamine concentrations reflect sympathetic activity in response to stimuli. In view of the demonstrated effects of opioid peptides to alter metabolism of catecholamines and other neurotransmitters in a number of brain regions,[95,96,133–137] we undertook a series of studies to examine possible effects of opioid peptides acting in brain to alter central sympathetic outflow, thus to alter plasma concentrations of catecholamines.[138–143]

Plasma epinephrine, norepinephrine, and dopamine increased in a dose-dependent manner after intracisternal injection of synthetic human β-endorphin in awake rats.[140] Catecholamine secretion was not stimulated by these doses of β-endorphin given systemically.[141] The epinephrine response was most sensitive and was stimulated by an intracisternal dose as low as 0.2 μg. The adrenomedullary catecholamine response appeared to be faster in onset than that from sympathetic nerve endings. Naloxone inhibited the plasma catecholamine responses when given before intracisternal β-endorphin or after at the time of the peak catecholamine response.[140,142]

The catecholamine responses to β-endorphin were inhibited by ganglionic blockade with chlorisondamine, supporting a brain site of action in this response. Bilateral adrenal denervation completely blocked the epinephrine response and partially blocked the norepinephrine and dopamine responses.[140] Guanethidine, which decreases norepinephrine release induced by sympathetic nerve stimulation, also inhibited the β-endorphin-induced increase in plasma norepinephrine, further evidence that β-endorphin increases catecholamine release from sympathetic nerve endings in addition to adrenal medulla.[139]

The specific brain site(s) of action mediating the opioid peptide effects on peripheral catecholamine secretion remain to be determined. A number of neurotransmitter mechanisms appear involved in modulating these effects. Hemicholinium-3, which interferes with high-affinity uptake of choline and markedly decreases brain concentration of acetylcholine, given intracisternally blocked the endorphin-induced increase in plasma catecholamines, suggesting that the effect of β-endorphin to increase central sympathetic outflow involves a cholinergic mechanism in brain that is caudal to (or at) the site of action of β-endorphin.[140]

Brain noradrenergic neurons appear to have an inhibitory influence on the stimulatory effect of opioid peptides on central sympathetic outflow, suggesting that the opioid neurons are caudal to the noradrenergic neurons in this interaction.[82] Intracisternal norepinephrine blunted and intracisternal 6-hydroxydopamine potentiated the plasma catecholamine responses to β-endorphin. Activation of angiotensin II receptors in brain potentiates the stimulating effect of endogenous opioid neurons on central sympathetic outflow.[143] Simultaneous intracisternal administration of angiotensin II potentiated and the angiotensin II receptor antagonist, saralasin, inhibited the plasma catecholamine responses to β-endorphin.

Somatostatin is another neuropeptide that functions as a neurotransmitter in several brain areas. Simultaneous intracisternal somatostatin markedly inhibited the plasma epinephrine response to β-endorphin, while decreasing the dopamine and norepinephrine responses only slightly. These data suggest that somatostatin neurons may interact with opioid peptide neurons in modulating central sympathetic outflow to the adrenal medulla, but do not affect outflow to sympathetic nerve endings.[139]

Plasma catecholamine responses to intracisternal administration of the enkephalin analog, D-ala²-metenkephalinamide, were markedly less than responses to a comparable molar dose of β-endorphin, and a dose of naloxone that inhibited the β-endorphin effects was ineffective in blocking the catecholamine responses to D-ala²-metenkephalinamide.[141] Thus, both μ and δ receptors may be involved in mediating in brain the opioid peptide-induced increases in catecholamine secretion. Administration of D-ala²-met-enkephalinamide intra-arterially, in the same or a four-fold greater dose than given intracisternally, did not alter plasma catecholamine concentrations.[141]

Naloxone administered systemically alone did not alter basal or stress-induced catecholamine secretion.[141,142] Naloxone also did not alter plasma catecholamine concentration in normotensive or hypertensive humans.[63]

These effects of administration of opioid peptides to increase plasma catecholamines reflect an increase in central sympathetic outflow. Such increases in sympathetic outflow clearly have implications not only for cardiovascular regulation, but also for a number of metabolic functions such as the regulation of glycemia.[144]

In keeping with our reports of the effects of opioid peptides to increase plasma catecholamines in awake rats, systemic morphine has been reported to increase plasma epinephrine in awake dogs; however, morphine did not affect plasma norepinephrine.[145] In contrast, these authors reported that morphine produced a naloxone-reversible inhibition of epinephrine and norepinephrine secretion in response to laparotomy in anesthetized dogs.[145,146] Since morphine did not affect the plasma catecholamine responses to 2-deoxy-D-glucose, the authors suggested that morphine suppression of laparotomy-induced catecholamine secretion is related to its analgesic properties rather than to inhibition of central sympathetic outflow.[146]

Following spinal injury in cats, there is a period of hypotension, which is blunted by naloxone. In these animals, naloxone administration increased plasma dopamine concentration without affecting plasma concentrations of either norepinephrine or epinephrine.[147]

Summary

The distribution of opioid peptides in brain areas known to be important for the regulation of cardiovascular function, and the known effects of morphine and other opiate drugs on blood pressure and heart rate, has led to a considerable number of studies on the effects of endogenous opioid peptides on arterial blood pressure. A number of genetically distinct classes of endogenous opioid peptides have been described, including β-endorphin, met- and leu-enkephalin, and dynorphin. Also, a number of different opioid receptor types including μ, δ, κ, and σ have been characterized.

Variable blood pressure responses including increases, decreases, or biphasic effects have been described following the administration of a number of synthetic opioid peptides. This variability relates to the specific peptide, dosage, route of administration, time after administration, state of consciousness, basal blood pressure, and species of animal. Many of these effects appear to be mediated at various brain sites, including the nucleus tractus solitarius and the anterior hypothalamus, but direct peripheral effects have also been described.

Endogenous opioid peptides have been implicated in the central regulation of blood pressure in the genetic spontaneously hypertensive rat and in other animal models of hypertension. It appears that endogenous opioids may contribute to the hypotension of experimental or clinical shock, since opiate receptor antagonists increase blood pressure in endotoxin, hypovolemic, or spinal shock. Finally, intracerebral administration of opioid peptides affects cardiovascular function not only directly but also increases catecholamine secretion by increasing central sympathetic outflow to sympathetic nerves and adrenal medulla.

References

1. Hill L: The influence of the force of gravity on the circulation of the blood. J Physiol (Lond) **18:**15–23, 1895
2. Pert CB, Snyder SH: Opiate receptor: demonstration in nervous tissue. Science **179:**1011–1014, 1973
3. Hughes J, Smith TW, Kosterlitz HW, Fothergill LA, Morgan BA, Morris HR: Identification of two related pentapeptides from the brain with potent opiate agonist activity. Nature **258:**577–580, 1975
4. Li CH: Lipotropin, a new active peptide from pituitary glands. Nature **201:**924, 1964
5. Ling N, Burgus R, Guillemin R: Isolation, primary structure and synthesis of γ-endorphin and α-endorphin, two peptides of hypothalamic hypophysial ori-

gin with morphinomimetic activity. Proc Natl Acad Sci (USA) **73**:3942–3946, 1976

6. Cox BM, Goldstein A, Li CH: Opioid activity of a peptide, β-lipotropin-(61-91), derived from β-lipotropin. Proc Natl Acad Sci (USA) **73** (6): 1821–1823, 1976
7. Eipper BA, Mains RE: Structure and biosynthesis of pro-ACTH/endorphin and related peptides. Endocrine Rev **1**:1–27, 1980
8. Noda M, Furutani Y, Takahashi H, Toyosato M, Hirose T, Inayama S, Nakanishi S, Numa S: Cloning and sequence analysis of cDNA for bovine adrenal preproenkephalin. Nature **295**:202–206, 1982.
9. Gubler U, Seeburg, P, Hoffman BJ, Gage LP, Udenfriend S: Molecular cloning establishes proenkephalin as precursor of enkephalin-containing peptides. Nature **295**:206–208, 1982
10. Goldstein A, Tachibana S, Lowney LI, Hunkapiller M, Hood L: Dynorphin-(1-13), an extraordinary potent opioid peptide. Proc Natl Acad Sci (USA) **76**:6666–6670, 1979
11. Kangawa K, Minamino N, Chino N, Sakakibara S, Matsuo H: The complete amino acid sequence of β-neo-endorphin. Biochem Biophys Res Commun **99**:871–878, 1981
12. Bloom F, Battenberg E, Rossier J, Ling N, Guillemin R: Neurons containing β-endorphin in rat brain exist separately from those containing enkephalin: immunocytochemical studies. Proc Natl Acad Sci USA **75**:1591–1595, 1978
13. Finley JCW, Maderdrut JL, Petrusz P: The immunocytochemical localization of enkephalin in the central nervous system of the rat. J Comp Neurol **198**:541–565, 1981
14. Watson SJ, Khachaturian H, Akil H, Coy DH, Goldstein A: Comparison of the distribution of dynorphin systems and enkephalin systems in brain. Science **218**:1134–1136, 1982
15. Lord JAH, Waterfield AA, Hughes J, Kosterlitz HW: Endogenous opioid peptides: multiple agonists and receptors. Nature **267**:495–499, 1977
16. Chang KJ, Cooper BR, Hazum E, Cuatrecasas P: Multiple opiate receptors: different regional distribution in the brain and differential binding of opiates and opiate peptides. Molec Pharmacol **16**:91–104, 1979
17. Imura H, Nakai Y, Nakao K, Oki S, Tanaka I: Control of biosynthesis and secretion of ACTH, endorphins and related peptides. *In* Neuroendocrine Perspectives, edited by Muller EE, MacLeod RM. Amsterdam, Elsevier Biomedical Press, 1982, pp 137–167
18. Clement-Jones V, Lowry PJ, Rees LH, Besser GM: Met-enkephalin circulates in human plasma. Nature **283**:295–297, 1980
19. Smith R, Grossman A, Gaillard R, Clement-Jones V, Ratter S, Mallinson J, Lowry PJ, Besser GM, Rees LH: Studies on circulating met-enkephalin and β-endorphin: normal subjects and patients with renal and adrenal disease. Clin Endocrinol **15**:291–300, 1981
20. Boarder MR, Erdelyi E, Barchas JD: Opioid peptides in human plasma: evidence for multiple forms. J Clin Endocrinol Metab **54**:715–720, 1982
21. Wilson SP, Chang KJ, Viveros OH: Proportional secretion of opioid peptides and catecholamines from adrenal chromaffin cells in culture. J Neurosci **2**:1150–1156, 1982
22. Hambrook JM, Morgan BA, Rance MJ, Smith CFC: Mode of deactivation of the enkephalins by rat and human plasma and rat brain homogenates. Nature **262**:782–783, 1976

23. Eckenhoff JE, Oech SR: The effects of narcotics and antagonists upon respiration and circulation in man. Clin Pharmacol Ther **1**:483–524, 1960

24. Feldberg W, Wei E: Cardiovascular effects of morphine and of opioid peptides in anesthetized cats. *In* Central Nervous System Mechanisms in Hypertension, edited by Buckley JP, Ferrario CM. New York, Raven Press, 1981, pp 229–233

25. Fennessy MR, Rattray JF: Cardiovascular effects of intravenous morphine in the anesthetized rat. Eur J Pharmacol **14**:1–8, 1971

26. Evans AGJ, Nasmyth PA, Stewart HC: The fall of blood pressure caused by intravenous morphine in the rat and cat. Brit J Pharmacol **7**:542–552, 1952

27. Willette RN, Sapru HN: Peripheral versus central cardiorespiratory effects of morphine. Neuropharmacol **21**:1019–1026, 1982

28. Dashwood MR, Feldberg W: A pressor response to naloxone. Evidence for release of endogenous opioid peptides. J Physiol (Lond) **281**:30P–31P, 1978

29. Byrd L: Cardiovascular effects of naloxone, naltrexone and morphine in the squirrel monkey. Life Sci **32**:391–398, 1983

30. Drew JH, Dripps RD, Comroe JH: Clinical studies on morphine. II. The effect of morphine upon the circulation of man and upon the circulatory and respiratory responses to tilting. Anesthesiology **7**:44–61, 1946

31. Lowenstein E, Hallowell P, Levine FH, Daggett WM, Austen WG, Laver MB: Cardiovascular response to large doses of intravenous morphine in man. New Eng J Med **281**:1389–1393, 1969

32. Mansour E, Capone R, Mason DT, Amsterdam EA, Zelis R: The mechanism of morphine-induced peripheral arteriolar dilatation—central nervous sympatholysis. Am J Cardiol **26**:648, 1970

33. Feldberg W, Wei E: The central origin and mechanism of cardiovascular effects of morphine as revealed by naloxone in cats. J Physiol (Lond) **272**:99P–100P, 1977

34. Bolme P, Fuxe K, Agnati L, Bradley R, Smythies J: Cardiovascular effects of morphine and opioid peptides following intracisternal administration in chloralose-anesthetized rats. Eur J Pharmacol **38**:319–324, 1978

35. Laubie M, Schmitt H, Canellas J, Roquebert J, Desmichel P: Centrally mediated bradycardia and hypotension induced by narcotic analgesics: dextromoramide and fentanyl. Eur J Pharmacol **28**:66–75, 1974

36. Laubie M, Schmitt H, Drouillat M: Central sites and mechanisms of the hypotensive and bradycardic effects of the narcotic analgesic agent fentanyl. Naunyn-Schmied Arch Pharmacol **296**:255–261, 1977

37. Freye E, Arndt JO: Perfusion of the fourth cerebral ventricle with fentanyl induces naloxone-reversible bradycardia, hypotension and EEG synchronisation in conscious dogs. Naunyn-Schmied Arch Pharmacol **304**:123–128, 1979

38. Laubie M, Schmitt H, Vincent M: Vagal bradycardia produced by microinjections of morphine-like drugs into the nucleus ambiguus in anesthetized dogs. Eur J Pharmacol **59**:287–291, 1979

39. Simon W, Schaz K, Ganten U, Stock G, Schlor KH, Ganton D: Effects of enkephalins on arterial blood pressure are reduced by propranolol. Clin Sci Mol Med **55**(Suppl 4):237s–241s, 1978

40. Schaz K, Stock G, Simon W, Schlor KH, Unger TL, Rockhold R, Ganten D: Enkephalin effects on blood pressure, heart rate and baroreceptor reflex. Hypertension **2**:395–407, 1980

41. Feldberg W, Wei E: Central cardiovascular effects of enkephalins and C-fragment of lipotropin. J Physiol (Lond) **280**:18P, 1978

42. Moore RH III, Dowling DA: Effects of intravenously administered leu- or met-enkephalin on arterial blood pressure. Regul Peptides **1**:77–87, 1980
43. Elghozi JL, Bellet M, Meyer P: Central pressor action of enkephalins in rats. *In* Central Nervous System Mechanisms in Hypertension, edited by Buckley JP, Ferrario CM. New York, Raven Press, 1981, pp 249–254
44. Bellet M, Elghozi, Meyer P: Implication des enkephalines dans la regulation cardiovasculaire centrale du rat. Arch Mal Coeur **75**:37–40, 1982
45. Yukimura T, Stock G, Stumpf H, Unger T, Ganten D: Effects of D-ala²-methionine-enkephalin on blood pressure, heart rate, and baroreceptor reflex sensitivity in conscious cats. Hypertension **3**:528–533, 1981
46. Laubie M, Schmitt H, Vincent M, Remond G: Central cardiovascular effects of morphinomimetic peptides in dogs. Eur J Pharmacol **46**:67–71, 1977
47. Florez J, Mediavilla A: Respiratory and cardiovascular effects of met-enkephalin applied to the ventral surface of the brain stem. Brain Res **138**:585–590, 1977
48. Yukimura T, Unger TL, Rascher W, Lang RE, Ganten D: Central peptidergic stimulation in blood pressure control: role of enkephalins in rats. Clin Sci **61**(Suppl 7):347s–350s, 1981
49. Wei E, Lee A, Chang JK: Cardiovascular effects of peptides related to the enkephalins and β-casomorphine. Life Sci **26**:1517–1522, 1981
50. Petty MA, Reid JL: Opiate analogs, substance P, and baroreceptor reflexes in the rabbit. Hypertension **3**:I142–I147, 1981
51. Ganten D, Unger TL, Simon W, Schaz K, Scholkens B, Mann JFE, Speck G, Lang R, Rascher W: Central peptidergic stimulation: focus on cardiovascular actions of angiotensin and opioid peptides. *In* Central Nervous System Mechanisms in Hypertension, edited by Buckley JP, Ferrario CM. New York, Raven Press, 1981, pp 265–282
52. Pfeiffer A, Feuerstein G, Faden A, Kopin IJ: Evidence for an involvement of μ-, but not γ- or κ-opiate receptors in sympathetically mediated cardiovascular responses to opiates upon anterior hypothalamic injection. Life Sci **31**:1279–1282, 1982
53. Feuerstein G, Faden AI: Differential cardiovascular effects of μ, δ and κ opiate agonists at discrete hypothalamic sites in the anesthetized rats. Life Sci **31**:2197–2200, 1982
54. Cowan A, Doxey JC, Metcalf G: A comparison of pharmacological effects produced by leucine-enkephaline, methionine-enkephaline, morphine and ketocyclazocine. *In* Opiates and Endogenous Opioid Peptides, edited by Kosterlitz H. Amsterdam, Elsevier/North Holland Press, 1976, pp 95–105
55. Von Graffenried B, del Pozo E, Roubicek J, Krebs E, Poldinger W, Burmeister P, Kerp L: Effects of the synthetic enkephalin analogue FK 33–824 in man. Nature **272**:729–730, 1978
56. Dockray GH, Vaillant C, Williams RG: New vertebrate brain-gut peptide related to a molluscan neuropeptide and an opioid peptide. Nature **293**:656–657, 1981
57. Price DA, Greenberg MG: Structure of a molluscan cardioexcitatory neuropeptide. Science **197**:670–671, 1977
58. Mues G, Fuchs I, Wei ET, Weber E, Evans CJ, Barchas JD, Chang JK: Blood pressure elevation in rats by peripheral administration of Tyr-Gly-Gly-Phe-Met-Arg-Phe and the invertebrate neuropeptide, Phe-Met-Arg-Phe-NH. Life Sci **31**:2555–2561, 1982
59. Van Loon GR, Appel NM, Ho D: Endorphin-induced stimulation of central

sympathetic outlow. *In* Advances in Physiological Sciences, Vol. 14, Endocrinology, Neuroendocrinology: Neuropeptides II, edited by Stark E, Makara GB, Halasz B, Rappay GY. Oxford, Pergamon Press, 1981, pp 289–293

60. Lemaire I, Tseng R, Lemaire S: Systemic administration of β-endorphin: potent hypotensive effect involving a serotonergic pathway. Proc Natl Acad Sci (USA) **75**:6240–6242, 1978

61. Lemaire I, Tseng R, Lemaire S: Modulation de l'effet hypotenseur de la beta-endorphine par les glandes surrenales. L'Union Med Canada **100**:1363–1367, 1980

62. Catlin DH, Gorelick DA, Gerner RH, Hui KK, Li CH: Clinical effects of β-endorphin infusions. Adv Biochem Psychopharmacol **22**:465–472, 1980

63. Pickar D, Cohen MR, Naber D, Cohen RH: Clinical studies of the endogenous opioid system. Biol Psychiat **17**:1243–1276, 1982

64. Estillo AE, Cottrell JE: Hemodynamic and catecholamine changes after administration of naloxone. Anesth Analg **61**:349–353, 1982

65. Moore RH III, Dowling DA: Effects of enkephalins on perfusion pressure in isolated hindlimb preparations. Life Sci **31**:1559–1566, 1982

66. Konturek SJ, Pawlik W, Walus KM, Coy DH, Schally AV: Methionine-enkephalin stimulates gastric secretion and gastric mucosal blood flow. Proc Soc Exp Biol Med **158**:156–160, 1980

67. Pawlik WW, Walus KM, Fondacaro JD: Effects of methionine-enkephalin on intestinal circulation and oxygen consumption. Proc Soc Exp Biol Med **165**:26–31, 1980

68. Palkovits M, Zaborszky L: Neuroanatomy of central cardiovascular control. Nucleus tractus solitarii: afferent and efferent neuronal connections in relation to the baroceptor reflex arc. Prog Brain Res **47**:9–34, 1977

69. Finley JC, Lindstrom P, Petrusz P: Immunocytochemical localization of β-endorphin-containing neurons in the rat brain. Neuroendocrinology **33**:28–42, 1981

70. Uhl GR, Goodman RR, Kuhar MJ, Childers SR, Snyder SH: Immunohistochemical mapping of enkephalin containing cell bodies, fibers and nerve terminals in the brain stem of the rat. Brain Res **166**:75–94, 1979

71. Law PY, Loh HH, Li CH: Properties and localization of β-endophin receptor in rat brain. Proc Natl Acad Sci (USA) **76**:5455-5459, 1979

72. Akil H, Hewlett WA, Barchas JD, Li CH: Binding of ^{3}H-β-endorphin to rat brain membranes: characterization of opiate properties and interaction with ACTH. Eur J Pharmacol **64**:1–8, 1980

73. Petty MA, De Jong W: Cardiovascular effects of β-endorphin after microinjection into the nucleus tractus solitarii of the anesthetised rat. Eur J Pharmacol **81**:449–457, 1982

74. Petty MA, De Jong W, de Wied D: An inhibitory role of β-endorphin in central cardiovascular regulation. Life Sci **30**:1835–1840, 1982

75. Petty MA, Sitsen JMA, De Jong W: β-endorphin, an endogenous depressor agent in the rat? Clin Sci **61**:339s–342s, 1981

76. Hassen AH, Feuerstein GZ, Faden AI: Cardiovascular responses to opioid agonists injected into the nucleus tractus solitarius of anesthetized cats. Life Sci **31**:2193–2196, 1982

77. Elde R, Hokfelt T, Johansson O, Terenius L: Immunohistochemical studies using antibodies to leucine-enkephalin. Initial observations on the nervous system of the rat. Neuroscience **1**:349–351, 1976

78. Laubie M, Schmitt H: Indication for central vagal endorphinergic control of heart rate in dogs. Eur J Pharmacol **71**:401–409, 1981
79. Farsang C, Ramirez-Gonzalez MD, Mucci L, Kunos G: Possible role of an endogenous opiate in the cardiovascular effects of central alpha adrenoceptor stimulation in spontaneously hypertensive rats. J Pharmacol Exp Ther **214**:203–208, 1980
80. Kunos G, Farsang C, Ramirez-Gonzales MD: β-endorphin: possible involvement in the antihypertensive effect of central α-receptor activation. Science **211**:82–84, 1981
81. Petty MA, De Jong W: Does β-endorphin contribute to the central antihypertensive action of α-methyldopa in rats? Clin Sci **63**:293s–295s, 1982
82. Appel NM, Van Loon GR: β-endorphin-induced increase in plasma epinephrine: inhibitory modulation by central noradrenergic neurons. Fed Proc **41**:1259, 1982
83. Bickerton RK, Buckley JP: Evidence for a central mechanism in angiotensin induced hypertension. Proc Soc Exp Biol Med **106**:834–836, 1961
84. Szilagyi JE, Ferrario CM: Central opiate system modulation of the area postrema pressor pathway. Hypertension **3**:313–317, 1981
85. Summy-Long JY, Keil LC, Deen K, Rosella L, Severs WB: Endogenous opioid peptide inhibition of the central actions of angiotensin. J Pharmacol Exp Ther **217**:619–629, 1981
86. Philbin DM, Moss J, Akins CW, Rosow CE, Kono K, Schneider RC, VerLee TR, Savarese JJ: The use of H$_1$ and H$_2$ histamine antagonists with morphine anesthesia: a double-blind study. Anesthesiology **55**:292–296, 1981
87. Saavedra JM: Central biogenic amines and neuropeptides in genetic hypertension. *In* Central Nervous System Mechanisms in Hypertension, edited by Buckley JP, Ferrario CM. New York, Raven Press, 1981, pp 129–139
88. Thoolen MJMC, Timmermans PBMWM, Van Zwieten PA: Morphine suppresses the blood pressure responses to clonidine withdrawal in the spontaneously hypertensive rat. Eur J Pharmacol **71**:351–353, 1981
89. Thoolen MJMC, Timmermans PBMWM, Van Zwieten PA: The influence of continuous infusion and sudden withdrawal of azepexole (G-HT 933) on blood pressure and heart rate in the spontaneously hypertensive and normotensive rat. Supression of the withdrawal responses by morphine. J Pharmacol Exp Ther **219**:786–791, 1981
90. Ramirez-Gonzalez M, Farsang C, Tchakarov L, Kunos G: Opiate antagonists reverse the centrally mediated antihypertensive action of propranolol in spontaneously hypertensive rats. Eur J Pharmacol **81**:167–170, 1982
91. Yao T, Anderson S, Thoren P: Long-lasting cardiovascular depressor responses following sciatic stimulation in spontaneously hypertensive rats. Evidence for the involvement of central endorphin and serotonin systems. Brain Res **244**:295–303, 1982
92. Coote JH, MacLeod VH: The influence of bulbospinal monoaminergic pathways on sympathetic nerve activity. J Physiol (Lond) **241**:453–475, 1974
93. Sole MJ, Shum A, Van Loon GR: Alterations in brain serotonin during congestive heart failure in the cardiomyopathic Syrian hamster. Cardiovasc Res **12**:373–375, 1978
94. Sole MJ, Van Loon GR, Shum A, Lixfield W, MacGregor DC: Left ventricular receptors inhibit brain serotonin neurons during coronary artery occlusion. Science **210**:620–622, 1978

95. Van Loon GR, De Souza EB: Effects of β-endorphin on brain serotonin metabolism. Life Sci **23:**971–978, 1978
96. Van Loon GR, De Souza EB, Kim C: Alterations in brain dopamine and serotonin metabolism during the development of tolerance to human β-endorphin in rats. Can J Physiol Pharmacol **56:**1067–1071, 1978
97. Rockhold RW, Crofton JT, Share L: Increased pressor responsiveness to enkephalin in spontaneously hypertensive rats: the role of vasopressin. Clin Sci **59:**235s–237s, 1980
98. Rockhold RW, Crofton JT, Share L: Vasopressin release does not contribute to pressor action of enkephalin in SHR. Hypertension **3:**410–415, 1981
99. Fu TC, Halenda S, Lawrence L, Chau-Pham TT, Martin BR, Dewey WL: Evidence for the blockade of the release of morphine-induced endogenous opiates by naloxone. Fed Proc **38:**364, 1979
100. Nakamura K, Hayashi T: Methionine enkephalinergic neuronal activity in cerebral nuclei of spontaneously hypertensive rats. Hypertension **4:**662–669, 1982
101. DiGuilio AM, Yang HYT, Fratta W, Costa E: Decreased content of immunoreactive enkephalin-like peptide in peripheral tissues of spontaneously hypertensive rats. Nature **278:**646–647, 1979
102. Morris M, Wren JA, Sundberg DK: Central neural peptides and catecholamines in spontaneous and DOCA/salt hypertension. Peptides **2:**207–211, 1981
103. Hutchinson JS, Di Nicolantonio R, Lim A, Clements J, Funder JW: Effects of bromocriptine on blood pressure and plasma β-endorphin in spontaneously hypertensive rats. Clin Sci **61:**343s–345s, 1981
104. Hutchinson JS, Kim A, Di Nicolantonio R, Clements JA, Funder JW: Immunoreactive β-endorphin levels in plasma and pituitary tissue from genetically hypertensive and normotensive rats. Clin Exp Pharmacol Physiol **8:**455–457, 1981
105. Zamir N, Segal M: Hypertension-induced analgesia: changes in pain sensitivity in experimental hypertensive rats. Brain Res **160:**170–173, 1979
106. Zamir N, Simantov R, Segal M: Pain sensitivity and opioid activity in genetically and experimentally hypertensive rats. Brain Res **184:**299–310, 1980
107. Dworkin BR, Filewich RJ, Miller NE, Criagmyle N, Pickering TG: Baroreceptor activation reduces reactivity to noxious stimulation: implications of hypertension. Science **205:**1299–1301, 1979
108. Zamir N, Shuber E: Altered pain perception in hypertensive humans. Brain Res **201:**471–474, 1980
109. Faden AI, Holaday JW: Naloxone treatment of endotoxic shock: stereospecificity of physiologic and pharmacologic effects in the rat. J Pharmacol Exp Ther **212:**441–447, 1980
110. Reynolds DG, Guill NJ, Vargish T, Lechner R, Faden AI, Holaday JW. Blockade of opiate receptors with naloxone improves survival and cardiac performance in canine endotoxic shock. Circ Shock **7:**39–48, 1980
111. Janssen HF, Lutherer LO: Ventriculocisternal administration of naloxone protects against severe hypotension during endotoxin shock. Brain Res **194:**608–612, 1980
112. Gahos FN, Chin RCJ, Hinchey EJ, Richards GK: Endorphins in septic shock. Hemodynamic and endocrine effects of an opiate receptor antagonist and agonist. Arch Surg **117:**1053–1057, 1982

113. Faden AI, Holaday JW: Opiate antagonists: a role in the treatment of hypovolemic shock. Science **205**:317–318, 1979
114. Isoyama T, Tanaka J, Sato T, Shatney CH: Effects of naloxone and morphine in hemorrhagic shock. Circ Shock **9**:375–382, 1982
115. Vargish T, Reynolds DG, Guill NJ, Lechner RB, Holaday JW, Faden AI: Naloxone reversal of hypovolemic shock in dogs. Circ Shock **7**:31–38, 1980
116. Holaday JW, Faden AI: Naloxone acts at central opiate receptors to reverse hypotension, hypothermia and hypoventilation in spinal shock. Brain Res **189**:295–299, 1980
117. Faden AI, Jacobs TP, Holaday JW: Endorphin-parasympathetic interaction in spinal shock. J Auton Nerv System **2**:295–304, 1980
118. Holaday JW, O'Hara M, Faden AI: Hypophysectomy alters cardiorespiratory variables: central effects of pituitary endorphins in shock. Am J Physiol **241**:H479–H485, 1981
119. Lang RE, Bruckner UB, Kempf B, Rascher W, Sturm V, Unger TL, Speck G, Ganten D: Opioid peptides and blood pressure regulation. Clin Exp Hypertension. Theory and Practice **A4**:249–269, 1982
120. Carr DB, Bergland R, Hamilton A, Blume H, Kasting N, Arnold M, Martin JB, Rosenblatt M: Endotoxin-stimulated opioid peptide secretion: two secretory pools and feedback control in vivo. Science **217**:845–848, 1982
121. De Souza EB, Van Loon GR: Plasma β-endorphin (β-END), β-lipotropin (LPH) and ACTH responses to stress in intact and adrenalectomized rats. Soc Neurosci **8**:54, 1982
122. Peters WP, Friedman PA, Johnson MW, Mitch WE: Pressor effect of naloxone in septic shock. Lancet **1**:529–532, 1981
123. Tiengo M: Naloxone in irreversible shock. Lancet **2**:690, 1980
124. Dirksen R, Otten MH, Wood GH, Verbaan CJ, Haalbebos MMP, Verdouw PV, Nijhuis GMM: Naloxone in shock. Lancet **2**:1360–1361, 1980
125. Higgins, TL, Sivak ED: Reversal of hypotension with naloxone. Cleve Clin Q **48**:283–288, 1981
126. Higgins, TL, Sivak ED, O'Neil DM, Graves JW, Foutch DG: Reversal of hypotension by continuous naloxone infusion in a ventilator-dependent patient. Ann Int Med **98**:47–48, 1982
127. Baskin DS, Hosobuchi Y: Naloxone reversal of ischemic neurological deficits in man. Lancet **2**:272–275, 1981
128. Rubin P, Blaschke TF, Guilleminault C: Effect of naloxone, a specific opioid inhibitor, on blood pressure fall during sleep. Circulation **63**:117–121, 1981
129. Reisin E, Abel R, Modan M, Silverberg DS, Eliahou HE, Modan B: Effect of weight loss without salt restriction on the reduction of blood pressure in overweight hypertensive patients. New Engl J Med **298**:1–6, 1978
130. Young JB, Mullen D, Landsberg L: Caloric restriction lowers blood pressure in the spontaneously hypertensive rat. Metabolism **27**:1711–1714, 1978
131. Einhorn D, Young JB, Landsberg L: Hypotensive effect of fasting: possible involvement of the sympathetic nervous system and endogenous opiates. Science **217**:727–729, 1982
132. Brasch H, Zetler G: Caerulein and morphine in a model of visceral pain. Effects on the hypotensive response to renal pelvis distension in the rat. Naunyn-Schmied Arch Pharmacol **319**:161–167, 1982
133. Loh HH, Brase DA, Sampath-Khanna S, Mar JB, Way EL, Li CH: β-endorphin in vitro inhibition of striatal dopamine release. Nature **264**:567–568, 1976

134. Subramanian N, Mitznegg P, Sprugel W, Domschke W, Domschke S, Wunsch E, Demling L: Influence of enkephalin on K$^+$-evoked efflux of putative neurotransmitters in rat brain. Selective inhibition of acetylcholine and dopamine release. Naunyn-Schmied Arch Pharmacol **299**:163–165, 1977
135. Moroni F, Cheney DL, Costa E: β-endorphin inhibits ACh turnover in nuclei of rat brain. Nature **267**:267–268, 1977
136. Van Loon GR, Kim C: β-endorphin-induced increase in striatal dopamine turnover. Life Sci **23**:961–970, 1978
137. Van Loon GR, Ho D, Kim C: β-endorphin-induced decrease in hypothalamic dopamine turnover. Endocrinology **106**:76–80, 1980
138. Van Loon GR, Appel NM: β-endorphin-induced increases in plasma dopamine, norepinephrine and epinephrine. Res Commun Chem Pathol Pharmacol **27**:607–610, 1980
139. Van Loon GR, Appel NM, Ho D: β-endorphin-induced increases in plasma epinephrine, norepinephrine and dopamine in rats: inhibition of the adrenomedullary response by intracerebral somatostatin. Brain Res **212**:207–214, 1981
140. Van Loon GR, Appel NM, Ho D: β-endorphin-induced stimulation of central sympathetic outflow: β-endorphin increases plasma concentrations of epinephrine, norepinephrine, and dopamine in rats. Endocrinology **109**:46–53, 1981
141. Van Loon GR, Appel NM: Plasma norepinephrine, epinephrine, and dopamine responses to intracerebral administration of a met-enkephalin analog, D-ala²-met-enkephalinamide, in rats. Neuroendocrinology **33**:153–157, 1981
142. Van Loon GR, Appel NM, Ho D: Regulation of catecholamine secretion by endogenous opioid peptides. Prog Clin Biol Res **74**:293–318, 1981
143. Appel NM, Van Loon GR: Activation of angiotensin II receptors in brain potentiates the stimulating effect of endogenous opioid neurons on central sympathetic outflow. Peptides **4**:59, 1983
144 Van Loon GR, Appel NM: β-endorphin-induced hyperglycemia is mediated by increased central sympathetic outflow to adrenal medulla. Brain Res **204**:236–241, 1981
145. Taborsky GJ Jr, Halter JB, Porte D Jr: Morphine: dual effects on plasma catecholamines. Endocrinology **109**:319–321, 1981
146. Taborsky GJ Jr, Halter JB, Porte D Jr: Morphine suppresses plasma catecholamine responses to surgical but not glucopemic stress. Am J Physiol **242**:E317–E322, 1982
147. Faden AI, Jacobs TP, Feuerstein G, Holaday JW: Dopamine partially mediates the cardiovascular effects of naloxone afer spinal injury. Brain Res **213**:415–421, 1981

Effects of Blood Pressure on the Brain

Chapter 8

Cerebral Blood Flow Regulation in Normotension and Hypertension

H. Richard Winn, E. Clarke Haley, Jr.,
and Robert M. Berne

Introduction

The cause of essential hypertension remains uncertain and controversial. However, effects of prolonged, severe systemic hypertension on most organs are clear and, in general, detrimental. For the brain, hypertension of a prolonged or short nature can result in sudden neurologic deterioration primarily due to alterations in the cerebral circulation. The changes in the cerebral circulation may be secondary to either anatomic or physiologic causes. Proper clinical management of patients with hypertension, therefore, requires an understanding of the physiology of cerebral blood flow (CBF).

This chapter reviews the mechanisms regulating cerebral blood flow in the normal and hypertensive brain. Although there has been much effort to define the factors regulating CBF in the normal state, a complete understanding remains to be defined. On the other hand, the regulation of CBF in the hypertensive state has received limited attention, and factors affecting blood flow in this case are, in general, unknown.

Like the heart, the brain receives a high percentage (15%) of the cardiac output in comparison to its weight (only 2% of total body weight). Similar disparities apply to total brain oxygen and glucose consumption. Thus, the brain receives a higher percentage of blood flow and nutrients than other organs, except for the heart. Whereas this flow/weight disparity is great in the human, CBF, as a percentage of cardiac output, is less in most laboratory animals (3% in dog, cat, rabbit, and rat).[1]

Another unique feature of the cerebral circulation is the blood-brain barrier.[2] The brain is, in general, isolated from the systemic circulation by this barrier, which is characterized by tight endothelial cell junctions and a high degree of metabolic activity in the endothelial cells.[3] The latter is exemplified by the presence of monoamine oxidase,[4,5] which effectively degrades arterial-borne catecholamines and prevents their entrance into, and action on, the central nervous system.[6] The blood-brain barrier under normal circumstances also prevents transport of protein and polar compounds into the extracellular space and cerebrospinal fluid.[2,6] Drugs that normally affect other circulatory beds, such as the kidney or skeletal muscle, may have no effect on CBF due to the blood-brain barrier.[2] Breakdown of the blood-brain barrier can occur by several means; one of the best documented is acute, transient systemic hypertension.[7] The mechanism by which the blood-brain barrier is altered in acute systemic hypertension appears to be by increased vesicular transport in the endothelial cells.[8] However, with chronic hypertension, the blood-brain barrier appears intact.

The vascular anatomy of the brain is also unique by comparison with other organs. In the human the two internal carotid arteries provide blood to the anterior circulation, while the vertebral-basilar system supplies to the hind brain. The relative contributions of these two systems varies significantly in other species.[1,9] For example, in goat, the vertebral-basilar system contributes little to brain circulation, whereas in the rat the vertebral-basilar contribution predominates. In cats the external carotid, not the internal, is the major contributor to the anterior circulation of the brain and feeds first into a rete mirabile, a complex network of vessels at the base of the brain that functions as a countercurrent cooling device.[10] Similar arterial arrangements exist in other species.[10]

The carotid and basilar vessels contribute to the formation of the circle of Willis, the completeness of which anatomically may vary considerably from individual to individual. Irrespective of the anatomic completeness of the circle of Willis, under normal circumstances, flow studies reveal little mixing of blood from the carotid and vertebral-basilar trunks, nor is there significant mixing of the blood across the midline. However, the circle of Willis provides collateral flow in the event of proximal occlusion.

Emanating from the circle of Willis are three large paired vessels—the anterior, posterior, and middle cerebral arteries—that provide the major flow to the cerebral cortex. The marginal regions of brain supplied by each of these three blood vessels are known as boundary zones. For many years it has been well known that these boundary zones are susceptible to ischemia during systemic hypotension.[11] Less well recognized is the susceptibility of these boundary zones to hemorrhage during systemic hypertension.[12,13] The susceptibility of the border zones to hemorrhage may be related to the breakdown in the blood-brain barrier.

In addition to the uniqueness of the blood-brain barrier and the arterial anatomy, the location and distribution of the vascular resistance vessels in brain appears somewhat different compared with other organs. The large extracranial and intracranial vessels are the site for a major portion of total cerebral vascular resistance.[14,15,16,17] In general, 40–50% of the total cerebral vascular resistance occurs upstream to the smaller penetrating brain vessels.[18] Consequently, these longer vessels, unlike large vessels in other beds, can serve to redistribute flow when local changes occur, thereby preventing "steal" phenomena. Moreover, the large arteries may also dampen the effects of systemic pressure changes on the smaller intracerebral vessels.[18] Thus, during systemic hypertension, vasoconstriction of these larger vessels will protect the brain from hypertensive-induced injury to the blood-brain barrier.

The blood vessels of the brain appear to be richly innervated, but the functional significance of these nerves and their anatomical origin and their neuropharmacologic description have not been fully defined.[19,20,21] The possible regulation of CBF by neuronal mechanisms will be discussed later but the anatomic details will be reviewed here. The larger cerebral vessels are innervated by nerves arising in the superior cervical ganglion.[22,23] These nerves have been demonstrated to have catecholamine endings, and to be, in general, unilaterally distributed, but with some bilateral innervation of the more medially placed vessels. Innervation includes both arteries and veins and extends down to pial and, to a lesser extent, parenchymal arteries.

Smaller intraparenchymal vessels and capillaries are associated with another catecholamine system arising in the locus ceruleus.[24] Although this system has been receiving much recent attention, its physiologic function remains unclear.[25] Some investigators have attributed a CBF regulator role to the cells arising in locus ceruleus,[26,27] whereas others have suggested a cell permeability regulatory function.[28] A direct regulatory role of intraparenchymal resistance vessels by this system appears unlikely, however, due to the distance that these nerves lie from the vascular smooth muscle of these vessels, the interposition of perivascular astrocytes,[18,29] and lack of innervation of cerebral resistance vessels.[25]

Lastly, an important feature of brain blood flow is its intimate coupling to cerebral metabolism and nerve cell activity. Whereas many other organs also display this flow/metabolism coupling, in the brain this link is very tight and is both temporally and spatially correlated.

General Characteristics of CBF

Some characteristics of brain blood flow are unique to the nervous tissue, whereas others are similar to responses in other circulatory beds.

Autoregulation

Autoregulation[30,31] is the physiological adaptation of an organ to maintain its blood flow relatively stable in response to changes in perfusion pressure. Thus, when cerebral perfusion pressure falls, cerebral vasodilation occurs; conversely, when cerebral perfusion pressure rises, cerebral vasoconstriction results (Figure 8-1). Cerebral perfusion pressure (CPP) is the difference between mean arterial pressure and intracranial venous pressure and represents the driving force for blood flow through the brain vascular bed. Since intracranial venous pressure and intracranial pressure (ICP) are practically identical in the clinical setting, CPP is defined as being equal to mean arterial blood pressure (MABP) minus ICP. Normal values range from 40 mm Hg to 80 mm Hg. Alterations in CPP can occur by either a change in MABP or ICP. For example, a decrease in CPP would result from either a decrease in MABP (e.g., systemic shock) or an increase in ICP (e.g., brain tumor or intracerebral hematoma).

The vasodilation (or vasoconstriction) in response to a decrease (or increase) in CPP results in relative constancy of CBF over a wide range of blood pressures. In general the limits of autoregulation are stated to ex-

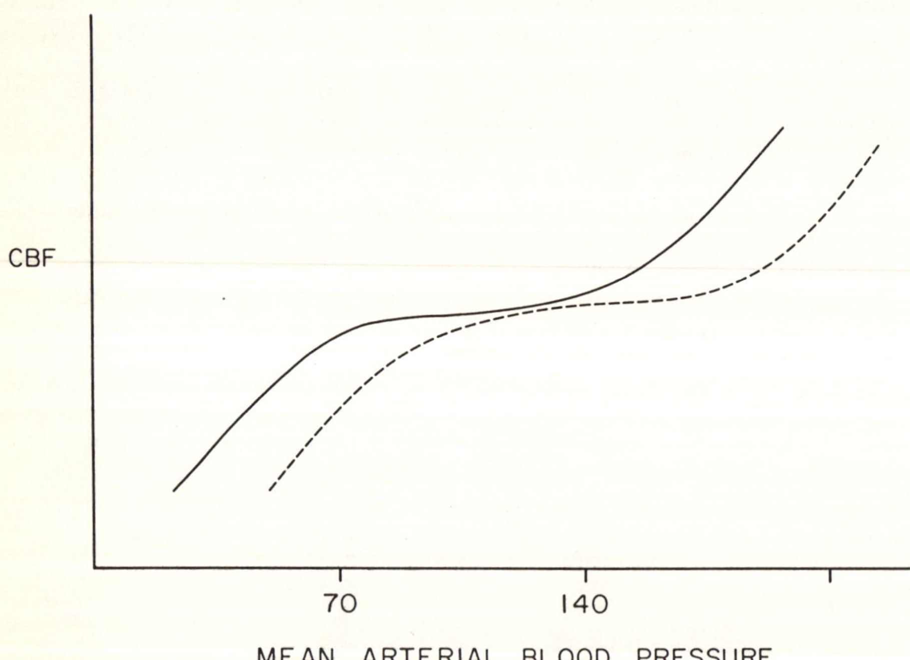

Figure 8-1. Autoregulation: change in cerebral blood flow in response to change in blood pressure. In the normotensive state there are minimal changes in blood flow between a mean arterial blood pressure (MABP) of 140 and 70 mm Hg (i.e., the "autoregulatory range"). Below 70 mm Hg, cerebral blood flow decreases as MABP decreases; above 140 mm Hg, blood flow directly correlates with blood pressure. In hypertensive individuals there is a shift of the curve to the right. Consequently, both the lower and upper limits of autoregulation are shifted to higher MABP.

tend from a mean arterial blood pressure of 140 mm Hg down to 70 mm Hg in the non-hypertensive individual[32] (Figure 8-1). The blood pressure at which CBF decreases to a significant extent is known as "the lower limit of autoregulation."[33] In actual fact, cerebral blood vessels continue to dilate even below this limit and cerebral vascular resistance continues to fall, but decreases in MABP exceed the decrease in resistance so that CBF decreases significantly.[15,34] Even in the autoregulatory part of the curve, blood flow is not perfectly stable but changes slightly (approximately 4–6% decrease in CBF per 10 mm Hg change in MABP).[18]

The upper limit of the autoregulatory curve (Figure 8-1) is that point where CBF begins to increase significantly (i.e., greater than 4–6%/10 mm Hg) with an increase in MABP.[35,36,37] In non-hypertensive humans and animals this point occurs at approximately a mean blood pressure of 140 mm Hg. In the hypertensive state the autoregulatory curve is shifted to the right so that CBF is not as well maintained at lower MABP; in contrast, CBF remains normal at higher blood pressures.[35,36,38] Eventually, in the hypertensive individual, further increases in MABP result in "breakthrough" and an increase in CBF.

When CPP changes, pial vessel response is noted within 3.5–7 sec and a new steady state is established in approximately 60 sec.[15] Any mechanism hypothesized to explain the autoregulatory phenomenon must therefore account for these temporal observations. Formerly, it was thought that the response time (3.5–7 sec) was too rapid for a metabolic mechanism, but recently changes in metabolic factors have been documented well within this time period.[39,40]

Response of the Cerebral Bed to Carbon Dioxide

The vascular bed of the central nervous system is uniquely sensitive to changes in arterial $PaCO_2$.[41,42] Hypercarbia causes cerebral vasodilation with resultant increases in CBF and blood volume, whereas hypocarbia causes cerebral vasoconstriction with resultant decreases in CBF and blood volume (Figure 8-2). By contrast, acute changes in arterial pH have little effect on CBF.[43] This non-responsiveness of the cerebral bed to changes in arterial pH is due to the presence of a blood-brain barrier to H^+ and HCO_3^-.

The response of CBF to alteration in $PaCO_2$ is described by a curvilinear relationship (Figure 8-2), with maximal changes noted in the midrange and lesser responses at the extremes.[44,45] Alterations in CBF are more marked in the cortical gray matter and the medulla. In general, between $PaCO_2$ of 30 mm Hg and 70 mm Hg, CBF increases 20–25% per 10 mm Hg increase in $PaCO_2$.

The response of the cerebral bed to alterations in $PaCO_2$ is very rapid and changes in CBF occur within seconds. Pial vascular response to changes in pH has also been shown to occur quickly.[46] With prolonged changes in $PaCO_2$, CBF returns to normal values within hours.

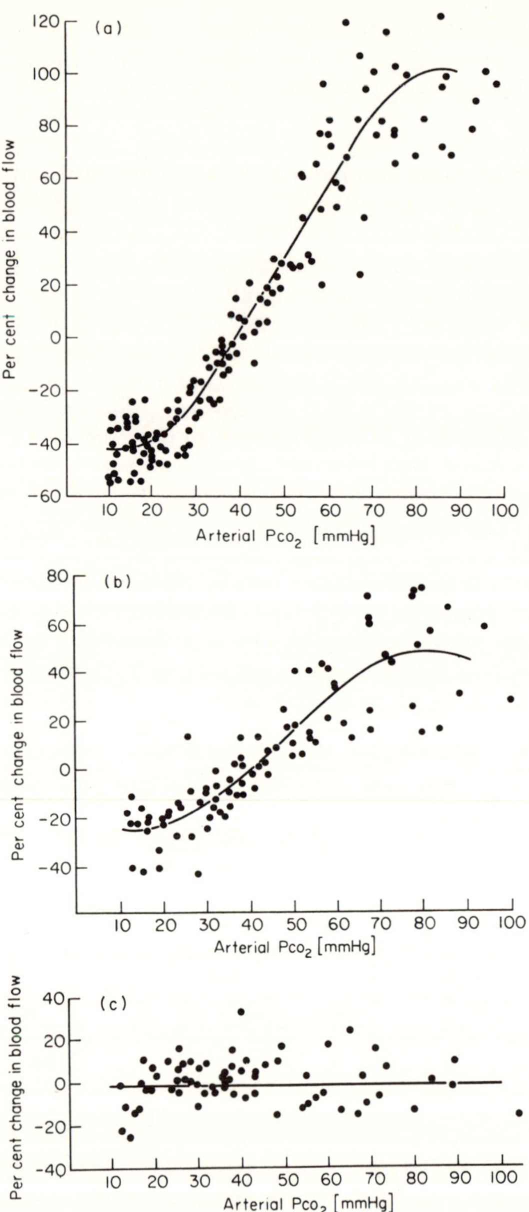

Figure 8-2. CBF/PaCO$_2$ response. The top figure represents the CBF/PaCO$_2$ relationship at normal blood pressures. The middle figure represents the CBF/PaCO$_2$ relationship when mean arterial blood pressure was lowered by hemorrhage to 100 mm Hg. The lower figure represents the CBF/CO$_2$ relationship with mean arterial blood pressure maintained at 50 mm Hg. Courtesy of The British Medical Association.[44]

The $PaCO_2$-CBF response is affected by several factors. Age may influence the responsiveness, with smaller changes being noted in older humans.[47] Decreasing the perfusion pressure, likewise, decreases the CO_2 response[44] (Figure 8-2). The vasodilatory response to a decrease in CPP limits the vasodilation elicited by an increase in $PaCO_2$[44] (Figure 8-3). Diminution in the CO_2 response has also been observed following the administration of various drugs such as atropine[48,49,50] and adrenergic blockers,[51] as well as denervation procedures[52,53] but contrary observations have also been noted.[54,55,56,57] Results are conflicting concerning the effects of indomethacin on CO_2-induced vasodilation of pial vessels.[58,59,60] The mechanism by which changes in $PaCO_2$ affect cerebral vascular muscle with resultant changes in CBF appears to be by means of changes in intracellular pH.

Response of the Cerebral Bed to Hypoxia and Hyperoxia

In contrast with carbon dioxide, alteration in PaO_2 has a less dramatic effect on CBF (Figure 8-3). Mild hypoxia (PaO_2 of 50 mm Hg) is associated with a two-fold increase in CBF, whereas hyperoxia (100% O_2) is accompanied by a small (11–14%) reduction in CBF.[61,62] Severe hypoxia (PaO_2 of 20–30 mm Hg) results in maximal vasodilation of a degree comparable to that seen with hypercarbia[63] (Figure 8-3). Although not extensively investigated, the effects of hypertension appear to be minimal on the PaO_2/CBF curve. A metabolic mechanism probably accounts for reaction of the cerebral bed to alterations in PaO_2, although neural factors have been suggested.[53,64] The most likely candidate for the chemical link controlling blood flow during hypoxia is adenosine, which is a potent cerebral vasodilator and is elevated in brain during hypoxia.[40]

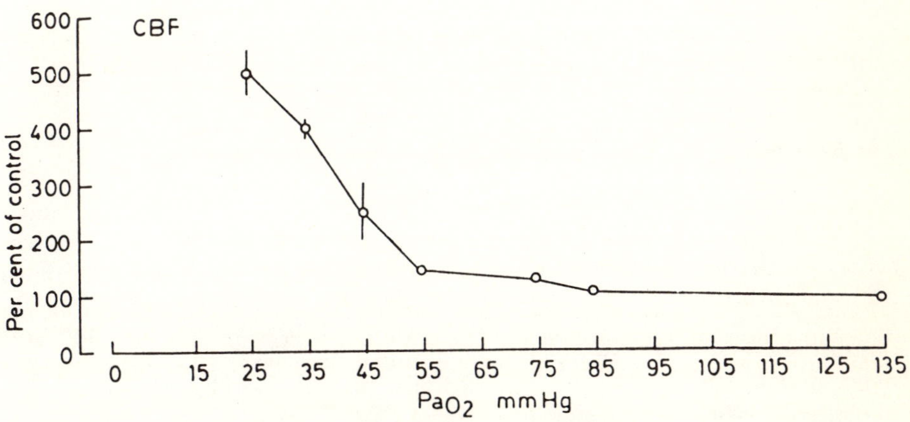

Figure 8-3. CBF/PaO_2 relationship.

The Response of the Cerebral Bed to Alteration in Brain Metabolism

The cerebral circulation is very sensitive to changes in brain metabolism. Cerebral blood flow is, under almost all physiologic circumstances, tightly coupled to cerebral metabolism. Generalized increases in cerebral metabolic rate produced by seizures or electrical stimulation result in increases in CBF, whereas depression of metabolism caused by drugs, or occurring in comatose states, results in decreases in CBF. The precision of the spatial coupling has been demonstrated by use of regional cerebral blood flow (rCBF) measurements in humans. These observations have clearly shown very localized increases in rCBF that correlate with appropriate regions of the cerebral cortex and deeper structures.[65,66,67,68] For example, volitional movement of the arm is associated with an increase in CBF in contralateral cerebral motor cortex,[67] while listening to music elicits an increase in CBF in auditory regions of the brain.[69]

In animals, 2-deoxy [14_C] glucose studies also have provided detailed localization for regional increases in metabolism that correlate closely with regional increases in CBF.[70,71] The 2-deoxy [14_C] glucose studies have demonstrated extremely detailed mapping of the alteration in glucose metabolism.[70,71] For example, increases in glucose uptake are noted in the dorsal horn of lumbar spinal cord during sciatic nerve stimulation,[71] and decreases in glucose uptake are observed in the cochlear nucleus and auditory cortex as well as intervening structures of the brain stem and thalamus with auditory deprivation.[72]

CBF is thus discreetly tied to metabolic changes in the brain, and metabolic changes can be localized with present techniques to extremely small volumes of the brain, perhaps consisting of a few hundred cells. The mechanism that accounts for this tight coupling between metabolism and CBF is unclear, but probably local production and release of vasoactive substances account for the phenomenon.[64] Some of the likely candidates that could serve as a chemical link between metabolism and CBF are considered in detail later. A linear relationship exists between O_2 consumption[73] and rCBF, so that factors linking CBF to metabolism are probably oxygen-sensitive or produced as a by-product of oxygen-sensitive reactions.

The Response of the Cerebral Bed to Alteration in Hematocrit

Changes in hematocrit influence CBF. Decreasing hematocrit causes an increase in CBF; an increase results in a decrease in CBF.[74,75,76,77] Both acute and chronic anemia result in alterations in CBF. Increases in CBF are minimal until hematocrit decreases below 30%. The most likely explanation for this increase is the associated alteration in arterial O_2 content, although changes in tissue oxygen metabolism due to a decrease in oxygen delivery may also play a role.[18] In addition, alteration in blood viscosity due to changes in hematocrit may also affect CBF.[18]

Proposed Mechanism Regulating CBF

Three general hypotheses have been proposed to explain the regulation of CBF: 1) metabolic, 2) neurogenic, and 3) myogenic. There is supportive data for each but, in general, the present consensus suggests that the dominant influence regulating CBF is local metabolic mechanisms. Modulating roles by neural and myogenic factors are likely. The various facets of each hypothesis will now be considered.

Metabolic Regulation of CBF

Metabolic regulation of a vascular bed implies that a chemical is locally produced (i.e., by the parenchyma) that is vasoactive. With a decrease in CBF and oxygen delivery, this vasoactive chemical causes vasodilation and thereby increases CBF and oxygen delivery. Alternatively, increased metabolic activity and oxygen demand may be the stimulus for production of the vasoactive chemical link whose actions would increase CBF and oxygen delivery. Thus, oxygen and metabolic supply equals oxygen and metabolic demand.

Potential Mediators of Metabolic Vasodilation of Cerebral Vessels: The identity of the transducer that adjusts the contractile state of cerebral arteriolar vascular smooth muscle to modify CBF to meet the needs of the brain parenchymal tissue has not been definitely established, although a number of candidates have been suggested. To serve as a mediator of metabolically induced vasodilation, a substance must meet the following criteria:[40]

1. The mediator must be a potent vasodilator that originates from an endogenous source.
2. The mediator must be released in response to an imbalance between parenchymal oxygen supply and need and have ready access to the arterioles.
3. The mediator must reach concentrations in the vicinity of the resistance vessels that will increase blood flow to the same degree as observed with identical concentrations of exogenously administered substance.
4. The mediator must show temporal changes in tissue concentration that closely follow the changes in blood flow.
5. Potentiators and inhibitors of the proposed mediator should have the appropriate effect on CBF.

Having described some of the general characteristics of the proposed metabolic mediator, we will now consider specific chemical factors and how well they fulfill the outlined criteria. The mediators to be discussed are oxygen, CO_2 + H^+ ion, potassium, adenosine, and prostaglandins.

Oxygen: Oxygen has been suggested as directly regulating cerebral blood flow.[78] Kety and Schmidt[61] demonstrated that hypoxia produced an increase in CBF that was reversible when PaO_2 was restored to normal values. In the rat, CBF was also increased when PaO_2 was reduced further to 50 mm Hg or less; a five-fold increase in CBF occurred when PaO_2 was reduced by 25 mm Hg[68] (Figure 8-3). Similar changes in CBF have been documented in other animals.[1]

Under normoxemic conditions, direct measurement of PaO_2 in the lumen of the pial vessels revealed a longitudinal gradient, indicating a loss of oxygen from precapillary vessels, presumably the site of cerebral vascular regulation.[79] With systemic hypoxia, the effect of the reduction in PaO_2 on the pial vessels is apparently a local one, since in cats equipped with a cranial window, pial arterial dilation induced by general hypoxia was reversed when CSF under the cranial window was replaced with oxygen-loaded mock CSF or oxygenated fluorocarbon.[80]

However, it is doubtful that the physiologic regulation of CBF occurs by the direct effects of oxygen, because CBF remains elevated following transient systemic hypoxia despite normalization of PaO_2.[81,82] Furthermore, a dissociation between CBF and PaO_2 is observed in the immediate vicinity of electrically stimulated neurons.[83] However, there are conflicting data as to whether PaO_2 decreases,[84,85,86] remains constant,[83] or increases[87] during electrical or chemical stimulation of the brain. These disparities may be related to differences in species or in techniques used to measure PaO_2. Decreases in cerebral vascular resistance observed in the auto-regulatory blood pressure range are also independent of the oxygen content of arterial blood, although the redox state of tissue cytochrome a,a3 is reduced with minimal decreases in mean arterial blood pressure.[88]

In addition to the disparities outlined, the presence of an oxygen receptor has not been established in the brain or in other tissues. In the hamster cheek pouch a clear distinction was noted between the vascular response confined to a small segment of a single arteriole and a generalized PaO_2 change over the tissue surface.[89] Minimal changes in arteriolar diameter were found in response to localized changes in surface PaO_2, whereas significant increases in arteriolar diameter occurred when changes in surface PaO_2 included parenchymal cells. In brain, Kontos et al.[80] noted a greater decrease of pial vessel diameter with oxygen-loaded fluorocarbon than with oxygen-loaded mock CSF. While the oxygen tension of the CSF and fluorocarbons was equal, the oxygen content of the fluorocarbon was much greater. These investigators[80] reasoned that the higher oxygen content of the fluorocarbon permitted more widespread diffusion of oxygen. The oxygen-loaded fluorocarbon would thus affect parenchymal as well as vascular smooth muscle tissue. It was concluded[80] that hypoxia in brain, as in hamster cheek pouch,[89] altered vascular diameter only indirectly by affecting the parenchymal tissue.

Carbon dioxide and hydrogen ion concentration: The possibility that H^+ regulated CBF was initially suggested because of the observations that CBF varied directly with changes in $PaCO_2$ and the general parallelism between extracellular H^+ activity and CBF.[41,90,91,92] Initially, a controversy existed as to whether CO_2 per se influenced cerebrovascular resistance, or whether the effects of CO_2 were secondary to CO_2-induced changes in pH. Application of mock CSF containing bicarbonate (25 meq/liter) to the pial arterioles resulted in a reduction in their diameter, whereas mock CSF without bicarbonate produced vasodilation[93,94] (Figure 8-4). These observations indicate the importance of pH on pial arteriolar tone. However, they do not rule out a separate and direct effect of CO_2 on the pial vessels.

Conclusive evidence for mediation of the CO_2 effect via changes in pH have been provided by the studies of Kontos et al.[95] In these experiments, cats were fitted with a cranial window with ports that enabled the investigator to change independently the PCO_2 and/or pH of the fluid under the window. Arteriolar diameter varied solely with changes in pH, regardless of the PCO_2. Hence, pH rather than PCO_2 is the primary determinant of vascular resistance with hypocapnia or hypercapnia. The response of the

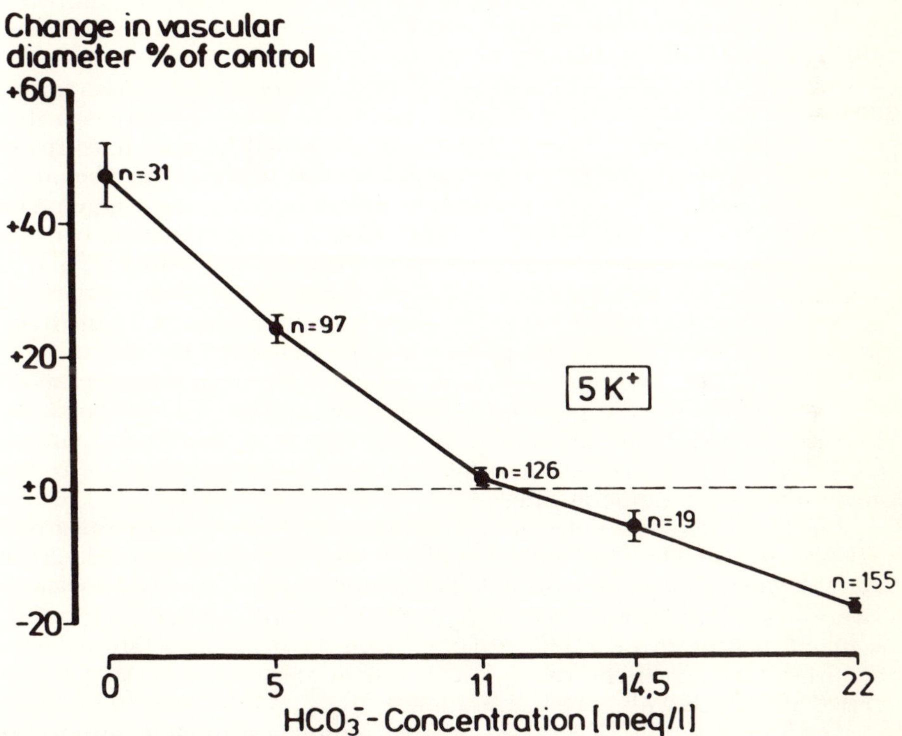

Figure 8-4. Concentration-response curve for bicarbonate in mock spinal fluid containing 5 meq/liter of K^+. Means $\pm$ SE were calculated from values obtained by random injection. Vascular diameters prior to the application were 24–260 μ. Courtesy of the American Heart Association.[94]

vessels to alterations in pH is rapid enough (10 sec or less) to explain the flow changes observed with hypercapnia.[46]

Whereas it is clear that pH can directly, and CO_2 indirectly, affect vascular diameter, some doubt has been cast on the earlier suggestion that these factors regulate CBF. The onset of changes in extracellular pH with local ischemia occurs after increases in vascular diameter are observed.[83] With hypoxia, an increase rather than a decrease in extracellular pH occurs.[96] Subsequently (about 20–30 sec and later) a decrease in pH takes place, and it is during this later phase that H^+ may be involved in CBF regulation. The initial increase in pH has been ascribed to the increase in CBF and resultant "wash-out" of CO_2 from the tissue.[96] A similar increase in pH that lasts 20 sec is observed with direct electrical stimulation of the cerebral cortex of cats.[97] Under these conditions, CBF started to rise within 1 sec and prior to the changes in extracellular pH.[97]

A recent study by Koehler and Traystman[98] also casts doubts on the role of pH as a CBF regulator during hypoxia. These investigators altered CSF and interstial fluid pH by ventriculo-peritoneal perfusion and determined that significant increases in CBF occurred in hypoxia despite alkalinization of the CSF and interstitial fluid pH.

The vasodilator response to alteration in blood pressure also occurs without change in cisternal CSF pH[99] or peripial pH.[100] Moreover, calculated intracellular pH remains stable[101] during mild hypotension. In baboons, cisterna magna CSF pH becomes elevated initially with prolonged hyperventilation, but returns toward control values over a period of 3 hr, whereas CBF remains depressed.[96] Similar observations were made in the cat subjected to hyperventilation for 1 hr. In these experiments, pH returned to control levels despite a persistent reduction in CBF.[102]

In seizures, when CBF is rapidly increased manyfold,[103] some investigators[96] have observed an increase in pH immediately after the onset of bicuculline-induced seizures, whereas others[104,105] have observed a decrease in pH during the same time period. In localized epileptogenic foci created by topical application of penicillin, CBF was increased equally in ipsilateral and contralateral hemispheres, but intracellular pH decreased only in the ipsilateral hemisphere.[106]

Lastly, further evidence against the role of H^+/CO_2 as a regulator of CBF was obtained by Maximillian et al.,[107] who measured regional CBF in acutely hypercarbic patients stressed by spatial reasoning tests. Despite increases in resting CBF caused by hypercarbia, further increases in rCBF occurred in postcentral regions of the brain during testing. However, in rats, more extreme hypercarbia did result in an attenuation of CBF increases associated with neural activation.[74]

In short, the role of H^+/CO_2 in CBF regulation remains unresolved despite intensive study, and although pH remains a plausible candidate for regulating CBF it does not appear to be the sole or initiating factor.

Potassium: The potassium ion has been postulated as a metabolic vasodilator in skeletal and cardiac muscle,[108,109] but the release of potassium is transitory and cannot account for the vasodilation that continues throughout the period of increased muscle activity. Early observations in neural tissue by Baylor and Nicholls[110] confirmed that an increase in K$^+$ concentrations occurs with neural activation.

In brain,[95] potassium is a dilator of pial arterioles when applied topically at constant bicarbonate levels. At potassium concentrations from 0–10 meq/liter, the change in vessel diameter varies directly with the concentration (Figure 8-5). Between 10 and 20 meq/liter, the vasodilator response is reduced; above 20 meq/liter, K$^+$ induces vasoconstriction. A complex interaction exists between K$^+$ and bicarbonate: the potassium-dependent vascular reaction at 0–10 meq/liter dominates the bicarbonate reaction in the range of 5–22 meq/liter; however, with low extracellular pH, the vasodilator effects of K$^+$ are diminished.[95] Unlike skeletal muscle, in which constant application of K$^+$ causes only a transient increase in vessel diameter,[111] brain pial vessels remain dilated during prolonged application of K$^+$.[32] Cameron and Caronna[112] demonstrated that hypothalamic

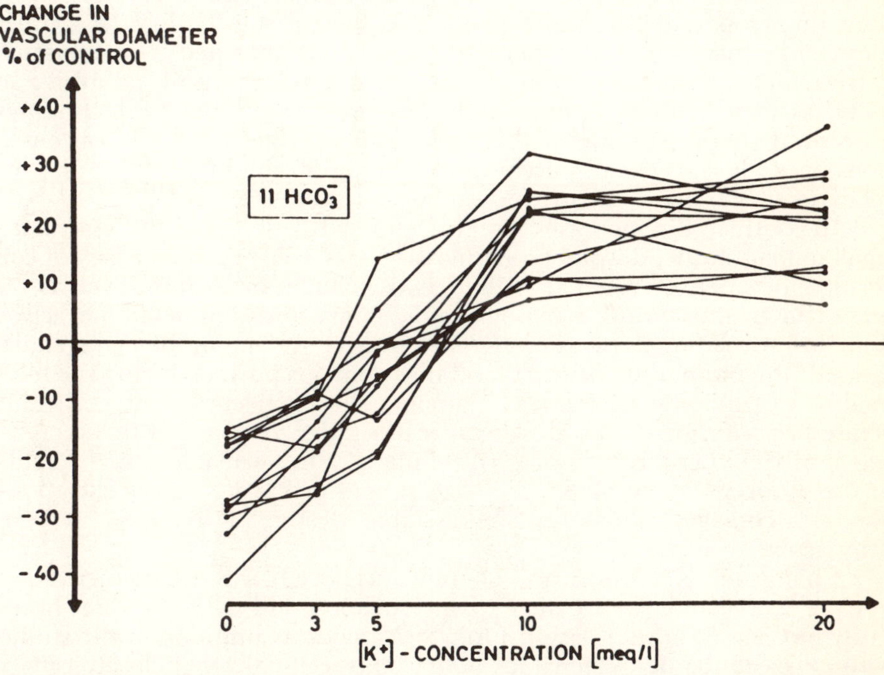

Figure 8-5. Concentration-response curves of individual pial arteries for K$^+$ applied in mock spinal fluid containing 11 meq/liter of bicarbonate. Vascular diameters prior to the application were 46–187 μ. Courtesy of the American Heart Association.[94]

blood flow was increased following an increase in local [K$^+$] (10 mmole/liter) caused by intraparenchymal injections.

A possible mechanism of action of K$^+$ on cerebral vascular smooth muscle was suggested by the findings of Harder,[113] who noted a higher resting membrane potential and K$^+$ conductance in the middle cerebral artery than in the mesenteric artery in the cat. This increased potassium conductance would make the membranes of the vascular smooth muscle cells in the middle cerebral artery more sensitive to changes in external K$^+$ concentrations. Moreover, with an increase in extracellular K$^+$ concentration from 4 to 8 mM, the resting membrane potential increases.

Whereas it is clear that cerebral vessels respond to changes in extracellular K$^+$ concentrations, conflicting data exist as to whether the changes in extracellular [K$^+$] are of sufficient magnitude or are sufficiently temporally related to account for observed changes in CBF and cerebrovascular resistance. Direct measurements of peripial CSF have demonstrated that during prolonged (1 hr) hyperventilation, K$^+$ concentrations paralleled the decreases in CBF.[102] However, only transient changes in extracellular K$^+$ levels were observed with direct cortical stimulation[114] or evoked cortical stimulation.[97] These transient increases in K$^+$ concentrations do not parallel the more prolonged increases in CBF.[97] In seizures induced by bicuculline, the increases in CBF are matched by increases in extracellular K$^+$ concentrations during the initial seconds of convulsive activity, as measured by either whole brain[96] or microflow[105] techniques. Moreover, the magnitude of the increases in extracellular K$^+$ concentrations would be sufficient to account for the significant increases in pial vessel diameter observed during bicuculline-induced seizures.[96]

In contrast, the increases in extracellular K$^+$ observed in hypoxia are small in magnitude, despite large increases in CBF.[96] A similar lack of correlation between elevated CBF and extracellular potassium levels is observed in insulin-induced hypoglycemic coma and amphetamine activation.[96] In spreading depression, K$^+$ briefly accumulates in the extracellular space of the brain, but cortical blood flow remains normal during the maximal rate of increase of extracellular potassium concentration.[115] CBF increased by a factor of two during spreading depression, but this increase was subsequent to a return of extracellular K$^+$ to normal levels.[115] Finally, in the autoregulatory blood pressure range, peripial K$^+$ concentrations, like H$^+$ concentrations, remained stable despite a decrease in cerebrovascular resistance.[100]

Changes in K$^+$ concentrations obviously occur with neural activation, but the "correlation between K$^+$ concentration and CBF does not necessarily indicate a causal relationship."[114] A major assumption in the studies with extracellular K$^+$ electrodes is that extracellular [K$^+$] closely reflects perivascular K$^+$ activity.[96] In view of the investiture of intracerebral vessels by glial cells[116] and the "spatial buffering" of K$^+$ by glial cells,[117] perivascular K$^+$ activity may not be reflected by extracellular K$^+$ concentrations. Hence, as in the case of pH, the role of potassium in the regulation of CBF is not clearly defined.

Adenosine: The purine nucleoside, adenosine, is a potent vasodilator that appears to play an important role in the regulation of coronary blood flow and possibly in several other tissues as well. In brain, topically applied adenosine causes pial vessel dilation,[118] and the smaller ($< 50 \mu$m) pial vessels are more reactive than are the larger pial vessels.[118] After topical micropipette application of adenosine, Wahl and Kuschinsky[119] found a sigmoid-shaped dose-response curve for feline pial vessels. In the presence of physiologic concentrations of bicarbonate, maximal dilation (approximately 20%) occurred between 10^{-5}M and 10^{-7}M adenosine, with an inflection point at 10^{-6}M. In acidic CSF the vasodilator response to adenosine was diminished.[120] Increasing concentrations of CSF potassium also attenuated the dilator effect of adenosine.[120] Changes in regional CBF can also be observed with increases in CSF concentrations of adenosine or 2-chloro-adenosine, a stable analog of adenosine.[121]

Whereas topical application causes vasodilation and an increase in rCBF, intracarotid injections in dog had no effect on brain blood flow.[118] Berne et al.[118] interpreted this lack of increase in CBF after intracarotid infusions as representing a relative blood-brain barrier for adenosine, which was in keeping with a lack of incorporation of labeled adenosine from blood into brain in both the dog[118] and the rat.[122] However, Heistad et al.[123] recently found a two-fold increase in cortical blood flow after intracarotid infusions of adenosine in the rabbit. These investigators[123] attributed the lack of an increase of CBF in dog following common carotid artery injections to an extracarotid steal phenomenon, which occurs in the dog due to anatomical peculiarities of its carotid architecture.[124]

Neither adenosine nor its metabolites, inosine and hypoxanthine, are metabolized in CSF; therefore, there is limited loss into the cerebral venous blood.[125] Adenosine is produced by dephosphorylation of AMP by 5'-nucleotidase that has been localized to the cell wall of the glial footplate.[126] These glial processes surround the intracerebral vessels, and thus adenosine may achieve high concentrations rapidly in the perivascular space, thereby affecting the vascular smooth muscle of intracerebral arterioles. Formerly, it was presumed that almost all of the adenosine existed in the extracellular space, but there is growing evidence that adenosine may be found in a second location, which is intracellular and associated with S-adenosylhomocysteine hydrolase.[127] This latter enzyme may thus serve as a second source for adenosine production.

Interventions that lead to an imbalance between oxygen demand and oxygen supply appear to result in rapid formation and release of adenosine from cerebral tissue. Ischemia,[39,118] hypoxemia,[128,129] a reduction in cerebral perfusion pressure[129,130,131] (Figure 8-6), or enhanced cerebral metabolic activity produced by electrical stimulation[128,132] or chemically induced seizures[133,134] all result in an increase in tissue adenosine levels. During ischemia,[39] hypoxia,[135] and seizures,[133] the increase in brain adenosine concentrations parallel, in a temporal fashion, the changes in cerebrovascular resistance (Figure 8-7). In addition, intracarotid infusion of dipyridamole, which blocks cellular uptake of adenosine and therefore would

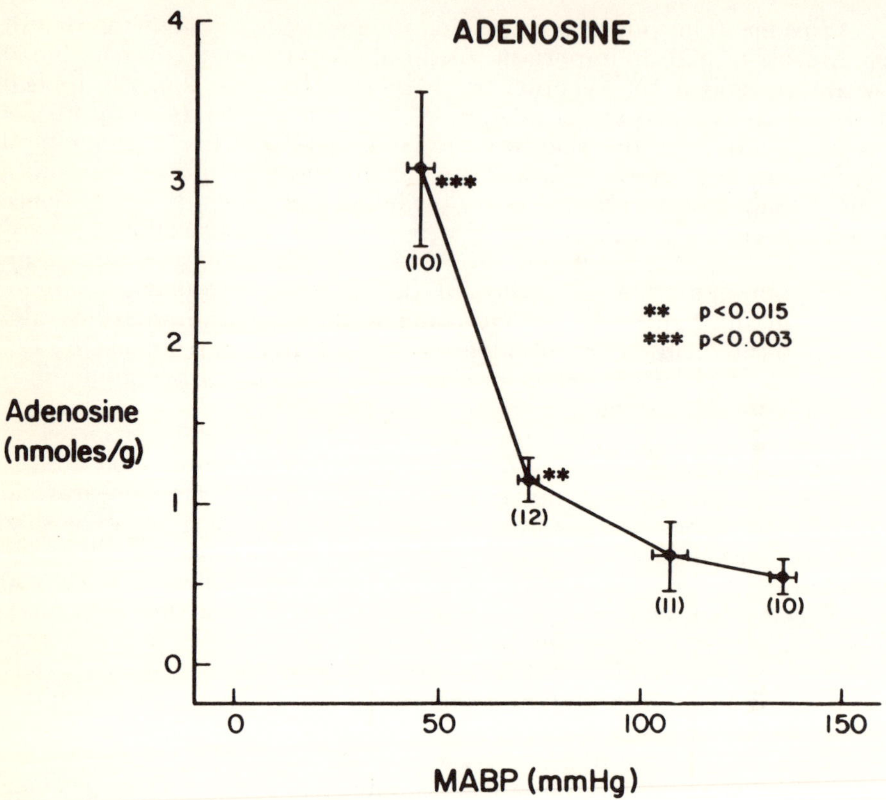

Figure 8-6. Effects of reduction in mean arterial blood pressure (MABP) on brain adenosine levels in the rat. Brain samples obtained by freeze-blowing technique. All values are mean ± SE. n = number of animals in each group.

increase extracellular adenosine levels, results in an increase in CBF.[123] When analyzing tissue for adenosine, rapid methods of freezing are required when sampling brain tissue in the rat under conditions of increased CBF.[129] The use of a slow method of freezing brain (i.e., in situ) may thus explain the failure of Rehncrona et al.[136] to document increases in adenosine in the rat during hypoxia and seizures.

In summary, adenosine, like K^+, appears to be a prime candidate for the regulation of CBF.[40] It is a potent vasodilator and is elevated in conditions in which CBF is increased. Moreover, the changes in brain adenosine concentration are temporally related to changes in CBF. A cause and effect relationship remains to be proven, although recent studies with adenosine blockers and agonists are consonant with the hypothesis that endogenous brain concentrations of adenosine are capable of affecting CBF and that

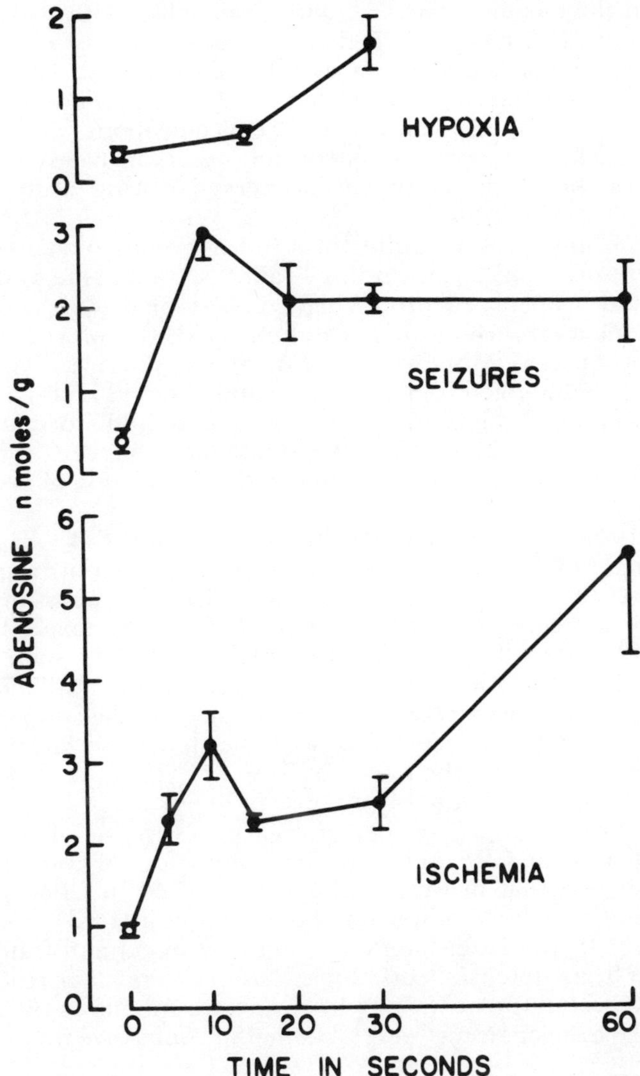

Figure 8-7. Changes in brain adenosine concentration in the rat during short-lasting hypoxia (PaO_2 = 21 mm Hg by 15 sec), bicuculline-induced seizures, and complete ischemia. Brain samples obtained by freeze-blowing technique. All values are mean ± SE. Closed circles differed from zero time values at $p < 0.05$.

adenosine is the metabolic factor linking metabolism with CBF. For example, Kontos et al.[137] have shown that the vasodilation of pial vessels that occurs with hypoxia can be reversed or blocked with CSF containing adenosine deaminase, an enzyme that catabolizes adenosine to inosine, a vasoactive substance. Finally, low concentrations of theophylline ($< 10^{-4}$M), which acts as an adenosine receptor blocker, significantly attenuates the increases in CBF observed during acute or chronic hypoxia.[138,139]

Prostaglandins: Prostaglandins have been proposed as a regulator of blood flow in many organs including brain.[140] Brain tissue as well as cerebral vessels are capable of producing a variety of prostaglandins,[141] and brain contains a large pool of arachidonic acid, the precursor for prostaglandin production. Moreover, most prostaglandins are dilators of cerebral vessels when applied topically.[18] Arachidonic acid is also a vasodilator and its effects can be blocked by cyclo-oxygenase inhibitors such as indomethacin.[142] This blocking effect of indomethacin suggests that the vasodilating effect of arachidonic acid is due to the stimulation of prostaglandin synthesis.[142]

Early studies suggested a role for prostaglandins in CBF regulation during changes in $PaCO_2$ but, as discussed previously, controversy exists as to the effect of indomethacin on CBF. After administration of indomethacin, a decrease in resting CBF levels with marked alteration in the carbon dioxide response has been noted by some investigators.[58,59,143,144,145,146] Other workers have been unable to demonstrate effects of moderate concentrations of indomethacin either on resting vessel diameter,[142,147] or CBF.[60] Very recent studies have also failed to confirm that indomethacin alters the CO_2 response.[60] Cyclo-oxygenase inhibitors do not affect the vasodilation in response to hypoxia[58] or hypotension.[144]

Whereas the data are unclear in regard to the role of prostaglandin in the regulation of CBF under normal physiological conditions,[140] the evidence suggests that prostaglandins are involved in CBF alteration in pathologic states such as complete ischemia, brain injury,[148] and acute hypertension.[149] In the latter condition, induced by administration of norepinephrine or angiotensin, pathologic changes in vascular reactivity were inhibited by pretreatment with cyclo-oxygenase inhibitors or free-radical scavengers.[149] Similar results were obtained in concussive brain injury.[150]

Neural Regulation of CBF

Although the role of neural mechanisms in the regulation of CBF has been intensively studied for many years, the exact contribution of neural factors to CBF regulation remains unclear. Under certain conditions, neural activitation or ablation appears to influence CBF in an independent fashion.[151] However, the present consensus is that neural factors contribute only in a limited fashion to CBF regulation.[19] Rather, the role of the nervous system appears to be as a modulator of CBF and to be more significant in the coordination of various circulatory systems.[152]

As discussed earlier, large extracranial and intracranial vessels receive input from cervical sympathetic sources.[1,22,157] These vessels have been shown responsive to neural activation or ablation under very specific circumstances. During normotension, sympathetic stimulation has no or little effect on CBF.[154,155] However, in conditions where CBF is increased (e.g., hypertension, hypercarbia, or seizures), sympathetic stimulation attenuates hyperemia.[21,154,156,157,158,159] Brain capillaries are associated with a different catecholamine system arising in the locus ceruleus.[24,29] The function of this system is unclear but may be involved in regulation of capillary permeability.[28]

Cholinergic nerve fibers are also associated with arteries of the brain surface but the origin and functional significance of these cholinergic fibers is unknown.[160] Acetylcholine when applied topically causes vasodilation, which is blocked by prior administration of atropine.[161] The effects of intra-arterial acetylcholine are unclear and may be species-dependent.[124,162] Some investigators[49,50] have claimed that atropine attenuates the CO_2 response, but other workers have failed to confirm this observation.[163,164]

In addition to the effects of catecholamine and acetylcholine, other neurotransmitters have been found to influence surface vessels of the brain. Vasoactive intestinal peptide (VIP) has been localized in cerebral vessels and causes dose-related vasodilation when applied topically to pial vessels.[165,166] CBF is also increased following intra-arterial infusions of VIP in rabbit,[124] but the anatomic source and pathways of this peptide are obscure.[167] Histamine, likewise, produces vasodilation when applied topically (in cats)[168] and intra-arterially (in humans).[169] Histamine-induced vasodilation appears to be mediated by H_2 receptors.[168] Nerves in cerebral vessels, however, do not appear to contain histamine.

The response of cerebral vessels and CBF to catecholamines varies depending on the state of the blood-brain barrier and the systemic response to the catecholamine. Intravenous infusions of norepinephrine provokes indirect autoregulatory cerebral vasoconstriction in response to systemic hypertension caused by the catecholamine infusion.[15,170] If the blood-brain barrier is disrupted, intra-arterial infusions will cause a secondary increase in CBF due to a primary increase in cerebral metabolism.[171] With an intact blood-brain barrier, intra-arterial changes in norepinephrine concentration have little direct effect on CBF.[171]

Although the previous comments indicate that the cerebral vascular bed responds to exogenous application of various neurotransmitters, the role of neural factors in CBF regulation is unknown. Most studied is the effect of sympathetic stimulation and ablation. Under normotensive, normocarbic conditions, stimulation or ablation of the cervical sympathetics results in minimal alteration of pial vessel diameter and little change in resting CBF.[154,155,172–176] In contrast, during severe acute and steady-state hypertension, sympathetic stimulation decreases the hyperemia ipsilateral to the site of stimulation.[21,83,154,157,158,177] During sudden increases in systemic arterial pressure, the brain is better protected by an intact nervous system.[83,176] In contrast, cervical sympathectomy does not alter autoregulatory phenomenon, but a shift of the autoregulatory curve to the left is observed.[178] Thus, the upper limit of autoregulation occurs at a lower blood pressure in the absence of sympathetic fibers.[83]

The blood-brain barrier is also preserved by the presence of sympathetic innervation.[83,154,157,159,179] Absence of sympathetic fibers results in increased passage of albumin into the brain from the vascular compartment and increases in frequency of associated hemorrhages. In addition, cerebral blood volume is increased with sympathetic denervation.[180] Extirpation of the superior cervical ganglion causes an increase in large vessel dilation[173] and an increase in CBF[52] during hypercarbia.

In summary, the major role of the sympathetic nerves appears to be one of protecting the brain against sudden increases in systemic blood pressure.

Myogenic Regulation of CBF

The myogenic hypothesis states that cerebral vessels respond to a change in transmural pressure to preserve a preset level of vascular tone. Increases in transmural pressure result in constriction, whereas decreases in transmural pressure produce vasodilation. Such a mechanism would be primarily utilized in the autoregulatory response. Separation of metabolic and myogenic influences are, however, difficult. Several studies, beginning with the early observations of Fog,[181] support the role of myogenic factors in regulating CBF. However, recent studies cast doubt on a significant role for myogenic influences on CBF during autoregulation.[182,183] Wei and Kontos[182] raised cerebral venous pressure in the cat. Such an increase in venous pressure should, according to the myogenic hypothesis, result in an increase in transmural pressures and result in vasoconstriction. However, Wei and Kontos observed vasodilation with an increase in cerebral venous pressure, implying the absence of myogenic factors in that paradigm. The role of a myogenic factor in CBF regulation thus appears limited but it may play a modulating role in some circumstances.

Cerebral Blood Flow Regulation in Hypertension

Regulation of CBF in the hypertensive state has received increasing attention, but the factors affecting CBF are, in general, unclear. Except for the autoregulatory response and neuronal influences, the differing effect of other factors, such as carbon dioxide, metabolic coupling, and oxygen delivery, on CBF in the hypertensive brain are either unknown or not different from the effect in normotensive conditions.[184,185]

Despite the lack of a comprehensive understanding of the factors involved in blood flow regulation in the hypertensive state, it is clear that systemic hypertension, either acute or chronic, has a profound influence on brain circulation. Hypertension is a major contributor to cerebral atherosclerosis and stroke. Kannel et al.[186,187] consider that hypertension is the most important predisposing factor for stroke, exceeding other important risk factors such as heart disease, diabetes, and oral contraceptives. Stroke incidence increases six-fold with hypertension, and this co-relationship is greater for brain infarction and hemorrhage. Systolic pressure may be a better predictor of stroke risk than diastolic pressure.[186,187]

Chronic hypertension contributes to pathologic changes in cerebral vessels and to an increased risk of stroke by a number of mechanisms. The major anatomic change observed in cerebral vessels is the development of vascular hypertrophy.[188] This cerebral vascular hypertrophy is reflected in an increase in wall-to-lumen ratio. In young spontaneously hypertensive rats the ratio is modest, but increases markedly with age.[12,189,190] Wall thickening presumably protects the vascular tissue and the brain from the increased systemic blood pressure but may alter the delivery of oxygen and other nutrients at low levels[189] of CBF. In addition, wall thickening would presumably affect the myogenic mechanism.

These structural changes in the wall of cerebral vessels may account for the alterations in the autoregulatory response and for the predisposition for stroke and cerebral hemorrhage in hypertension. The effects of acute hypertension can be distinctly different from those caused by chronic hypertension. Whereas during chronic hypertension the thicker cerebral walls protect the brain, in acute hypertension the vessels will passively dilate and the blood-brain barrier will be disrupted.[35,36]

As outlined briefly in previous sections of this chapter, the clinical and pathological manifestations and influences of hypertension in and on the brain are well described, yet the influences of physiological factors on CBF regulation during hypertension are incomplete. However, some data are available and are outlined briefly next.

During acute transient hypertension, breakdown of the blood-brain barrier occurs[7] and the mechanism responsible is alteration of vesicular transport in endothelial cells[8] and disruption of tight junctions.[192] In contrast, in chronic hypertension, the blood-brain barrier remains intact. Moreover, the presence of intact sympathetic nerves arising from the cervical ganglion appears to protect the brain from the effects of acute and chronic hypertension.[12,159,179]

The marginal vascular regions of the brain ("boundary zones") are susceptible areas for hemorrhage during systemic hypertension,[12] and neural innervation protects against hypertensive hemorrhages.[13,176]

With chronic hypertension in both human and animals the autoregulatory curve is shifted to the right[35,36,190] (Figure 8-1), but medical therapy may improve cerebral dysautoregulation.[193] CBF is not as well maintained at lower MABP in the hypertensive state, whereas at high

MABP, CBF is normal. The explanation for this alteration in the auto-regulatory curve is unknown. However, thickening and alteration of the walls of cerebral vessels, including capillaries,[194] may affect the delivery of oxygen and other nutrients at lower levels of CBF and account for the shift of the lower end of the autoregulatory curve. The etiology of the changes in the vessel wall is also unclear, but if cerebral vessels respond as periph-eral vessels, alterations in hypertension may be secondary to changes in excitation-contraction or inhibition-relaxation coupling and may precede development of high blood pressure.[195]

Spontaneous hypertensive rats (SHR) are more susceptible to cerebral ischemia than are normotensive rats.[196,197,198,199] This increased sensitivity to alteration in perfusion pressure reflects the shift to the right of the auto-regulatory curve. In contrast, SHR respond to hypocarbia with a decrease in CBF similar to that observed in normotensive animals.

Patients with intracerebral hematomas may present with acute sys-temic hypertension, often of an alarming degree. Such hypertension should not be aggressively treated since it is a response to the elevated intracranial pressure and a defensive reflex (Cushing reflex) designed to maintain cerebral perfusion at an adequate level. Precipitous lowering of the blood pressure may severely compromise blood flow to the brain, re-sulting in cerebral infarction. A recent study in patients with intracerebral hematomas and systemic hypertension indicates that a 20% reduction in blood pressure should be the desired goal of blood pressure therapy be-cause this percentage reduction in MABP will not compromise cerebral blood flow.[200]

In conclusion, whereas systemic hypertension profoundly influences the pathology of cerebral circulation, further studies are required to better define the factors in the hypertensive state that affect the physiology of CBF. The presence of an appropriate animal model such as the SHR allows for further investigations, although such an animal model may not be suit-able for studying "essential" human hypertension.[201] Moreover, future in-vestigators should be aware of the differences in the response of the brain circulation and metabolism between the SHR and the renovascular hyper-tensive model.[202,203]

References

1. Purves MJ: The Physiology of the Cerebral Circulation. New York, Cambridge University Press, 1972, p 1–414
2. Bradbury M: The concept of a blood-brain barrier. New York, Wiley, 1979
3. Reese TS, Karnovsky MJ: Fine structural localization of a blood-brain barrier to exogenous peroxidase. J Cell Biol **34:**207–217, 1967
4. Bertler A, Falck B, Owman CH, Rosengren E: The localization of mono-aminergic blood-brain barrier mechanisms. Pharmacol Rev **18:**369–385, 1966
5. Hardebo JE, Owman C: Barrier mechanisms for neurotransmitter mono-amines and their precursors at the blood-brain interface. Ann Neurol **8:**1–11, 1980

6. Oldendorf WH: Brain uptake of radiolabeled amino acids, amines and hexoses after arterial injection. Am J Physiol **221**:1629–1639, 1971

7. Westergaard E: The blood-brain barrier to horseradish peroxidase under normal and experimental conditions. Acta Neuropathol **39**:181–187, 1977

8. Beggs JL, Waggener JL: Transendothelial vesicular transport of protein following compression injury to the spinal cord. Lab Invest **34**:428–439, 1976

9. Schmidt CF: The cerebral circulation in health and disease. Springfield, Thomas, 1950, p 1–86

10. Hayward JN, Baker MA: A comparative study of the role of the cerebral arterial blood in the regulation of brain temperature in five mammals. Brain Res **16**:417–440, 1969

11. Brierly JB, Brown AW, Excell BJ, Meldrum BS: Brain damage in the rhesus monkey resulting from profound arterial hypotension. I. Its nature, distribution and general physiological correlates. Brain Res **13**:68–100, 1969

12. Sadoshima S, Busija D, Brody M, Heistad DD: Sympathetic nerves protect against stroke in stroke-prone hypertensive rats: a preliminary report. Hypertension **3**, Suppl I:I124–I127, 1981

13. Graham DI, Grome JJ, Kelly PAT, MacKenzie ET, McCulloch J, Reis DJ, Talman WT: Cerebral circulatory effect of fulminating neurogenic hypertension. *In* Cerebral Blood Flow: Effects of Nerves and Neurotransmitters, edited by Heistad D, Marcus M. New York, Elsevier, 1982, pp 493–508

14. Heistad DD, Marcus ML, Abboud FM: Role of large arteries in regulation of cerebral blood flow in dogs. Clin Invest **62**:761–768, 1978

15. Kontos HA, Wei EP, Navari RM, Levasseur JE, Rosenblum WI, Patterson JL Jr: Responses of cerebral arteries and arterioles to acute hypotension and hypertension. Am J Physiol **234** (Heart Circ Physiol 3):H371–II383, 1978

16. Shapiro HM, Stromberg DD, Lee DR, Wiederhielm CA: Dynamic pressures in the pial arterial microcirculation. Am J Physiol **221**:279–283, 1971

17. Symon LA: A comparative study of middle cerebral pressure in dogs and macaques. J Physiol (Lond) **191**:449–465, 1967

18. Heistad DD, Kontos HA: Handbook of Physiology (in press)

19. Heistad DD, Marcus ML: Evidence that neural mechanisms do not have important effects on cerebral blood flow. Circ Res **42**:295–302, 1978

20. Purves MJ: Do vasomotor nerves significantly regulate cerebral blood flow? Circ Res **43**:485–493, 1978

21. Edvinsson L, Owman C, Siesjo B: Physiological role of cerebrovascular sympathetic nerves in the autoregulation of cerebral blood flow. Brain Res **117**:518–523, 1976

22. Iwayama T, Furness JB, Burnstock G: Dual adrenergic and cholinergic innervation of the cerebral arteries of the rat. Circ Res **26**:635–646, 1970

23. Nielsen KC, Owman CH: Adrenergic innervation of pial arteries related to the circle of Willis in the cat. Brain Res **6**:773–776, 1967

24. Hartman BK, Zide D, Udenfriend D: The use of dopamine beta hydroxylase as a marker for the central noradrenergic nervous system in rat brain. Proc Natl Acad Sci (USA) **69**:2722–2726, 1972

25. Edvinsson L, Lindvall M, Nielsen KC, Owman C: Are brain vessels innervated also by central (non-sympathetic) adrenergic neurones? Brain Res **63**:496–499, 1973

26. Bates D, Weinshilboum RM, Campbell RJ, Sundt TM Jr: The effect of lesions in the locus coeruleus on the physiological responses of the cerebral blood vessels in cats. Brain Res **136**:431–443, 1977

27. Langfitt TW, Kassell NF: Cerebral vasodilatation produced by brain-stem stimulation: neurogenic control vs. autoregulation. Am J Physiol **215**:90–97, 1968
28. Raichle ME, Hartman BK, Eichling JO, Sharpe LG: Central noradrenergic regulation of cerebral blood flow and vascular permeability. Proc Natl Acad Sci (USA) **72**:3726–3730, 1975
29. Rennels ML, Forbes MS, Anders JJ, Nelson E: Innervation of the microcirculation in the central nervous system and other tissues. *In* Neurogenic Control of the Brain Circulation, edited by Owman CH, Edvinsson L. New York, Pergamon, 1977, p 91–104
30. Rapela CE, Green HD, Denison AB Jr: Baroreceptor reflexes and autoregulation of cerebral blood flow in the dog. Circ Res **21**:559–568, 1967
31. Harper AM: Autoregulation of cerebral blood flow: influence of the arterial pressure on the blood flow through the cerebral cortex. J Neurol Neurosurg Psychiatry **29**:398–403, 1966
32. Kuschinsky W, Wahl W: Local chemical and neurogenic regulation of cerebral vascular resistance. Physiological Reviews **58**:656–689, 1978
33. Jones JV, Fitch W, MacKenzie ET, Strandgaard S, Harper AM: Lower limit of cerebral blood flow autoregulation in experimental renovascular hypertension in the baboon. Circ Res **39**:555–557, 1976
34. MacKenzie ET, Farrar JK, Fitch W, Graham DI, Gregory PC, Harper AM: Effects of hemorrhagic hypotension on the cerebral circulation. Stroke **10**:711–718, 1979
35. Strandgaard S, Olesen J, Skinhoj E, Lassen NA: Autoregulation of brain circulation in severe arterial hypertension. Br Med J **1**:507–510, 1973
36. Strandgaard S, Jones JV, MacKenzie ET, Harper AM: Upper limit of cerebral blood flow autoregulation in experimental renovascular hypertension in the baboon. Circ Res **37**:164–167, 1975
37. Lassen NA, Agnoli A: The upper limit of autoregulation of cerebral blood flow. On the pathogenesis of hypertensive encephalopathy. Scand J Clin Lab Invest **30**:113–116, 1972
38. Barry DI, Strandgaard S, Svendsen UG, Braendstrup O, Graham DI, Hemmingsen R, Bolwig TG: Adaptive changes in the lower limit of cerebral blood flow autoregulation in hypertensive rats. J Cerebral Blood Flow Metab **1**:40, 1981
39. Winn HR, Rubio R, Berne RM: Brain adenosine production in the rat during 60 seconds of ischemia. Circ Res **45**:486–492, 1979
40. Winn HR, Rubio GR, Berne RM: The role of adenosine in the regulation of cerebral blood flow. J Cerebral Blood Flow Metab **1**:239–244, 1981
41. Gotoh F, Tazaki Y, Meyer JS: Transport of gases through brain and their extravascular vasomotor action. Exp Neurol **4**:48–58, 1961
42. Spagnuolo C, Sautebin L, Galli G, Racagni G, Galli C, Mazzari S, Finesso M: PGF_2, thromboxane B_2 and HETE levels in gerbil brain cortex after ligation of common carotid arteries and decapitation. Prostaglandins **18**:53–61, 1979
43. McDowall DG, Harper AM: The relationship between blood flow and the extracellular pH of the cerebral cortex. *In* Blood Flow Through Organs and Tissues, edited by Bain W, Harper AM. Baltimore, Williams and Wilkins, 1967, p 261–278
44. Harper AM, Glass HI: Effect of alterations in the arterial carbon dioxide tension on the blood flow through the cerebral cortex at normal and low arterial blood pressures. J Neurol Neurosurg Psychiatry **28**:449–452, 1965

45. Reivich M: Arterial PCO_2 and cerebral hemodynamics. Am J Physiol **206**:25–35, 1964
46. Greenberg JH, Reivich M: Response time of cerebral arterioles to alterations in extravascular fluid pH. Microvasc Res **14**:383–393, 1977
47. Fazekas JR, Alman RW, Bessman AN: Cerebral physiology of the aged. Am J Med Sci **223**:245–257, 1952
48. Kawamura Y, Meyer JS, Hiromoto H, Aoyagi M, Tagashira Y, Ott EO: Neurogenic control of cerebral blood flow in the baboon. J Neurosurg **43**:676–688, 1975
49. Rovere AA, Scremin OU, Beresi MR, Raynald AC, Giardini A: Cholinergic mechanism in the cerebrovascular action of carbon dioxide. Stroke **4**:969–972, 1973
50. Schremin OU, Rubinstein EH, Sonnenschein RR: Cerebrovascular reactivity: role of a cholinergic mechanism modulated by anesthesia. Stroke **9**:160–165, 1978
51. Corbett JL, Eidelman BH, Debarge O: Modification of cerebral vasoconstriction with hyperventilation in normal man by thymoxamine. Lancet **2**:461–463, 1972
52. James IM, Millar RA, Purves MJ: Observations on the extrinsic neural control of cerebral blood flow in the baboon. Circ Res **25**:77–93, 1969
53. Ponte J, Purves MJ: The role of the carotid body chemoreceptors and carotid sinus baroreceptors in the control of cerebral blood vessels. J Physiol (Lond) **237**:315–340, 1974
54. Hoff JT, Harper M, Sengupta D, Jennett B: Effect of alpha-adrenergic blockade in response of cerebral circulation to hypocapnia in the baboon. Lancet **2**:1337–1339, 1972
55. Hoff JT, MacKenzie ET, Harper AM: Responses of the cerebral circulation to hypercapnia and hypoxia after 7th cranial nerve transection in baboons. Circ Res **40**:258–262, 1977
56. Busija DW, Heistad DD: Effects of cholinergic nerves on cerebral blood flow in cats. Circ Res **48**:62–69, 1981
57. Skinhoj E: Sympathetic nervous system and the regulation of cerebral blood flow in man. Stroke **3**:711–716, 1972
58. Sakabe T, Siesjo BK: The effect of indomethacin on the blood flow-metabolism couple in the brain under normal, hypercapnic and hypoxic conditions. Acta Physiol Scand **107**:283–284, 1979
59. Pickard JD, MacKenzie ET: Inhibition of prostaglandin synthesis and the response of baboon cerebral circulation to carbon dioxide. Nature London New Biol **245**:187–188, 1973
60. Busija DW, Heistad DD: Effects of indomethacin on cerebral blood flow during hypercapnia in cats. Am J Physiol **244**:H519–H524, 1983
61. Kety SS, Schmidt CF: Effects of altered arterial tensions of carbon dioxide and oxygen on cerebral blood flow and cerebral oxygen consumption of normal young men. J Clin Invest **27**:484–492, 1948
62. Lambertson CJ, Kough RH, Cooper DY, Emmel GL, Loeschcke HH, Schmidt CF: Oxygen toxicity: effects in man of oxygen inhalation at 1 and 3.5 atmospheres upon blood gas transport, cerebral circulation and cerebral metabolism. J Appl Physiol **5**:471–486, 1953
63. Borgstrom L, Johannsson H, Siesjo BK: The relationship between arterial pO_2 and cerebral blood flow in hypoxic hypoxia. Acta Physiol Scand **93**:423–432, 1975

64. Berne RM, Winn HR, Rubio R: The local regulation of cerebral blood flow. Progress in Cardiovascular Diseases **24**(3):243–260, 1981
65. Halsey JH Jr, Blauenstein UW, Wilson EM, Willia EH: Regional cerebral blood flow comparison of right and left hand movement. Neurology **29**:21–28, 1979
66. Ingvar EH: Functional landscapes of the dominant hemisphere. Brain Res **107**:181–197, 1976
67. Olesen J: Contralateral focal increase of cerebral blood flow in man during arm work. Brain **94**:635–646, 1971
68. Lassen NA, Ingvar DH, Skinhoj E: Brain function and blood flow. Sci Am **239**:62–71, 1978
69. Kuschinsky W, Wahl M: Interactions between perivascular norepinephrine and potassium or osmolarity on pial arteries of cats. Microvasc Res **14**:173–180, 1977
70. Sokoloff L, Reivich M, Kennedy C, Des Rosiers CS, Patlak KD, Pettigrew KD, Sakurada O, Shinohara M: The [^{14}C] deoxyglucose method for the measurement of local cerebral glucose utilization: theory, procedure, and normal values in the conscious and anesthetized albino rat. J Neurochem **28**:897–916, 1977
71. Kennedy C, Des Rosiers MH, Jehle JW, Reivich M, Sharpe F, Sokoloff L: Mapping of functional neural pathways by autoradiographic survey of local metabolic rate with ^{14}C deoxyglucose. Science **187**:850–853, 1975
72. Sokoloff L: Relation between physiological function and energy metabolism in the central nervous system. J Neurochem **29**:13–26, 1977
73. Raichle ME, Grubb RL, Gado MH, Eichling JO, Ter-Pogossian MM: Correlation between regional cerebral blood flow and oxidative metabolism. Arch Neurol Chicago **33**:523–526, 1976
74. Borgstrom L, Johannsson H, Siesjo BK: The influence of acute normovolemic anemia on cerebral blood flow and oxygen consumption of anesthetized rats. Acta Physiol Scand **93**:505–514, 1975
75. Paulson OB, Parving HH, Olesen J, Skinhoj E: Influence of carbon monoxide and of hemodilution on cerebral blood flow and blood gases in man. J Appl Physiol **35**:111–116, 1973
76. Heyman A, Patterson JL Jr, Duke TW: Cerebral circulation and metabolism in sickle cell and other chronic anemias, with observations on the effects of oxygen inhalation. J Clin Invest **37**:824–828, 1952
77. Scheinberg P: Cerebral blood flow and metabolism in pernicious anemia. Blood **6**:213–227, 1951
78. Bicher HI: Brain oxygen autoregulation: A protective reflex to hypoxia? Microvasc Res **8**:291–313, 1974
79. Duling BR, Kuschinsky W, Wahl M: Measurements of the perivascular pO$_2$ in the vicinity of the pial vessels of the cat. Pflugers Arch **383**:29–34, 1979
80. Kontos HA, Wei EP, Raper AJ, Rosenblum WI, Navari RM, Patterson JL Jr: Role of tissue hypoxia on local regulation of cerebral microcirculation. Am J Physiol **234**:H582–H591, 1978
81. Betz E: pH-abhangige regulationen der lokalen gehirndurchblutung. *In* Hydrodynamik, Elektrolyt und Saure-Basen-Haushalt im Liquor und Nervensystem, edited by Kienle G. Stuttgart, Thieme, 1967, pp 17–25
82. Kogure K, Scheinberg P, Reinmuth OH, Fugishima M, Busto R: Mechanisms of cerebral vasodilatation in hypoxia. J Appl Physiol **29**:223–229, 1970
83. Silver IA: Cellular microenvironment in relation to local blood flow. *In* Cere-

bral Vascular Smooth Muscle and Its Control, edited by Purves MJ. Ciba Foundation Symposium **56**:49–61, 1978

84. Ingvar DH, Lubbers DW, Siesjo BK: Normal and epileptic EEG patterns related to cortical oxygen tension in the cat. Acta Physiol Scand **55**:210–244, 1962

85. Metzger H: Effects of direct stimulation on cerebral cortex oxygen tension level. Microvasc Res **17**:80–89, 1979

86. Caspers H, Speckmann EJ: Cerebral pO_2, pCO_2, and pH: changes during convulsive activity and their significance for spontaneous arrest of seizures. Epilepsia **13**:699–725, 1972

87. Leniger-Follert E, Lubbers DW: Behavior of microflow and local pO_2 of the brain cortex during and after direct electrical stimulation. Pflugers Arch **366**:39–44, 1976

88. Hempel FG, Jobsis FF: Comparison of cerebral NADH and cytochrome a,a_3 redox shifts during anoxia or hemorrhagic hypotension. Life Sci **25**:1145–1151, 1979

89. Duling BR: Oxygen sensitivity of vascular smooth muscle. II. In vivo studies. Am J Physiol **227**:42–49, 1974

90. Skinhoj E: Regulation of cerebral blood flow as a single function of the interstitial pH. Acta Neurol Scand **42**:604–607, 1966

91. Lassen NA: Brain extracellular pH: the main factor controlling cerebral blood flow. Scand J Clin Lab Invest **22**:247–251, 1968

92. McDowall DG, Harper AM: Cerebral blood flow and CSF pH during hyperventilation. Prog Anesthesiol, Excerpta Medica International Congress Series **200**:542–545, 1968

93. Wahl M, Deetjen P, Thurau K, Ingvar DH, Lassen NA: Micropuncture evaluation of the importance of perivascular pH for the arteriolar diameter on the brain surface. Pflugers Arch **316**:152–163, 1970

94. Kuschinsky W, Wahl M, Bosse O, Thurau K: Perivascular potassium and pH as determinants of local pial arterial diameter in cats. Circ Res **31**:240–247, 1972

95. Kontos HA, Raper AJ, Patterson JL Jr: Analysis of vasoactivity of local pH, pCO_2, and bicarbonate on pial vessels. Stroke **8**:358–360, 1977

96. Astrup J, Heuser D, Lassen NA, Nilsson B, Norberg K, Siesjo BK: Evidence against H^+ and K^+ as main factors for the control of cerebral blood flow: a microelectrode study. *In* Cerebral Vascular Smooth Muscle and Its Control, edited by Purves MJ. Ciba Foundation Symposium **56**:313–337, 1978

97. Leniger-Follert E, Urbanics R, Lubbers DW: Behavior of extracellular H^+ and K^+ activities during functional hyperemia of microcirculation in the brain cortex. Adv Neurol **20**:97–101, 1978

98. Koehler RC, Traystman RJ: Bicarbonate ion modulation of cerebral blood flow during hypoxia and hypercapnia. Am J Physiol **243**:H33–H40, 1982

99. Hernandez-Perez MJ, Anderson DK: Autoregulation of cerebral blood flow and its relation to cerebrospinal fluid pH. Am J Physiol **231**:929–935, 1976

100. Wahl M, Kuschinsky W: Unimportance of perivascular H^+ and K^+ activities for the adjustment of pial arterial diameter during changes of arterial blood pressure in cats. Pflugers Arch **382**:203–208, 1979

101. Eklof B, MacMillan V, Siesjo BK: Cerebral energy state and cerebral venous pO_2 in experimental hypotension caused by bleeding. Acta Physiol Scand **86**:515–527, 1972

102. Heuser D, Nabe U, Gebert G, Betz E: Reactions of pial vessels during varia-

tion of local perivascular ionic composition of the CSF. Eur Neurol **6**:96–99, 1971/72

103. Meldrum BS, Nilsson B: Cerebral blood flow and metabolic rate early and late in prolonged epileptic seizures induced in rats by bicuculline. Brain **99**:523–542, 1976

104. Kuschinsky W, Wahl M: Perivascular pH and pial arterial diameter during bicuculline induced seizures in cats. Pflugers Arch **382**:81–85, 1979

105. Leniger-Follert E: Mechanisms of regulation of cerebral microcirculation during bicuculline induced seizures. Proc Int Union Physiol Sci **14**:545, 1980 (abstr)

106. Tenny RT, Sharbrough FW, Anderson RE, Sundt TM: Correlation of intracellular redox states and pH with blood flow in primary and secondary seizure foci. Ann Neurol **8**:564–573, 1980

107. Maximillian VA, Prohovnik I, Risberg J: Cerebral hemodynamic response to mental activation in normo- and hypercapnia. Stroke **11**:342–347, 1980

108. Kjellmer I: Potassium as a vasodilator during muscular exercise. Acta Physiol Scand **63**:460–468, 1965

109. Murray PA, Belloni FL, Sparks HV: The role of potassium in the metabolic control of coronary vascular resistance of the dog. Circ Res **44**:767–780, 1979

110. Baylor DA, Nicholls JG: Changes in extracellular potassium concentration produced by neuronal activity in the central nervous system of the leech. J Physiol (Lond) **203**:555–569, 1969

111. Duling BR: Effects of potassium ion on the microcirculation of the hamster. Circ Res **37**:325–332, 1975

112. Cameron IR, Caronna J: The effect of local changes in potassium and bicarbonate concentration of hypothalamic blood flow in the rabbit. J Physiol **262**:415–430, 1976

113. Harder DR: Comparison of electrical properties of middle cerebral and mesenteric artery in cat. Am J Physiol **239**:C23–C26, 1980

114. Branston NM, Symon L, Strong AJ, Hope DT: Measurements of regional cortical blood flow during changes in extracellular potassium activity evoked by direct cortical stimulation in the primate. Exp Neurol **59**:243–253, 1978

115. Hansen AJ, Quistorff B, Gjedde A: Relationship between local changes in cortical blood flow and extracellular K^+ during spreading depression. Acta Physiol Scand **109**:1–6, 1980

116. Maynard EA, Schulta RL, Pease DC: Electron microscopy of the vascular bed of the rat cerebral cortex. Am J Anat **100**:409–433, 1957

117. Orkland RK, Nicholls JG, Kuffler SW: Effects of nerve impulses on the membrane potential of glial cells in the central nervous system of amphibia. J Neurophysiol **29**:788–806, 1966

118. Berne RM, Rubio R, Curnish RR: Release of adenosine from ischemic brain: effect on cerebral vascular resistance and incorporation into cerebral adenine nucleotides. Circ Res **35**:262–271, 1974

119. Wahl M, Kuschinsky W: The dilatory action of adenosine on pial arteries of cats and its inhibition by theophylline. Pflugers Arch **362**:55–59, 1976

120. Wahl M, Kuschinsky W: Dependency of the dilatory action of adenosine on the perivascular H^+ and K^+ at pial arteries of cats. CBF VIII: Copenhagen, Cerebral Function, Metabolism and Circulation, 1977, pp 218–219

121. Winn HR, Rubio R, Curnish RR, Berne RM: Changes in regional cerebral blood flow (rCBF) caused by increases in CSF concentrations of adenosine and

2-chloroadenosine (CHL-ADO). J Cerebral Blood Flow Metab **1** (Suppl 1): S401–S402, 1981

122. Cornforde EM, Oldendork WH: Independent blood-brain barrier transport systems for nucleic acid precursors. Biochim Biophys Acta **394:**211–219, 1975

123. Heistad DD, Marcus ML, Gourley JK, and Busija DW: Effect of adenosine and dipyridamole on cerebral blood flow. Am J Physiol **240** (Heart Circ Physiol):H775–H780, 1981

124. Heistad DD, Marcus ML, Said SI, Gross PM: Effect of acetylcholine and vasoactive intestinal peptide on cerebral blood flow. Am J Physiol **239:**H73–H80, 1980

125. Winn HR, Park TS, Curnish RR, Rubio R, Berne RM: Incorporation of adenosine and its metabolites into brain nucleotides. Am J Physiol **239:**H212–H219, 1980

126. Kreutzberg GW, Barron KD, Schubert P: Cytochemical localization of 5′-nucleotidase in glial plasma membranes. Brain Res **158:**247–257, 1978

127. Schatz RA, Vunnam CR, Sellinger OZ: S-adenosyl-L-homocysteine hydrolase from rat brain: Purification and some properties. *In* Transmethylation, edited by Usdin E, Borchardt RT, Creveling CR. New York, Elsevier-North Holland, 1978, pp 143–153

128. Rubio R, Berne RM, Bockman EL, Curnish RR: Relationship between adenosine concentration and oxygen supply in rat brain. Am J Physiol **228:**1896–1902, 1975

129. Winn HR, Bowe AB, Welsh JE, Rubio R, Berne RM: Changes in adenosine during sustained hypoxia. Acta Neurol Scand **30** (Suppl 72):330–332, 1979

130. Winn HR, Welsh JE, Rubio R, Berne RM: Brain adenosine production in rat during sustained alteration in systemic blood pressure. Am J Physiol **239:**H636–H641, 1980

131. Bockman EL, Fritschka E, Ferguson JL, Spitzer JJ: Increased adenosine in cerebrospinal fluid during the autoregulatory response to mild hypotension. *In* Cerebral Microcirculation and Metabolism: Erwin Riesch Symposium, edited by Cervos-Navarro J. New York, Raven, 1981, pp 243–248

132. Schultz V, Lowenstein JM: The purine nucleotide cycle. J Biol Chem **253:**1938–1943, 1978

133. Winn HR, Welsh JE, Rubio R, Berne RM: Changes in brain adenosine during bicuculline-induced seizures in rats. Circ Res **47:**568–577, 1980

134. Schrader J, Wahl M, Kuschinsky W, Kreutzberg GW: Increase of adenosine content in cerebral cortex of the cat during bicuculline-induced seizures. Pflugers Arch **387:**245–251, 1980

135. Winn HR, Rubio R, Berne RM: Brain adenosine concentration during hypoxia in rat. Am J Physiol **241:**H235–H242, 1981

136. Rehncrona S, Siesjo BK, Westerberg E: Adenosine and cyclic AMP in cerebral cortex of rats in hypoxia, status epilepticus and hypercapnia. Acta Physiol Scand **104:**453–463, 1978

137. Kontos HA, Wei EP: Role of adenosine in cerebral arteriolar dilation from arterial hypoxia. Fed Proc **40:**454–1981 (abstr)

138. Emerson TE Jr, Raymond RM: Involvement of adenosine in cerebral hypoxic hyperemia in the dog. Am J Physiol **241:**H134–H138, 1981

139. Winn HR, Morii S, Ngai AC, Berne RM: Effects of theophylline (T) on cerebral blood flow (CBF). Physiologist **25:**256, 1982

140. Kontos HA, Wei EP, Ellis EF, Dietrick WD, Povlishock JT: Prostaglandins in

physiological and in certain pathological responses of the cerebral circulation. Fed Proc **40:**2326–2330, 1981
141. Wolfe LS: Possible roles of prostaglandins in the nervous system. *In* Advances in Neurochemistry, edited by Agranoff BW, Aprison MH. Plenum, New York, 1975, pp 1–49
142. Wei EP, Ellis EF, Kontos HA: Role of prostaglandins in pial arteriolar response to CO_2 and hypoxia. Am J Physiol **238** (Heart Circ Physiol 7):H226–H230, 1980
143. Bill A: Effects of indomethacin on regional blood flow in conscious rabbits—a microsphere study. Acta Physiol Scand **105:**437–442, 1979
144. Pickard JD, MacDonell LA, MacKenzie ET, Harper AM: Response of the cerebral circulation in baboons to changing perfusion pressure after indomethacin. Circ Res **40:**198–203, 1977
145. Pickard J, Tamura A, Steward M, McGeorge A, Fitch W: Prostacyclin, indomethacin and the cerebral circulation. Brain Res **197:**425–431, 1980
146. Rapela CE, Green HD: Autoregulation of canine cerebral blood flow. Circ Res **14,** Suppl 1:205–211, 1964
147. Vlahov V, Betz E: Effects of indomethacin and D600 on the smooth muscles of pial vessels. *In* Pathology of Cerebral Microcirculation, edited by Cervos-Navarro J. Berlin, De Guyta, 1974, p 130–1360
148. Yoshida S, Inoh S, Asano T, Sano K, Kubota M, Shimazaki H, Ueta N: Effect of transient ischemia on free fatty acids and phospholipids in the gerbil brain. J Neurosurg **53:**323–331, 1980
149. Kontos HA, Wei EP, Dietrich WD, Navari RM, Povlishock JT, Ghatak NR, Ellis EF, Patterson JL Jr: Mechanism of cerebral arteriolar abnormalities after acute hypertension. Am J Physiol **240** (Heart Circ Physiol 9):H511–H527, 1981
150. Wei EP, Dietrich WD, Povlishock JT, Navari RM, Kontos HA: Functional, morphological, and metabolic abnormalities of the cerebral microcirculation after concussive brain injury in cats. Circ Res **46:**37–47, 1980
151. Nakai M, Iadecola C, Reis DJ: Global cerebral vasodilation by stimulation of rat fastigial cerebellar nucleus. Am J Physiol **243:**H226–H235, 1982
152. Hughes MJ, Barnes CD: Neural control of circulation. *In* Research Topics in Physiology, edited by Barnes CD. Academic Press, New York, 1980, pp 1–175
153. Purdy RE, Bevan JA: Adrenergic innervation of large cerebral blood vessels of the rabbit studied by fluorescence microscopy: absence of features that might contribute to non-uniform change in cerebral blood flow. Stroke **8:**82–87, 1977
154. Heistad DD, Marcus ML, Gross PM: Effects of sympathetic nerves on cerebral vessels in dog, cat and monkey. Am J Physiol **235** (Heart Circ Physiol 4):H544–H552, 1978
155. Sercombe R, Lacombe P, Aubineau P, Mamo H, Pinard E, Reyneir-Rebuffel AM, Seylaz J: Is there an active mechanism limiting the influence of the sympathetic system on the cerebral vascular bed? Evidence for vasomotor escape from sympathetic stimulation in the rabbit. Brain Res **164:**81–102, 1979
156. Bill A, Linder J: Sympathetic control of cerebral blood flow in acute arterial hypertension. Acta Physiol Scand **96:**114–121, 1976
157. Heistad DD, Marcus ML: Effect of sympathetic stimulation on permeability of the blood-brain barrier to albumin during acute hypertension in cats. Circ Res **45:**331–338, 1979
158. MacKenzie ET, McGeorge AP, Graham DI, Fitch W, Edvinsson L, Harper

AM: Effects of increasing arterial pressure on cerebral blood flow in the baboon: influence of the sympathetic nervous system. Pflugers Arch **378**:189–195, 1979

159. Mueller SM, Heistad DD, Marcus ML: Effect of sympathetic nerves on cerebral vessels during seizures. Am J Physiol **237** (Heart Circ Physiol 6):H178–H184, 1979

160. Vasquez J, Purves MJ: The cholinergic pathway to cerebral blood vessels. I. Morphological studies. Pflugers Arch **379**:157–163, 1979

161. Kuschinsky W, Wahl M, Weiss A: Evidence for cholinergic dilatory receptors in pial arteries of cat: a microapplication study. Pflugers Arch **347**:199–208, 1974

162. Matsuda M, Meyer JS, Deshmukh JD, Tagashira Y: Effects of acetycholine on cerebral circulation. J Neurosurg **45**:423–431, 1976

163. Busija DW, Heistad DD: Atropine does not attenuate cerebral vasodilatation during hypercapnia. Am J Physiol **242** (Heart Circ Physiol 11):H683–H687, 1982

164. Matsuda M, Yoneda S, Gotoh H, Handa J, Handa H: Effect of atropine on cerebrovascular responsiveness to carbon dioxide. J Neurosurg **48**:417–422, 1978

165. McCulloch J, Edvinsson L: Cerebral circulatory and metabolic effects of vasoactive intestinal polypeptide. Am J Physiol **238** (Heart Circ Physiol 7):H449–H456, 1980

166. Wei EP, Kontos HA, Said SI: Mechanism of action of vasoactive intestinal polypeptide on cerebral arterioles. Am J Physiol **239** (Heart Circ Physiol 8):H765–H768, 1980

167. Larsson LI, Edvinsson L, Fahrenkrug J, Hakanson R, Owman C, Schaffalitzky De Musckadell O, Sundler F: Immunohistochemical localization of a vasodilatory polypeptide (VIP) in cerebrovascular nerves. Brain Res **113**:400–404, 1976

168. Wahl M, Kuschinsky W: The dilating effect of histamine on pial arteries of cats and its mediation by H_2 receptors. Circ Res **44**:161–165, 1979

169. Tindall GT, Greenfield JC Jr: The effects of intra-arterial histamine on blood flow in the internal and external carotid artery of man. Stroke **4**:46–49, 1973

170. Wei EP, Raper AJ, Kontos HA, Patterson JL Jr: Determinants of response of pial arteries to norepinephrine and sympathetic nerve stimulation. Stroke **6**:654–658, 1975

171. MacKenzie ET, McCulloch J, OKeane M, Pickard JD, Harper AM: Cerebral circulation and norepinephrine: relevance of the blood-brain barrier. Am J Physiol **231**:483–488, 1976

172. Kuschinsky W, Wahl M: Alpha-receptor stimulation by endogenous and exogenous norepinephrine and blockade by phentolamine in pial arteries of cats. Circ Res **37**:168–174, 1975

173. Wei EP, Kontos HA, Patterson JL Jr: Dependence of pial arteriolar response to hypercapnia on vessel size. Am J Physiol **238** (Heart Circ Physiol 7):H697–H703, 1980

174. Marcus ML, Heistad DD: Effects of sympathetic nerves on cerebral blood flow in awake dogs. Am J Physiol **236** (Heart Circ Physiol 5):H549–H553, 1979

175. Mueller SM, Heistad DD, Marcus ML: Total and regional cerebral blood flow during hypotension, hypertension, and hypocapnia: effect of sympathetic denervation in dogs. Circ Res **41**:350–356, 1977

176. Sadoshima S, Thames M, Heistad D: Cerebral blood flow during elevation of

intracranial pressure: role of sympathetic nerves. Am J Physiol **241** (Heart Circ Physiol 10):H78–H84, 1981

177. Busija DW, Heistad DD, Marcus ML: Effects of sympathetic nerves on cerebral vessels during acute, moderate increases in arterial pressure in dogs and cats. Circ Res **46**:696–702, 1980

178. Fitch W, MacKenzie ET, Harper AM: Effects of decreasing arterial blood pressure on cerebral blood flow in the baboon. Circ Res **37**:550–557, 1975

179. Mueller SM, Heistad DD: Effect of chronic hypertension on the blood-brain barrier. Hypertension **2**:809–812, 1980

180. Edvinsson L, Owman C, West KA: Changes in cerebral blood volume of mice at various time-periods after superior cervical sympathectomy. Acta Physiol Scand **82**:521–526, 1971

181. Fog M: Cerebral circulation II: reaction of pial arteries to increase in blood pressure. Arch Neurol Psychiatry **41**:260–268, 1939

182. Wei EP, Kontos HA: Responses of cerebral arterioles to increased venous pressure. Am J Physiol **243**:H442–H447, 1982

183. Wagner EM, Traystman RJ: Cerebral venous outflow and arterial microsphere flow with elevated venous pressure. Am J Physiol **244**:H505–H512, 1983

184. Kety SS, Hafkenschiel JH, Jeffers WA, Leopold IH, Shenkin HA: The blood flow, vascular resistance and oxygen consumption of the brain in essential hypertension. J Clin Invest **27**:511–526, 1948

185. Ishitsuka T, Fujishima M, Nakatomi Y, Tamaki K, Omae T: Effects of hyperventilation on cerebral blood flow and brain tissue metabolism in normotensive and spontaneously hypertensive rats. Stroke **13**(5):687–692, 1982

186. Kannel WB, Dawbar TR, Sorlie P, Wolf PA: Components of blood pressure and risk of atherothrombotic brain infarction. The Framingham Study. Stroke **7**:327–331, 1976

187. Kannel WB, Wolf P, Dawbar TR: Hypertension cardiac impairments increase stroke risk. Geriatrics **33** (Sept) 71–83, 1978

188. Folkow B, Hallback M, Lundgren Y, Weiss L: Structurally based increase of flow resistance in spontaneously hypertensive rats. Acta Physiol. Scand **79**:373–391, 1970

189. Hart M, Heistad DD, Brody MJ: Effect of chronic hypertension and sympathetic denervation on wall/lumen ratio of cerebral arteries. Hypertension **2**:410–423, 1980

190. Nordborg C, Johansson B: Morphometric study on cerebral vessels in spontaneously hypertensive rats. Stroke **11**:266–270, 1980

191. Strandgaard W, MacKenzie ET, Sengupta D, Rowam JO, Lassen NA, Harper AM: Upper limit of autoregulation of cerebral blood flow in the baboon. Circ Res **34**:435–550, 1974

192. Nagy Z, Mathieson G, Huttner I: Blood-brain barrier opening to horseradish peroxidase in acute arterial hypertension. Acta Neuropathologica (Berl) **48**:45–53, 1979

193. Hoffman WE, Miletich DJ, Albrecht RF: The influence of antihypertensive therapy on cerebral autoregulation in aged hypertensive rats. Stroke **13**:701–704, 1982

194. Garcia JH, Ben-David E, Conger KA, Geer JC, Hollander W: Arterial hypertension injures brain capillaries. Definition of the lesions. Possible pathogenesis. Stroke **12** (4):410–413, 1981

195. Winquist RJ, Webb RC, Bohr DF: Vascular smooth muscle in hypertension. Fed Proc **41**:2387–2393, 1982
196. Fujishima M, Sugi T, Morotomi Y, Omae T: Effects of bilateral carotid artery ligation on brain lactate and pyruvate concentrations in normotensive and spontaneously hypertensive rats. Stroke **6**:62–66, 1975
197. Fujishima M, Ogata J, Sugi T, Omae T: Mortality and cerebral metabolism after bilateral carotid artery ligation in normotensive and spontaneously hypertensive rats. J Neurol Neurosurg Psychiat **39**:212–217, 1976
198. Fujishima M, Nakatomi Y, Tamaki K, Ogata J, Omae T: Cerebral ischemia induced by bilateral carotid occlusion in spontaneously hypertensive rats. J Neurol Sci **333**:1–11, 1977
199. Fujishima M, Omae T: Carotid back pressure following bilateral carotid occlusion in normotensive and spontaneously hypertensive rats. Experientia (Basel) **32**:1021–1022, 1976
200. Kaneko T, Sawada T, Niimi T, Naritomi H, Kuriyama Y, Kinugawa H: Lower limit of blood pressure in treatment of acute hypertensive intracranial hemorrhage (AHCH). J Cerebral Blood Flow Metab **3** (Suppl 1):S51–S52, 1983
201. McGiff JC, Quilley CP: The rat with spontaneous genetic hypertension is not a suitable model of human essential hypertension. Circ Res **48** (4):455–463, 1981
202. Mueller SM, Luft FC: The blood-brain barrier in renovascular hypertension. Stroke **13** (2):229–234, 1982
203. Fujishima M, Okoyama K, Oniki H, Ogata J, Omae T: The effects of acute hypertension on brain metabolism in normotensive, renovascular hypertensive and spontaneous hypertensive rats. Stroke **9**:349, 1978

Chapter 9

Hypertensive Encephalopathy

Theodore A. Kotchen and Mark W. Roy

Although decreasing in frequency, malignant hypertension with encephalopathy is a life-threatening emergency that requires prompt reduction of arterial pressure. This chapter reviews mechanisms that may be involved in the pathogenesis of malignant hypertension, particularly hypertensive encephalopathy. Most evidence suggests that encephalopathy is related to altered cerebral blood flow. Consequently, we will review alterations in its regulation that occur in acute and chronic hypertension. The therapeutic implications of these observations will be discussed.

Clinical Syndrome

Malignant hypertension is a syndrome associated with an abrupt increase of blood pressure in a patient with underlying hypertension or related to the sudden onset of hypertension in a previously normotensive individual.[1-3] Clinically, the syndrome is recognized by progressing retinopathy (arteriolar spasm, hemorrhages, exudates, papilledema), encephalopathy, deteriorating renal function with proteinuria and hematuria, and, frequently, microangiographic hemolytic anemia. Patients with long-standing hypertension are better able to tolerate acute elevations of blood pressure than previously normotensive patients. For example, children with acute glomerulonephritis and women with eclampsia may exhibit all the features of malignant hypertension at blood pressure levels of 160/100 mm Hg, whereas patients with chronic hypertension may have no detectable clinical changes with blood pressure levels of 250/150 mm Hg or higher.

Consequently, malignant hypertension cannot be defined in terms of any one arbitrary blood pressure level. Malignant hypertension may be a complication of acute or chronic hypertension of virtually any etiology, although the most frequent clinical setting is in patients with essential hypertension who have discontinued drug therapy. Blacks, in particular black men, are particularly prone to developing malignant hypertension. With the widespread availability of antihypertensive drug therapy, malignant hypertension has become a relatively uncommon disorder.

Hypertensive encephalopathy may be recognized by severe headache, nausea and vomiting (often of a projectile nature), and alterations in mental status ranging from confusion and disorientation to coma.[1–6] Focal neurologic signs may be transient and may include cranial nerve palsies, hemiparesis, aphasia, asymmetric reflexes, Babinski's sign, nystagmus, and visual disturbances (ranging from blurred vision to transient blindness). Signs of neuromuscular hyper-irritability (focal twitching, myoclonic movements) may also be present. Untreated, hypertensive encephalopathy may progress to stupor, coma, seizures, and death within hours.

Both clinically and in terms of pathophysiology, it is important to distinguish malignant hypertension from other neurologic syndromes that may be associated with hypertension—e.g., uremic encephalopathy, cerebral ischemia, hemorrhagic or thrombotic stroke, seizure disorder, cerebral embolus, subarachnoid bleed, intracerebral tumors (particularly of the posterior fossa), pseudotumor cerebri, delerium tremens, meningitis, acute intermittent porphyria, and traumatic or chemical (lead, carbon monoxide) injury to the brain.[1,3,6–8]

A diagnosis of hypertensive encephalopathy can be established only if there is no identifiable cause for cerebral malfunction other than hypertension. Occasionally this distinction may be difficult. Hypertensive encephalopathy can be prevented with adequate treatment of hypertension; when available, simple historical information about compliance to antihypertensive therapy is extremely helpful. In the patient with renal insufficiency, encephalopathy associated with asterixis or myoclonus and metabolic acidosis suggests uremic encephalopathy. Although hypertensive encephalopathy may appear within 12–24 hours of uncontrolled hypertension, the abrupt onset of neurologic signs and symptoms suggests some other acute intracerebral event. In the encephalopathic patient with hypertension and papilledema, arteriolar spasm of retinal vessels and other features of malignant hypertension (progressive nephropathy, microangiopathic hemolytic anemia) suggest that brain dysfunction is related to hypertensive encephalopathy.

In the absence of these findings, serious consideration should be given to the possibility that hypertension and papilledema are the consequence of some other intracerebral event, such as tumor or hemorrhage. Conversely, the absence of papilledema does not definitely exclude a diagnosis of malignant hypertension; in its early phases, if retinal arteriolar spasm is present, malignant hypertension (sometimes referred to as accelerated or premalignant hypertension) may be diagnosed before papilledema appears.

Other than measurement of renal function and evidence of microangiopathic hemolytic anemia, laboratory tests are generally of limited benefit in establishing a diagnosis of hypertensive encephalopathy, although they may detect other disorders involving the brain. In patients with hypertensive encephalopathy, skull films, brain scans, and echoencephalograms are normal. Cerebrospinal fluid pressure and protein concentration may be normal or increased. Generalized and/or focal EEG disturbances may be present.

Appropriate antihypertensive therapy depends on the cause of brain dysfunction. There is an increased risk of aggressive antihypertensive therapy in patients with disorders other than hypertensive encephalopathy, particularly in patients with stroke and cerebral arterial occlusive disease.[4,9] Nevertheless, because of the acute life-threatening nature of hypertensive encephalopathy, if the diagnosis is suspected, antihypertensive therapy should not be delayed until other disorders are excluded by extensive laboratory testing. Occasionally, confirmation of the diagnosis of hypertensive encephalopathy depends on the prompt response of brain dysfunction to a reduction of blood pressure. If such a response does not occur, it is probable that the neurologic disturbance is related to some other disorder, to a second complication of hypertension, or to overly aggressive antihypertensive therapy. However, in elderly patients, recovery from hypertensive encephalopathy may be delayed.

Pathology

Based on study of tissue obtained by biopsy or autopsy, malignant hypertension is associated with a diffuse necrotizing vasculitis, arteriolar thrombi, and fibrin deposition in arteriolar walls.[2,6] Fibrinoid necrosis has been observed in arterioles of brain, retina, choroid, kidney, and other organs. Additional vascular alterations include hyalinization, medial hypertrophy, and arteriosclerosis; these latter alterations are probably related to chronic hypertension rather than to the acute and severe blood-pressure elevation of malignant hypertension.

In the brain a number of parenchymal changes have also been observed in patients with hypertensive encephalopathy.[5,6] Microscopic foci of infarction and petechial hemorrhages are the most characteristic parenchymal changes and are presumably secondary to the vascular lesions. Although microscopic infarcts are not specific for hypertensive encephalopathy, in encephalopathic patients the most distinctive feature is their preferential localization in the basis pontis. Compared to autopsy studies in patients with chronic hypertension, patients with malignant hypertension do not have an increased incidence of other parenchymal lesions such as large infarcts, lacunar infarcts, and large hemorrhages. Although the older literature suggests that cerebral edema is important in the pathogenesis of hypertensive encephalopathy, the pathologic documentation of cerebral edema is not convincing.

Mechanisms of Malignant Hypertension

The mechanisms for the initiation of malignant hypertension are not well understood. Renin and aldosterone are generally markedly elevated in experimental animals and man with malignant hypertension. The onset of the malignant phase of hypertension coincides with a pressure-induced natriuresis, raising the possibility that sodium loss activates the renin-angiotensin system.[10] Alternatively, severe hypertension associated with necrotizing vasculitis may result in renal ischemia and consequent stimulation of renin secretion and increased angiotensin II production. Thus, a vicious cycle may become established whereby severe hypertension results in excessive renin secretion, which may further aggravate hypertension. Therapeutically, two approaches are available for interrupting this cycle: a) drugs that specifically inhibit renin-angiotensin, or b) potent antihypertensive agents that lower blood pressure by other mechanisms.

It has been suggested that the vascular damage in malignant hypertension is the consequence of a direct vasculotoxic effect of renin and/or aldosterone excess.[11] This seems unlikely for several reasons. Other high renin states are not associated with fibrinoid necrosis, and the angiotensin-converting enzyme inhibitor, captopril, is an effective acute and long-term therapy for patients with malignant hypertension, despite a reactive hyperreninemia.[12] In addition, necrosis is not found in vessels protected from severe hypertension—e.g., the clipped kidney in rats with experimental hypertension and the kidney distal to renal artery stenosis in man. Thus, vascular damage seems to be related to high arterial pressure per se rather than to a toxic effect of a circulating substance.

Plasma vasopressin concentrations are elevated in clinical and experimental models of malignant hypertension, possibly due to hypovolemia and to increased angiotensin II levels.[13] This raises the possibility that the vasoconstrictor action of vasopressin contributes to elevated arterial pressure in the malignant phase of hypertension. However, injection of vasopressin antiserum into rats with malignant renal hypertension has relatively little or no effect on blood pressure.[13] In patients with malignant hypertension, blood pressure does not correlate with vasopressin levels.[14] Despite comparable or higher elevations of plasma vasopressin in patients with the syndrome of inappropriate ADH excess and in normal subjects infused with vasopressin, blood pressure is not elevated. Consequently, it is unlikely that a direct vasoconstrictor action of vasopressin is the cause of malignant hypertension.

Alterations of the vasodepressor kallikrein-kinin system have also been described.[15] The plasma concentrations of both kininogen and a kinin-potentiating factor are decreased in patients with malignant hypertension, but not in patients with mild to moderate hypertension. The significance of these alterations in malignant hypertension remains to be determined.

Microangiopathic hemolytic anemia has been proposed as another factor that may be important in the production of vascular lesions.[6,16] Similar vascular lesions develop in association with intravascular coagulation in other states at a time when blood pressure is normal, although blood pressure may rapidly increase after the lesions appear. Thus, a cycle may become established whereby extremely high arterial pressures induce vascular damage, which in turn further increases blood pressure.

The acute vascular lesions in the kidney are similar to those observed in renal homograft rejection, suggesting that an immunologic factor may contribute to the vascular lesions in malignant hypertension. Furthermore, several immunologic changes have recently been described in patients with a history of malignant essential hypertension.[17] Compared to a matched control group, serum immunoglobulin concentrations (IgG, IgM) and the prevalence of auto-antibodies (predominantly antinuclear antibodies) are higher, and increased T-lymphocyte reactivity against human arterial antigen is more common. It remains to be determined whether these immunologic changes are primary or secondary to the previous pressure-induced vascular damage.

Although secondary parenchymal lesions in the brain may contribute to hypertensive encephalopathy, the rapidity with which cerebral function improves following reduction of arterial pressure suggests that alterations of blood flow per se are the primary cause of encephalopathy.

Cerebral Blood Flow and Hypertension

In the resting state, most studies indicate that cerebral blood flow is normal in the experimental animal and in man with chronic hypertension.[18] Cerebral blood flow may be decreased in older hypertensive patients with arteriosclerotic disease, and in one prospective study, decreased cerebral blood flow was associated with an increased incidence of stroke.[19] There is at least one report of decreased resting cerebral blood flow (particularly in the frontal cortex) in the stroke-prone SHR.[20] Decreased cerebral blood flow is also a predictor of stroke in this animal model, and pharmacologic control of hypertension prevents both the reduction of cerebral blood flow and stroke. Both normal and impaired cerebral vasodilator responses to carbon dioxide have been described in rats and man with chronic hypertension.[18,20–22]

Both the lower and upper limits of autoregulation of cerebral blood flow are shifted to higher levels of arterial pressure in the hypertensive baboon, rat, and man.[9,23–27] This resetting of autoregulation limits occurs within two to three months of the onset of hypertension.[25,28] Prolonged antihypertensive therapy may shift the lower limit toward normal.[29] Impaired autoregulation may be related to structural changes (hypertrophy) in the walls of resistance vessels. When arterial pressure increases acutely, autoregulatory constriction of arterioles and small arteries may be overridden, and an increase of cerebral blood flow will result.[9,23,30] In response to hypotension, cerebral blood flow decreases because of inadequate vasodilation. The brain compensates for decreased blood flow by increasing its extraction of oxygen, but when arterial pressure falls below 40 mm Hg, even this mechanism fails, and symptoms of brain hypoxia develop.

Hypertensive encephalopathy appears to be related to failure of autoregulation of cerebral blood flow at the upper pressure limit.[31,32] The earlier literature suggested that breakthrough of autoregulation resulted in cerebral vasospasm with subsequent hypoperfusion and ischemia of brain tissue.[33–40] However, recent studies of cerebral blood flow have failed to confirm the concept of vasospasm as the initiating event. Recent evidence also suggests that failure of autoregulation causes a forced vasodilation and hyperperfusion.[31,41] The increase of cerebral blood flow in response to hypercapnia is also exaggerated.[42] This "breakthrough" of autoregulation may cause vascular necrosis and disruption of the blood brain barrier to water soluble ions and to protein.[43,44] Increased permeability has also been observed in retinal vessels.[45]

These hemoresponses and alterations of vascular permeability may induce cerebral dysfunction and secondary parenchymal lesions in brain. Both experimental animals and patients with chronic hypertension may be relatively protected from the cerebral consequences of acute elevations of arterial pressure because the upper limit of autoregulation is shifted to a higher level of pressure. In the SHR, cerebral vessels are relatively resistant to blood brain barrier disruption during acute phenylephrine-induced hypertension.[46] These protective effects of chronic hypertension may be due to hypertrophy of cerebral vessels, resulting in attenuation of the increase in wall stress during acute hypertension.

Despite some evidence to the contrary, it appears that autoregulation of cerebral blood flow is not dependent on sympathetic nervous system activity.[47] Autoregulation to both increased and decreased arterial pressures is maintained following either surgical or pharmacologic sympathectomy. Nevertheless, sympathetic nerves may protect against the hemodynamic alterations and disruption of the blood brain barrier (particularly in cortical gray matter) that result from acute elevations of arterial pressure.[48–51]

Cerebral vasoconstrictor responses to electrical stimulation of sympathetic pathways and to activation of sympathetic nerves by sinoaortic deafferentation are augmented in cats and dogs with severe hypertension.[50] Although activation of the sympathetic nerves raises the upper limit of the autoregulatory range,[48,52–54] neither sympathetic blockade[30] nor chronic sympathetic denervation[30,55,56] alters the upper or lower limits of autoregulation. Thus activation of the sympathetic nerves protects the cerebral vasculature from large increases in blood pressure, but interference with or loss of the nerves does not impair autoregulation. However, in the stroke-prone SHR, sympathetic denervation attenuates the development of vascular hypertrophy in cerebral vessels, and increases susceptibility to both stroke and to disruption of the blood brain barrier.[57,58]

In contrast to its protective effect in acute hypertension, adrenergic activity appears to contribute to decreased cerebral blood flow in the anesthetized baboon subjected to hemorrhagic hypotension.[59] Both surgical and pharmacologic sympathectomy enhance the maintenance of cerebral blood flow in this model. Thus, sympathetic activity shifts both the upper and lower limits of autoregulation to higher levels of arterial pressure and prevents cerebral blood vessels from dilating at both blood pressure extremes.

Therapeutic Approaches

The rapidity and level to which blood pressure should be lowered in patients with malignant hypertension is an issue based more on clinical judgment than scientific fact. Hypertensive encephalopathy is an acute life threatening emergency requiring hospitalization and prompt reduction of blood pressure. Nevertheless, there are inherent risks in overly aggressive therapy, and the risk of normalizing blood pressure within minutes must be weighed against the risk of a major cardiovascular event occurring during that time period. Rapid lowering of blood pressure to below the lower limit of autoregulation may precipitate cerebral ischemia or even infarction.[60] In addition to potential complications of decreasing cerebral blood flow, abrupt lowering of blood pressure may precipitate a transient decrement of renal function (sometimes requiring dialysis), and in patients with a coronary artery disease, acute coronary insufficiency.[1,4]

Consequently, in the absence of encephalopathy or some other catastrophic event (e.g., pulmonary edema, dissecting aortic aneurysm) it is preferable to reduce blood pressure over hours or longer rather than minutes. Indeed, before antihypertensive drugs were available, Newborg and Kempner[61] reported a one-year survival of 57% in 120 patients with hypertensive vascular disease and papilledema who were treated with a rice diet only (low sodium, high potassium). Most of the deaths were attributed to non-compliance with the diet. By comparison, the one-year mortality in patients with untreated malignant hypertension approaches 90%.

Ledingham et al. have recently described a series of 10 patients with malignant hypertension who developed abnormal neurologic signs following rapid reduction of arterial pressure into the normotensive range.[62] We have observed a similar phenomenon in several patients. Finnerty found that normotensive subjects developed symptoms of cerebral ischemia only when mean arterial pressure was reduced to 30 mm Hg, whereas hypertensive patients became symptomatic when mean arterial pressure fell to 80 mm Hg.[63] It has recently been reported that oral nifedipine increases cerebral blood flow in patients with hypertensive emergencies, in contrast to a decrease following intravenous clonidine.[64]

The hypertensive rat is more prone to ischemic brain lesions following hypotension than the normotensive rat.[48] The decreased tolerance of hypertensive patients to acute reductions of blood pressure is most likely related to the fact that the lower blood-pressure limit for autoregulation of cerebral blood flow is set at a higher level in hypertensive patients. In acute stroke, autoregulation may be impaired to an even greater extent, or indeed abolished in the zone of cerebral ischemia.[9,23] Consequently, patients with cerebral infarction are particularly prone to further deterioration of brain function following precipitous reduction of blood pressure. Loss of autoregulation in ischemic brain may also permit passive increases of cerebral blood flow and local brain edema in response to elevations of systemic pressure. Unfortunately, there are no controlled studies that define the ideal level to which blood pressure should be reduced acutely in patients with hypertensive encephalopathy or cerebral infarction.

Empirically, our approach is to lower blood pressure acutely with parenteral drugs in patients with hypertensive encephalopathy, but not to normotensive levels in older patients or patients with a history of chronic hypertension. After the patient has stabilized, further gradual reduction of blood pressure with oral drugs is generally appropriate. In the acute therapy of hypertensive encephalopathy it is important to determine if reduction of blood pressure results in improvement or deterioration of brain function. Consequently, we avoid the use of antihypertensive drugs with central nervous system side effects.

References

1. Gifford RW, Westbrook E: Hypertensive encephalopathy: mechanisms, clinical features, and treatment. Prog in Cardiovasc Dis **17:**115–124, 1974
2. Dranov J, Skyler JS, Gunnells JC: Malignant hypertension: current modes of therapy. Arch Int Med **133:**791–801, 1974
3. Bennett C: The syndrome of accelerated or malignant hypertension. Cardiovasc Med **4:**1141–1161, 1979
4. Koch-Weser J: Hypertensive emergencies. New Engl J Med **290:**211–214, 1974
5. Healton EB, Brust JC, Feinfeld DA, Thomson GE: Hypertensive encephalopathy and the neurologic manifestations of malignant hypertension. Neurol **32:**127–132, 1982
6. Chester EM, Agamanolis DP, Banker BQ, Victor M: Hypertensive encephalopathy: a clinicopathologic study of 20 patients. Neurol **28:**928–939, 1978
7. Keith TA: Hypertension crisis: recognition and management. JAMA **237:**1570–1577, 1977
8. Ram CVS: Hypertensive encephalopathy: recognition and management. Arch Int Med **138:**1851–1853, 1978
9. Scheinberg P: Cerebral blood flow. *In* The Nervous System, edited by Tower DB. Vol 2: The Clinical Neurosciences. New York, Raven Press, 1975, pp 157–166
10. Mohring J, Mohring B, Naumann HJ, Philippi A, Homsy E, Orth H, Dauda G,

Kazda S, Gross F: Salt and water balance and renin activity in renal hypertension of rats. Am J Physiol **228**:1847–1855, 1975

11. Brunner HR, Laragh JH, Baer L, Newton MA, Goodwin FT, Krakoff LR, Bard RH, Buhler FR: Essential hypertension: renin and aldosterone, heart attack and stroke. New Engl J Med **286**:441–449, 1972

12. Case DB, Atlas SA, Sullivan PA, Laragh JH: Acute and chronic treatment of severe and malignant hypertension with oral angiotensin-converting enzyme inhibitor captopril. Circulation **64**:765–771, 1981

13. Mohring J, Mohring B, Petri M, Haack D: Plasma vasopressin concentrations and effects of vasopressin antiserum on blood pressure in rats with malignant two-kidney Goldblatt hypertension. Circulat Res **42**:17–22, 1978

14. Padfield PL, Brown JJ, Lever AF, Morton JJ, Robertson JIS: Blood pressure in acute and chronic vasopressin excess. New Engl J Med **304**:1067–1070, 1981

15. Almeida FA, Stella RCR, Voos A, Ajzen H, Ribeiro AB: Malignant hypertension: a syndrome associated with low plasma kininogen and kinin potentiating factor. Hypertension **3**(suppl II):46–49, 1981

16. Linton AL, Garvas H, Gleadle RI, Hutchinson HE, Lawson DH, Lever AF, Macadam RF, McNicol GP, Robertson JIS: Microangiopathic hemolytic anemia and the pathogenesis of malignant hypertension. Lancet **1**:1277–1282, 1969

17. Gudbrandsson T, Hansson L, Herlitz H, Lindholm L, Nilsson LA: Immunological changes in patients with previous malignant essential hypertension. Lancet **1**:406–407, 1981

18. Report of the Hypertension Task Force of the National Heart, Lung and Blood Institute: current research and recommendations from the subgroup on local hemodynamics. Hypertension **2**:342–369, 1980

19. Terashi A, Atarashi J: Cerebral circulation in cerebral stroke. **3**:69–82, 1976

20. Yamori Y, Horie R: Developmental course of hypertension and regional cerebral blood flow in stroke-prone spontaneously hypertensive rats. Stroke **8**:456–461, 1977

21. Tominaga S, Strandgaard S, Umeura K, Ito K, Kutsuzawa T, Lassen NA, MaKamura T: Cerebrovascular CO reactivity in normotensive and hypertensive man. Stroke **7**:507–510, 1976

22. Griffith DNW, James IM, Newburg PA, Woollard ML: Abnormal cerebrovascular regulation in hypertensive patients. Brit Med J **2**:740, 1978

23. Scheinberg P: Cerebral blood flow. *In* The Nervous System, edited by Tower DB. Vol 2: The Clinical Neurosciences. New York, Raven Press, 1975, pp 147–156

24. Strandgaard S, Jones JV, MacKenzie ET, Harper AM: Upper limit of cerebral blood flow autoregulation in experimental renovascular hypertension in the baboon. Circulat Res **37**:164–167, 1975

25. Jones JV, Fitch W, MacKenzie ET, Strandgaard S, Harper AM: Lower limit of cerebral blood flow autoregulation in experimental renovascular hypertension in the baboon. Circulat Res **39**:555–557, 1976

26. Strandgaard S, Olesen J, Skinhoj E, Lassen NA: Autoregulation of brain circulation in severe arterial hypertension. Brit Med J **1**:507–510, 1973

27. Strandgaard S: Autoregulation of cerebral circulation in hypertension. Acta Neurol Scand **57** (Suppl 66):1–82, 1978

28. Barry DI, Strandgaard S, Graham DI, Braendstrup O, Svendsen UG, Vorstrup S, Hemmingsen R, Bolwig TG: Cerebral blood flow in rats with renal and spontaneous hypertension: Resetting of the lower limit of autoregulation. J Cerebral Blood Flow Metab **2**:347–353, 1982

29. Strandgaard S: Autoregulation of cerebral blood flow in hypertensive patients. The modifying influence of prolonged antihypertensive treatment on the tolerance to acute drug induced hypertension. Circulation **53**:720–727, 1976

30. Strandgaard S, MacKenzie ET, Sengupta D, Rowan JO, Lassen NA, Harper AM: Upper limit of autoregulation of cerebral blood flow in the baboon. Circ Res **34**:435–440, 1974

31. Farrar JK, Jones JV, Graham DI, Strandgaard S, MacKenzie: Evidence against cerebral vasospasm during acutely induced hypertension. Brain Res **104**:176–180, 1976

32. Farrar JK, Jones JV, Graham DI, Strandgaard S, MacKenzie ET: Evidence against cerebral vasospasm during acutely induced hypertension. Brain Res **104**:176–180, 1976

33. Lassen NA, Agnoli A: The upper limit of autoregulation of cerebral blood flow on the pathogenesis of hypertensive encephalopathy. Scand J Clin Lab Invest **30**:113–116, 1973

34. Auer L, Walter GF: Reactions of pial vessels to acute arterial hypertension at various levels of arterial pH and carbon dioxide tension. Adv Neurol **20**:371–380, 1978

35. Johansson B: Regional cerebral blood flow in acute arterial hypertension. Acta Neurol Scand **50**:366–372, 1974

36. Strandgaard S: Studies on the cerebral circulation of the baboon in acutely induced hypertension. Stroke **7**:287–290, 1976

37. Johansson B, Strandgaard S, Lassen NA: The hypertensive "breakthrough" of autoregulation of cerebral blood flow with forced vasodilation, flow increase, and blood-brain-barrier damage. Circ Res (Suppl I) **34/35**:167–171, 1974

38. Byrom FB: The pathogenesis of hypertensive encephalopathy and its relation to the malignant phase of hypertension. Lancet **2**:201–211, 1954

39. Meyer JS, Waltz AG, Gotoh F: Pathogenesis of cerebral vasospasm in hypertensive encephalopathy. Neurol **10**:735–744, 1960

40. Dinsdale HB, Robertson DM, Haas RA: Cerebral blood flow in acute hypertension. Arch Neurol **31**:80–87, 1974

41. Johansson B, Li CL, Olsson Y, Klatzo I: The effect of acute arterial hypertension on the blood brain barrier to protein tracers. Acta Neuropath **16**:117, 1970

42. Ekstrom-Jodal B, Haggendal E, Linder LE and Nillson NJ: Cerebral blood flow autoregulation at high arterial pressures and different levels of carbon dioxide tension. Europ Neurol **6**:6–10, 1971

43. Johansson B, Linder LE: Blood brain barrier dysfunction in acute arterial hypertension induced by clamping of the thoracic aorta. Acta Neurol Scand **50**:360–365, 1974

44. Huggendal E: On the pathophysiology of increased cerebrovascular permeability in acute arterial hypertension in cats. Acta Neurol Scand **48**:265–270, 1972

45. Scarpelli PT, Brancato R, Menchini U, Santoro P, Lamanna S: The close interrelationship between increased vascular retinal permeability and blood pressure level. Evidence from retinal fluoroangiography. Ophthalmol **175**:309–320, 1977

46. Mueller SM, Heistad DD: Effect of chronic hypertension on the blood brain barrier. Hypertension **2**:809–812, 1980

47. Heistad DD, Marcus ML: Evidence that neural mechanisms do not have important effects on cerebral blood flow. Circ Res **42**:295–302, 1978

48. Bill A, Linder J: Sympathetic control of cerebral blood flow in acute arterial hypertension. Acta Physiol Scand **96:**114–121, 1976
49. MacKenzie ET, McGeorge AP, Graham DI, Fitch W, Edvinsson L, Harper AM: Effects of increasing arterial pressure on cerebral blood flow in the baboon: influence of sympathetic nervous system. Pflugers Arch **378:**189–195, 1979
50. Heistad DD, Marcus ML: Effect of sympathetic stimulation on permeability of the blood brain barrier to albumin during acute hypertension in cats. Circulat Res **45:**331–338, 1979
51. Sadoshima S, Heistad D: Sympathetic nerves protect the blood brain barrier in stroke-prone spontaneously hypertensive rats. Hypertension **4:**907–970, 1982
52. Edvinsson L, Owman C, Siesjo BK: Physiological role of the cerebrovascular sympathetic nerves in the autoregulation of cerebral blood flow. Brain Res **117:**519–523, 1976
53. MacKenzie ET, McGeorge AP, Graham DI, Fitch W, Edvinsson L, Harper AM: Breakthrough of cerebral autoregulation and the sympathetic nervous system. Acta Neurol Scand **56**(Suppl 64):10–11, 1977
54. Boisvert DJP, Jones JV, Harper AM: Cerebral blood flow autoregulation to acutely increasing blood pressure during sympathetic stimulation. Acta Neurol Scand **56**(Suppl 64):8–9, 1977
55. Waltz AG, Yamaguchi T, Regli F: Regulatory responses of cerebral vasculature after sympathetic denervation. Am J Physiol **221:**298–302, 1971
56. Eklof B, Ingvas DH, Koigstrom E, Olin T: Persistence of cerebral blood flow autoregulation following chronic bilateral cervical sympathectomy in the monkey. Acta Physiol Scand **82:**172–176, 1971
57. Hart MN, Heistad DD, Brody MJ: Effect of chronic hypertension and sympathetic denervation on wall/lumen ratio of cerebral vessels. Hypertension **2:**419–423, 1980
58. Sadoshima S, Busija D, Brody M, Heistad D: Sympathetic nerves protect against stroke in stroke-prone hypertensive rats. Hypertension **3**(Suppl I):124–127, 1981
59. Fitch W, MacKenzie ET, Harper AM: Effects of decreasing arterial pressure on cerebral blood flow in the baboon: influence of the sympathetic nervous system. Circulat Res **37:**550–557, 1975
60. Graham DI: Ischemic brain damage of cerebral perfusion failure type after treatment of severe hypertension. Brit Med J **4:**739, 1975
61. Newborg B, Kempner W: Analysis of 177 cases of hypertensive vascular disease with papilledema: 126 patients treated with rice diet. Am J Med **19:**33–47, 1955
62. Ledingham JGG, Rajagopalan B: Cerebral complications in the treatment of accelerated hypertension. Quart J Med **48:**25–41, 1979
63. Finnerty FA, Witkin W, Fazekas JF: Cerebral hemodynamics during cerebral ischemia induced by acute hypotension. J Clin Invest **33:**1227–1232, 1954
64. Bertel O, Coner D, Radu EW, Muller J, Lang C, Dubach VC: Nifedipine in hypertensive emergencies. Brit Med J **286:**19, 1983

Chapter 10

Consequences of Elevated Arterial Pressure in Brain

Henry B. Dinsdale

Hypertension is the most important risk factor leading to the major types of cerebrovascular disease. A discussion of the consequences to the brain of elevated arterial pressure must therefore be concerned mainly with the pathology of cerebral arterial disease. Most cerebrovascular disease associated with hypertension results from long-sustained elevations of blood pressure, the effects of which are manifest more in the brain than in any other body organ. This chapter deals with the consequences to the brain of chronic hypertension. Hypertensive encephalopathy, the most dramatic and serious consequence of severe acute arterial hypertension, is dealt with elsewhere in this book. The effect of hypertension on cerebral blood flow is mentioned only briefly here.

The Neurologic Symptoms of Hypertension

Few clinicians would deny that patients with malignant or accelerated hypertension usually show such symptoms as severe early morning headache, visual blurring, dyspnea, and the symptoms of uremia. But whether or not these symptoms are associated with milder forms of hypertension remains a debatable topic. The notion is held by much of the laity that high blood pressure causes a variety of physical symptoms including headache and dizziness. That this correlation exists in the minds of patients is supported by studies such as that by Haynes et al.[1] documenting that patients experience a significant increase in number of work days lost due to an increase in somatic complaints after being told they have elevated blood pressure. Although hypertension is rarely the explanation for the common complaints of headache and dizziness, there is evidence of an association between elevated blood pressure and such symptoms in some patients. The course of these symptoms in hypertensive patients will depend to a considerable degree on the physician's aptitude for counselling patients, including the ability to provide reassurance about the nature of the drugs prescribed.

Dizziness

Dizziness is a common complaint that requires a careful history for its correct interpretation and management. Rarely do patients with the complaint of "dizziness" describe vertigo—i.e., a distinct sense of rotation or disorientation of the body in space. In a report providing details of over 6500 health examinations the complaint of dizziness was increased in hypertensive subjects and significantly elevated in those patients with elevated diastolic pressures and hypertensive retinopathy.[2] Dizziness was a common complaint in another group of hypertensive patients and was one of two symptoms (the other was headache) that decreased significantly following treatment of hypertension in the study by Bullpitt et al.[3] They followed 178 patients, referred to a hospital clinic with a diagnosis of hypertension, before and after treatment with diuretics and adrenergic-beta-blocking drugs. There was an improvement in symptoms following treatment. Hypertensive patients tended to lose complaints of unsteadiness and headache but gained symptoms of vivid dreams and diarrhea.

Mechanisms listed by the authors as relevant to symptoms in undertreated hypertensive patients aware of their diagnosis were: (1) the raised blood pressure, (2) the hypertensive patient's concept of symptoms to be expected, (3) the referring doctor's concept of hypertension-related symptoms that led to the diagnosis, and (4) neurosis associated with hypertension.

Dizziness was not a complaint in a study assessing 100 children with severe and persistent hypertension.[4] Headache and tiredness were the commonest complaints in these children, although more than 50% were asymptomatic at the time their hypertension was detected.

Available data suggest that the complaint of dizziness may be due to elevated blood pressure per se and that it may be improved with treatment of hypertension. Conversely, the complaint may also of course be caused by treatment for hypertension. The view that elderly people are especially susceptible to the adverse effects of anti-hypertensive agents appears to be without foundation.[5] Dizziness is a common complaint in the clinic and may be due to any one of a number of diseases. A causal relationship with elevated blood pressure is documented in only a minority of elderly patients.

Headache

Widely divergent opinions are held about the association of headache with arterial blood pressure. Some knowledgeable authors[6,7] believe that headache is a common symptom in hypertension, while others[8] state that "it is generally believed that moderate hypertension alone does not cause headache." One community study documented similar blood pressures in patients complaining of headache and in those free of headache. Family doctors tend to record the blood pressure in patients with headache primarily to allay the patient's concern rather than in the expectation of finding hypertension.[9]

If headache in an individual patient is to be ascribed to hypertension, it should have clinical characteristics distinguishing it from other forms of headache and should be relieved by adequate treatment of hypertension. Untreated hypertension can be causally associated with headache,[10] especially early morning headache, which tends to be located in the occipital region and improve when the patient gets up, usually disappearing within an hour or two. The headache is generally mild unless associated with severely elevated levels of hypertension. The response of this early morning headache to treatment was demonstrated in a double blind study of patients with diastolic blood pressures between 115–129 mm Hg.[11] In the treated group, 8% complained of headache versus 21% of those given placebos.

The mechanism of the hypertensive headache remains unclear. When groups of patients are studied there is a positive correlation between increasing cerebrospinal fluid and systemic arterial pressures but no correlation in individual hypertensive patients between CSF pressure and headache.[12,13] Nevertheless, characteristics of the hypertensive headache suggest that it arises from a disturbance of intracranial structures.

Most individuals with muscle contraction, vascular, and migraine headache have blood pressures similar to those without headaches.[10] However, within the hypertensive population there is a group that complains of a headache that increases as levels of blood pressure rise and declines significantly following treatment of hypertension. As with the symptom dizziness, an elevated blood pressure is rarely the explanation for the common symptom headache, but hypertension is included justifiably in the list of conditions that can cause headache.

Hypertension and Cerebral Arterial Disease

The fact that little can be done to modify the brain damage of an ischemic or hemorrhagic stroke should be a compelling reason for physicians to deal effectively with any treatable risk factor for stroke. Hypertension is the major determinant of stroke occurrence;[14] therefore, the most effective measure to be taken to diminish the incidence of stroke is adequate and continuous treatment of patients with hypertension.[14–17] Cerebral infarction or hemorrhage is often the final incident in a series of vascular events that began for the patient many years earlier with the onset of hypertension.

Hypertension is strongly related to atherothrombotic brain infarction, transient ischemic attacks, and intracranial hemorrhage, which together account for approximately 85% of all strokes. The essential pathology in those conditions is located in medium and small-sized arteries and a few specific sites in larger vessels such as the origin of the internal carotid artery. Cerebral embolism, in which cardiac disease is the major factor, accounts for most of the remaining 15% of patients with stroke.

Cerebral Blood Flow and Hypertension

Cerebral blood flow remains relatively constant under normal circumstances in spite of wide variations of systemic blood pressure. This autoregulation arises mainly from a myogenic response in the walls of brain resistance vessels to the stretch caused by elevations in systemic arterial pressure. It is essentially independent of autonomic control except under circumstances of extreme stress or in the presence of brain pathology. The mean systemic arterial blood pressure is 90 mm Hg in a healthy adult; the average lower limit of cerebral autoregulation is approximately 60 mm Hg.

When hypertension is chronic, there is a shift of the cerebral blood flow/blood pressure curve to the right due presumably to thickening of vessel walls and decreased responsiveness of resistance vessels.[18] Consequently, the blood pressure levels unnecessary to produce hypertensive encephalopathy in a patient with chronic hypertension are higher than those in normotensive individuals. The flow/pressure curve is shifted to the left in children, which makes them more susceptible than adults to the development of hypertensive encephalopathy following sudden hypertension.[19] The extent and rate of elevation of blood pressure are the two most important factors determining the development of hypertensive encephalopathy, but clinically and experimentally it is difficult to evaluate them independently of each other.

Experimental evidence can be found to support either the narrowing (spasm)[20] or dilation[21] theories for the changes in cerebral blood flow and vascular permeability in acute hypertension. Demonstration of a "breakthrough of autoregulation" in patients following acute angiotensin-induced hypertension[22] provides support for the proponents of the dilation theory. However, studies in animals using high-resolution autoradiographic techniques demonstrate that patterns of cerebral blood flow during acute hypertension are complex, with both high and low flow areas coexisting in adjacent cortical regions, suggesting that both mechanisms may be important.[23]

By far the largest component of cerebrovascular resistance is provided by penetrating, parenchymal arterioles. These vessels show abnormal permeability associated with enhanced pinocytosis in vascular endothelial cells beginning as early as 90 seconds after the onset of hypertension.[24] Such pinocytosis can provide rapid transport for macromolecules from blood through vessel walls to the neuropil and may be an important mechanism producing brain edema in the presence of acute hypertension. Brain edema can occur in such circumstances without structural damage to cerebral vessels (Figure 10-1).

Because pH changes limited to the blood do not alter cerebrovascular resistance, the vasodilation accompanying high $PaCO_2$ presumably results from pH changes in the perivascular tissues. Tissue damage, as occurs with stroke or trauma, leads to local accumulation of lactic acid, excessive local blood flow, and loss of autoregulation.[25]

Hypertension and Atherosclerosis

Hypertension is an accelerator of atherosclerosis. An all-encompassing theory of the etiology of atherosclerosis must explain the appearance of lipid in vessel walls, proliferation of arterial smooth muscle cells, develop-

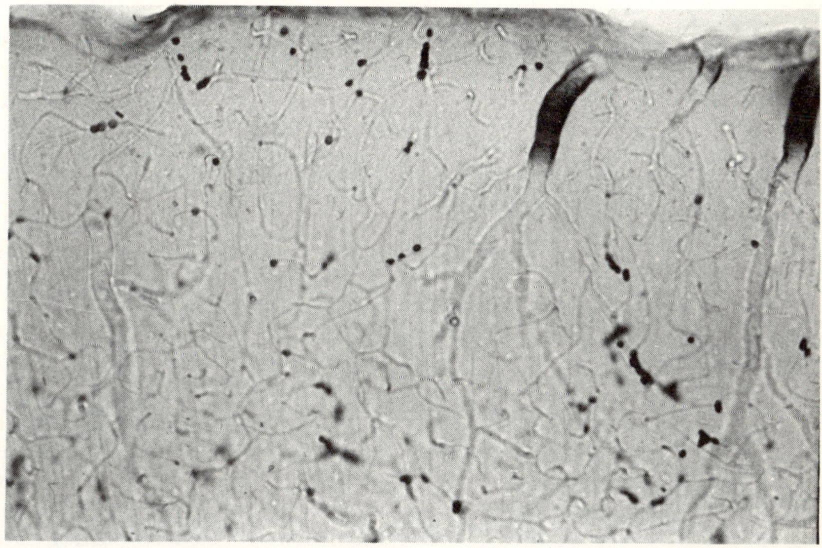

Figure 10-1. Rat cerebral cortex 90 seconds after onset of hypertension. Horseradish peroxidase has permeated the walls of focal segments of penetrating cortical arterioles (without evidence of mechanical damage by electron microsurgery) ($\times$ 110).

ment of mural thrombi, and the accumulation of collagen and proteo-glycans in the extra-cellular matrix.[26] Atheroma tend to develop in large arteries and therefore are more prominent in carotid than vertebral arteries and more prominent in the extracranial than intracranial circulation.[27]

The symptomatic atherosclerotic plaque is a mixture of smooth muscle cells; a connective tissue complex of elastin, collagen, and glycosamino-glycans that may produce a "cap"; and lipid deposits consisting of aggregates of cholesterol, triglycerides, and phospholipids.[28] Cell necrosis, calcification, and hemorrhage from small ingrowing vessels are frequent developments. Platelet clumps or thrombus may appear on the surface of the plaque and produce local or embolic complications, including such distinctive clinical symptoms as amaurosis fugax[29] (Figure 10-2).

Large cerebral infarcts were found by Cole and Yates[30] to occur with approximately the same frequency in hypertensive and normotensive patients, but there is a difference in the size of artery involved. In one study reviewing angiograms in patients with cerebrovascular disease, carotid occlusion was found in 25% of normotensive patients but in only 9% of hypertensive patients, a significant difference.[31] Such observations indicate that factors in addition to hypertension are major determinants of atherothrombotic brain infarction due to large vessel (carotid) disease. By contrast, large and small intracerebral hemorrhages and small infarcts were found almost exclusively in the brains of hypertensive patients, indicating

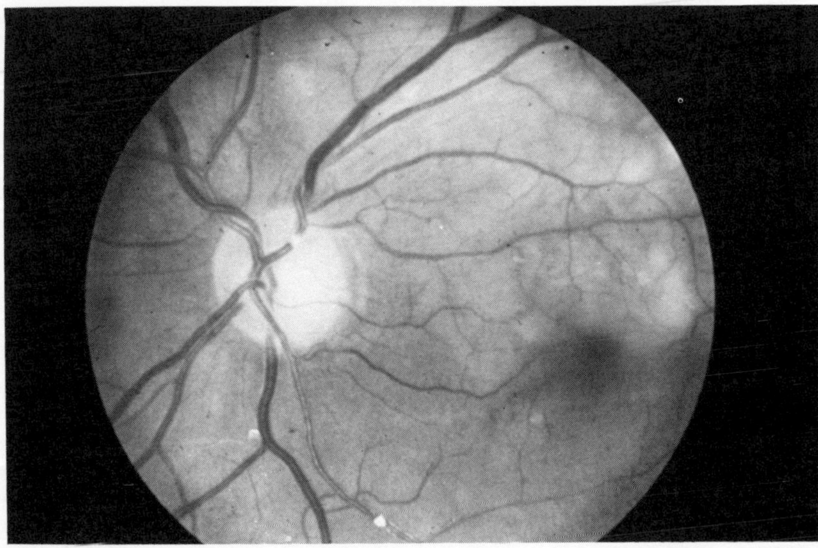

Figure 10-2. Fundus of 53-year-old male with history of seven attacks of transient left-eye blindness. Note cholesterol emboli over optic disc and in inferior temporal artery.

that hypertension is the major factor leading to disease in medium and small-sized arteries.

Cole and Yates described the autopsy findings in the brains of 100 hypertensive patients (diastolic blood pressure >110 mm Hg) and compared them with 100 normotensive patients. The brains of 50% of the hypertensive patients showed either ischemic or hemorrhagic lesions, compared with 25% of the normotensive brains. Ischemic infarcts were distributed equally between the two groups, but hemorrhages, either large or small, were confined almost exclusively to the hypertensive group. Such studies demonstrate that hypertensive patients are more liable to cerebrovascular disease than normotensive patients because of an increased incidence of pathology in medium and small-sized cerebral arteries. The limited effect of hypertension in accelerating atheroma in larger arteries such as the aorta and carotid is demonstrated in angiographic and post-mortem studies.[32,33]

Cerebral atherosclerosis may become symptomatic through a variety of mechanisms. A common one is recurring cholesterol or platelet-fibrin emboli arising from an ulcerated atherosclerotic plaque located either at the origin of the internal carotid artery or in an adjacent region of the bifurcation of the common carotid. The association between the passage of such emboli through the retinal circulation and transient visual symptoms is well established. It is reasonable to assume that similar emboli reaching cerebral arteries can produce transient neurologic symptoms. However, the cerebral circulation, unlike the retinal, is unavailable for routine visual inspection, thereby denying the opportunity to demonstrate an association between fibrin-platelet or cholesterol emboli and transient neurologic symptoms, although clinical experience often justifies a strong presumption of such an explanation.

The true frequency of emboli from the carotid or, less often, the vertebrobasilar circulation as the cause of transient ischemic attack therefore must remain unknown. A variety of other mechanisms such as emboli from the heart, mechanical compression of neck vessels, cardiac arrhythmias, postural hypotension, etc. will enter the differential diagnosis of many patients with transient ischemic attacks.

Emboli arising from neck vessels presumably lodge on occasion in a cerebral artery, cause tissue infarction, and leave a permanent neurologic deficit. Again, the frequency of such events is difficult to document at autopsy for a number of reasons including pre-mortem fragmentation of the embolus, difficulty in locating emboli due to the multiple sectioning required, or the failure to search for them (Figure 10-3).

Atheroma also produce completed strokes by thrombus formation in an atherosclerotic, stenosed carotid, or vertebral artery. Such an occlusion by itself may produce cerebral infarction in the territory of distal arterial tributaries. Occasionally, the distal part of a thrombus breaks off and produces an artery-to-artery embolus, causing occlusion of a distal cerebral artery (Figure 10-4).

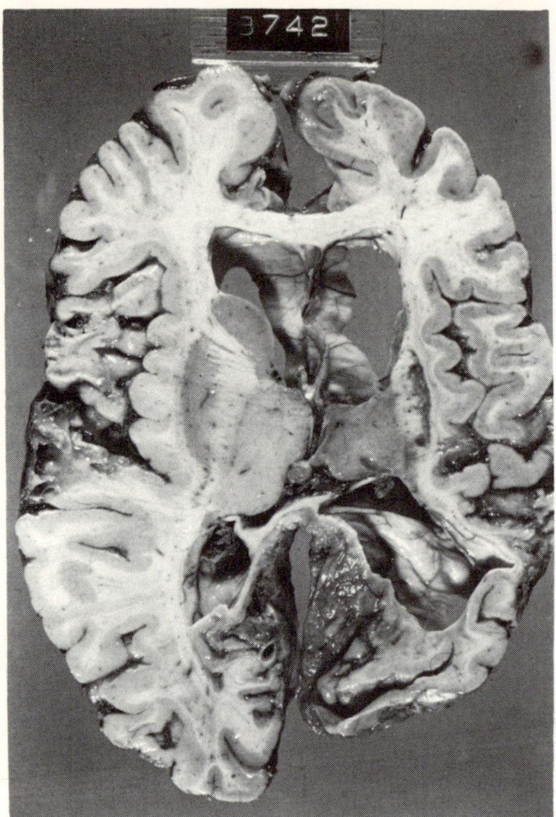

Figure 10-3. Multiple embolic cerebral infarctions, several years old, in patient with chronic atrial fibrillation. Both right and left posterior and middle cerebral artery territories are involved.

Hypertensive Changes in Medium and Small Cerebral Arteries

The penetrating cerebral arteries are smaller than the arteries of the neck and the base of the brain and are less affected by atherosclerosis. However, like small penetrating arteries elsewhere in the body, they develop a variety of hypertensive changes including hyalinization, hyperplastic sclerosis, medial degeneration, and fibrinoid necrosis. In some patients the fibrinoid form of hyalinosis may be limited almost entirely to the cerebral vessels.[34] Fisher has coined the term "lipohyalinosis" to emphasize the fatty component of the lesion and what he believes is a relationship between these hypertensive lesions and the fatty plaque of atherosclero-

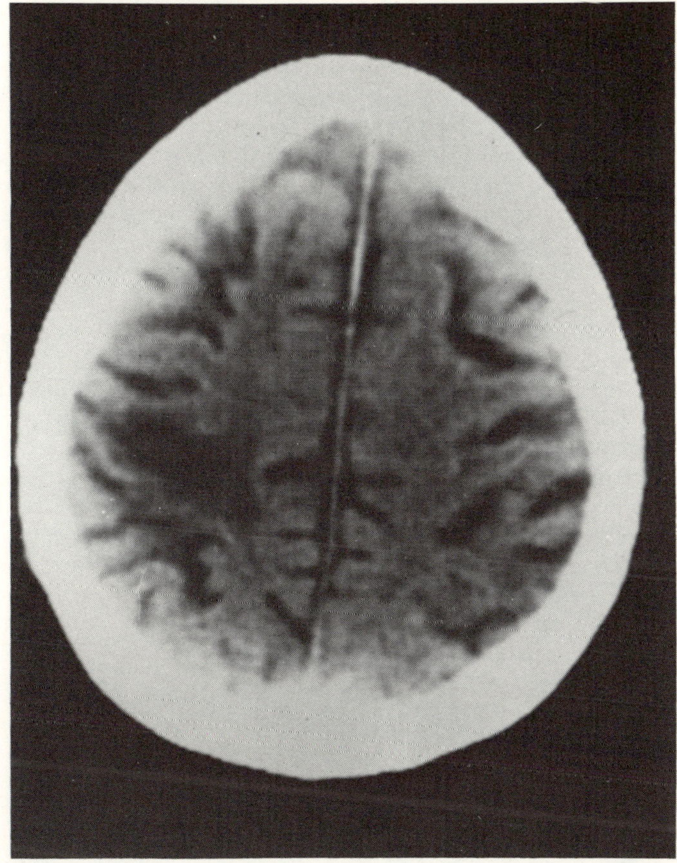

Figure 10-4. CAT scan demonstrating infarct in territory of left middle cerebral artery in 82-year-old man.

sis.[35] However, there appear to be fundamental differences between the development and composition of the atherosclerotic plaque and hypertensive lesions in smaller arteries.

The development of hypertensive arterial changes have been well studied in the hypertensive rat.[36,37] Intimal proliferation is followed by splitting of the internal elastic lamina and an increase in the number of smooth muscle cells, some of which migrate into the intima. Amorphous material then accumulates in the intima, smooth muscle cells become disorganized, and excessive adventitial collagen appears, all leading eventually to fibrinoid necrosis. This lesion differs considerably from the atherosclerotic plaque described earlier.

Lacunes

The term "lacune" was coined by Durant-Fardel[38] and used in the early part of this century to describe small cavitations in the brain caused by ischemia or, occasionally, hemorrhagic infarction. Fibrinoid necrosis, severe sclerosis, embolism, inflammation, and intravascular coagulation in perforating arteries are all mechanisms that can produce single or multiple infarcts widely distributed throughout the brain. The loss of tissue or "lacune" that may remain as the residue of a small infarct is most commonly seen in the putamen, globus pallidus, cerebral white matter, or brain stem. Such cystic cavities contain occasional macrophages and have a surrounding glial scar. The term "lacune" is descriptive and intended to describe a pathologic lesion that requires a few weeks to develop. It has been used recently as a clinical diagnosis, with subsequent confusion both in the literature and at the bedside (Figure 10-5).

As with most ischemic lesions, the extent of ischemic tissue during the acute phase is probably considerably greater than the area of the residual cavity. It has been suggested[39] that the term lacune should be limited to lesions due to permanent or transient occlusion of intracerebral arteries. Others use adjectives according to the size of the cavity—e.g., "giant" for those greater than 10 mm.[40] General usage refers to a cystic cavity measuring up to 15 mm in diameter. Painstaking pathologic studies have been

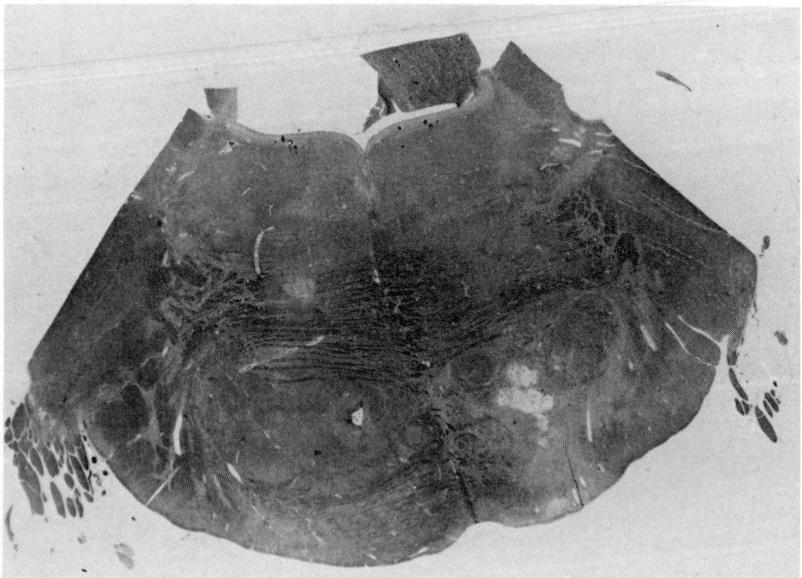

Figure 10-5. Lacunes. Small cystic cavities present in pons in area supplied by penetrating paramedian arteries (LFB-HE stain).

reported by a variety of authors, most recently Fisher, in which occlusive disease of a small penetrating artery is demonstrated as the cause of an individual lacune.[41] Some have suggested that small hemorrhages are the major cause of lacunes, but the expanding experience with CAT scan images[42] suggests that ischemia is the usual initial event in the development of a lacune.

Because the amount of brain tissue damaged in the process leading to a lacune is usually small, the corresponding clinical deficit is also limited; therefore, lacunes may be clinically silent. Attention has been drawn to the so called "lacunar syndromes" of motor hemiparesis, pure sensory stroke, ataxic hemiparesis, and dysarthria. But it must be remembered that such syndromes may result from a variety of pathologic mechanisms. The clinician must be aware that a hypertensive patient with limited neurologic deficit presenting with a history suggestive of vascular disease may have pathology limited to small penetrating cerebral arteries. This knowledge will influence the investigation and management of these patients.[43]

Intracerebral Hemorrhage

Spontaneous intracerebral hemorrhage is much more common in hypertensive than normotensive patients. The basal ganglia, cerebellum, and pons are the sites of most spontaneous hypertensive intracerebral hemorrhages. The destructive force of these hemorrhages is in keeping with an arterial source, although occasionally they may be caused by small arteriovenous malformations. Evidence favors rupture of intracerebral microaneurysms as the usual cause of spontaneous intracerebral hemorrhage. These microaneurysms were described first by Charcot and Bouchard in 1868,[44] misinterpreted or ignored for a number of years thereafter,[45,46] but then brought back to prominence by the report of Ross Russell in 1963.[47]

Using a micropaque post-mortem technique, Ross Russell found saccular dilations in intracerebral arteries in 15 of 16 hypertensive patients and 13 of 38 normotensive patients. Microaneurysms measuring 200-900 μm in diameter were found preferentially at points of bifurcation along branches of striate arteries measuring 100-300 μm. The aneurysmal wall was composed mainly of fibrous material with fragments of endothelium and elastica. One microaneurysm had ruptured at its thinnest point. Thrombus was found in a number of vessels and occlusion of the parent vessel was sometimes seen adjacent to the microaneurysm.

These microaneurysms are occasionally found in normotensive patients but their development is enhanced by hypertension. Spontaneous hemorrhage arising in the brain in a location other than the basal ganglia, pons, or cerebellum, the sites of microaneurysms, should alert the physician to other possible causes for hemorrhage such as clotting disorders or trauma (Figure 10-6).

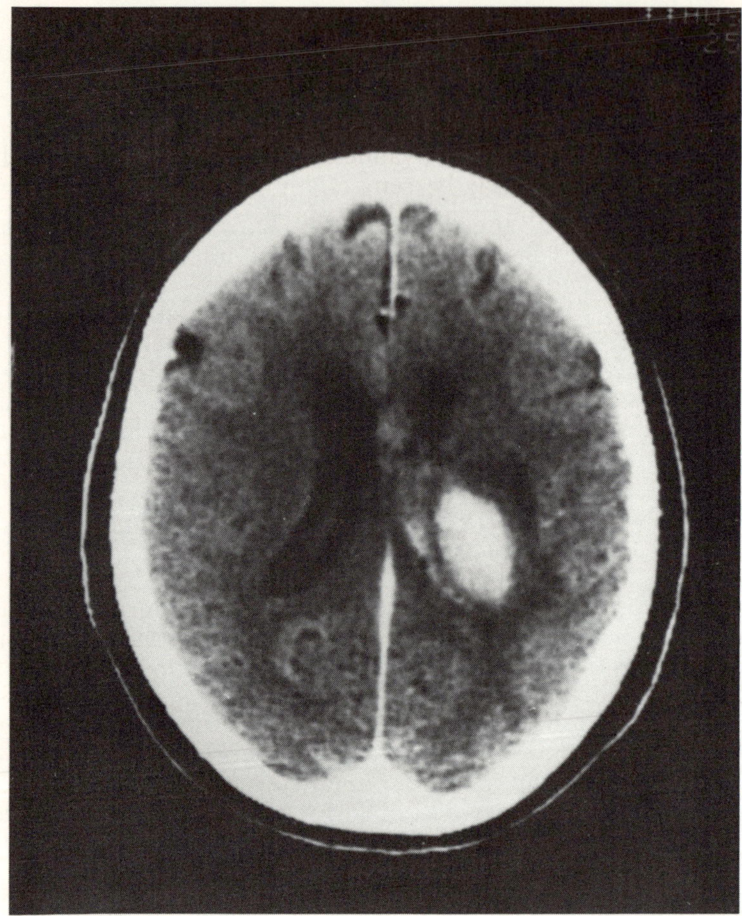

Figure 10-6. Hypertensive intracerebral hemorrhage arising from region of left thalamus with some bleeding into adjacent lateral ventricle.

Subcortical Arteriosclerotic Encephalopathy (Binswanger's Type)

Evidence has accumulated in recent years[48,49] supporting the early description by Binswanger[50] of a progressive neurologic syndrome comprised of focal neurologic deficits and disturbances in the mental state, including dementia, due to multiple small infarcts of the white matter caused by hyaline arteriosclerosis of small intracerebral arteries. This syndrome usually, but not always,[51] occurs in hypertensive patients.

The white matter of the cerebral hemispheres is reduced in amount, usually most pronounced in the occipital and temporal lobes. At times the process may be severe, with extensive dilatation of the lateral ventricles. Areas of demyelination may be sharply outlined in the white matter, with the cortex and subcortical arcuate fibers remaining intact. The arteries of the white matter show extensive hyaline change, with considerable thickening of the media. There may be remarkably little atherosclerotic involvement of the arteries of the base of the brain.

A variety of untested hypotheses have been proposed to explain such demyelination and subcortical arteriolar lesions, including a redistribution of cerebral blood flow,[52] the effects of local edema,[53] hypoxia,[54] or disturbed blood flow in the border zones between penetrating arteries.[48]

Binswanger's encephalopathy is an uncommon condition but its prevalence may have been underestimated. It has special pathologic features, so that a recent tendency to lump it under the general heading of multi-infarct dementia[55] will not assist efforts to identify specific etiologic factors. Future clinicopathologic correlation with CAT scan and nuclear magnetic resonance (NMR) images should improve the detection of Binswanger's disease during life.

Dementia and Arterial Disease

Senile dementia of the Alzheimer type[56] is now belatedly being recognized as the most frequent cause of severe dementia. For many years, arteriosclerosis was the unsubstantiated diagnosis in the majority of demented patients not otherwise assigned the uninformative diagnosis of "senile dementia." Dementia and stroke, two common clinical problems, rarely coexist in the same patient.

It is necessary to evaluate carefully what is meant by the term *dementia* in reports addressing the presumed role of vascular disease as a cause of dementia. Dementia implies an irreversible, usually progressive, form of mental disorder in which cognitive and intellectual functions are predominantly affected. Impairment of memory is usually one of the earliest signs. Clinical findings in patients with atherothrombotic brain infarction are dominated by motor, sensory, or aphasic defects which, although they may be cumulative, rarely produce the global disturbance of mental function characteristic of Alzheimer disease or other conditions causing general cognitive defects such as thyroid disease and vitamin B12, folate, or thiamine deficiency. On rare occasions, vascular disease in the form of multiple occlusions of major neck arteries will produce a slowly progressive dementia.

Aware of the lack of correlation between atherosclerosis of major neck vessels and dementia, some investigators have tried to determine if there is an association between disease of smaller cerebral vessels, as occurs with hypertension, and cognitive function. A study comparing intellectual function in 20 newly diagnosed untreated hypertensive men (diastolic blood pressure > 105 mm Hg) with 20 normotensive controls found a significant impairment of vigilance and attention span in the hypertensive group.[57] Intellectual loss, measured over a 10-year period, was significantly greater in a group of patients with diastolic blood pressure > 105 mm Hg when compared with matched, normotensive controls.[58]

Hypertension was the only risk factor significantly associated with dementia in a study comparing stroke patients free of intellectual deficit with those manifesting both stroke and dementia.[59] Further studies are needed to determine if deficits in performance by hypertensive subjects are due to factors such as disturbances in cerebral blood flow, changes in the oxygen extraction ratio, or the direct effect on neural function of pathologic change in cerebral blood vessels. Oxygen extraction ratios are unchanged in Alzheimer disease, indicating that ischemia is not a factor in that condition.[60]

Roth suggested[60] that

"arteriosclerotic psychosis could be differentiated from senile psychosis (Alzheimer disease) because the former presents as (1) dementia . . . associated with focal signs and symptoms of cerebrovascular disease or (2) . . . a remittent and markedly fluctuating course at some stage in the dementing process . . . combined with any one of the following features: emotional incontinence, the preservation of insight, or epileptiform seizures."

Neither neurologists nor psychiatrists conducting epidemiologic studies documenting the incidence and type of patients with dementia[62] derived much diagnostic confidence from such guidelines.

The designation of a group of patients with "multi-infarct dementia"[63] has the merit of directing attention to the primary problem of cerebral infarction in the relatively small group of patients with progressive intellectual decline as the dominant clinical problem but who also have evidence of multiple strokes.

Unfortunately, the notion of multi-infarct dementia has been promoted with unjustified enthusiasm as an explanation for dementia. For instance, a study claiming to demonstrate that 60% of patients with "vascular dementia" had multiple infarcts[64] actually provides evidence that the occurrence of multiple infarcts limited to one cerebral hemisphere is the same in patients with ischemic stroke without intellectual impairment as in demented patients. Another report started with the unjustified premise that a history of stroke and hypertension in the same patient was sufficient evidence to incriminate vascular disease as an explanation for accompanying dementia.[65] The relative importance of vascular disease as a cause for dementia remains unsettled.

What is needed for clinical precision in this area is an available objective marker for Alzheimer disease (preferably biochemical) and continuing careful clinical, metabolic, and pathologic examination of patients with intellectual decline and cerebrovascular disease.

Summary

Hypertension thus alters the function of the brain in diverse ways, ranging from subjective abnormalities such as dizziness and headache to severe events such as cerebral infarction, hemorrhage, and dementia. The close link between elevated blood pressure and these insults to the brain emphasizes the importance of blood pressure control to their prevention.

References

1. Haynes RB, Sackett DL, Taylor DW, Gibson ES, Johnson AL: Increased absenteeism from work after detection and labeling of hypertensive patients. N Eng J Med **299:**741, 1978
2. Weiss NS: Relation of high blood pressure to headache, epistaxis and selected other symptoms. New Eng J Med **287:**631, 1972
3. Bulpitt CJ, Dollery CT, Caine S: Change in symptoms of hypertensive patients after referral to hospital clinic. Brit Heart J **38:**121, 1976
4. Gill DG, Mendes da Costa B, Cameron JS, Joseph MC, Ogg CS, Chantler C: Analysis of one hundred (100) children with severe and persistent hypertension. Arch Dis Child **51:**951, 1976
5. Ameny A, Berthaux P, Birkenhager W: Antihypertensive therapy in patients above 60 years (4th interim report of the European Working Party on High Blood Pressure in the Elderly (EWPHE). Clin Sci (Suppl) **55:**263s, 1978
6. Wolff HG: Headache and Other Head Pain: New York, Oxford University Press, 1966
7. Pickering G: High Blood Pressure: Second edition, London, Churchill, 1968, p 324
8. Selby G, Lance JW: Observations on 500 cases of migraine and allied vascular headache. J Neurol Neurosurg Psychiat **23:**23, 1960
9. Robinson JO: Symptoms and the discovery of high blood pressure. J Psychosom Res **13:**157, 1969
10. Waters WE: Headache and blood pressure in the community. Brit Med J **1:**142, 1971
11. Veterans Administration Co-operative Study Group on Antihypertensive Agents I: results in patients with diastolic blood pressure averaging 115–129 monthly. JAMA **202:**1028, 1967
12. Pickering GW: The cerebrospinal fluid pressure in arterial hypertension. Clin Sci **3:**397, 1934
13. Taylor RD, Corcoran AC, Page IH: Increased cerebrospinal pressure and papilledema in malignant hypertension. Arch Int Med **93:**818, 1954
14. Wolf PA, Kannel WB, Verter J: Current Status of Risk Factors for Stroke in Neurology Clinics, Symposium on Cerebrovascular Disease, edited by Barnett HJM, Philadelphia, Saunders, 1983, p 317
15. Carter A: Hypertensive therapy in stroke survivors. Lancet **1:**485, 1970
16. Wolf FW, Lindeman RD: Effects of treatment in hypertension: results of a controlled study. J Chronic Dis **19:**227, 1966

17. Management Committee: The Australian Therapeutic Trial in Mild Hypertension. Lancet **1:**1261, 1980
18. Strandgaard S, Olesen J, Skinhoj E, Lassen NA: Autoregulation of brain circulation in severe arterial hypertension. Br Med J **1:**507, 1973
19. Hulse JA, Taylor VSI, Dillon MJ: Blindness and paraplegia in severe childhood hypertension. Lancet **2:**553, 1979
20. Rodda R, Denny-Brown D: The cerebral arteries in experimental hypertension. I. The nature of arteriolar constriction and its effects on the collateral circulation. Am J Pathol **49:**53, 1966
21. Haggendal E, Johansson B: On the pathophysiology of the increased cerebrovascular permeability in acute arterial hypertension in cats. Acta Neurol Scand **48:**265, 1972
22. Lassen NA, Agnoli A: Upper limit of autoregulation of cerebral blood flow in the pathogenesis of acute hypertensive encephalopathy. Scand J Clin Lab Invest **30:**113, 1972
23. Dinsdale HB, Robertson DM, Haas RA: Cerebral blood flow in acute hypertension. Arch Neurol **31:**80, 1974
24. Nag S, Robertson DM, Dinsdale HB: Cerebral cortical changes in acute experimental hypertension: an ultrastructural study. Lab Invest **36:**150, 1977
25. Lassen NA: The luxury perfusion syndrome and its possible relation to acute metabolic acidosis localized within the brain. Lancet **2:**1113, 1966
26. Ross R, Glomset JA: Atherosclerosis in the arterial smooth muscle cells. Science **180:**1332, 1973
27. Fisher CM, Gore I, Okabe N, White TD: Atherosclerosis of the carotid and vertebral arteries—extracranial and intracranial. J Neuropath Exp Neurol **24:**455, 1965
28. Wissler RW, Vesselinovith D, Getz GS: Abnormalities of the arterial wall and its metabolism in atherogenesis. Cardiovasc Dis **18:**331, 1976
29. Russel RWR: The source of retinal emboli. Lancet **2:**789, 1968
30. Cole FM, Yates PO: Comparative incidence of cerebrovascular lesions in normotensive and hypertensive patients. Neurology (Minneapolis) **18:**255, 1968
31. Harrison MJG, Marshall J: The results of carotid angiography and cerebral infarction in normotensive and hypertensive subjects. J Neurol Sci **24:**243, 1975
32. Harrison MJG, Wilson LA: Effect of blood pressure on prevalence of carotid atheroma. Stroke **14:**550, 1983
33. Metro JRA, Schwartz CJ, Zinger A: Relationship between aortic plaques and age, sex and blood pressure. Brit Med J **1:**205, 1964
34. Feigin I, Budzilovich GN: The general pathology of cerebrovascular disease. *In* Handbook of Clinical Neurology, Vascular Disease of the Nervous System, Part I, edited by Vinken RJ, Druin GW. Amsterdam, North-Holland, 1972, p 128
35. Fisher CM: Cerebral miliary aneurysms in hypertension. Am J Pathol **66:**313, 1972
36. Spiro D, Lattes RG, Wiener J: The cellular pathology of experimental hypertension. I. Hyperplastic arteriolarsclerosis. Am J Pathol **47:**19, 1965
37. Gardner VL, Matthews MA: Ultrastructure of the wall of small arteries in early experimental rat hypertension. J Pathol **97:**51, 1969
38. Durant-Fardel M: Traité du ramollissement du cerveau. Paris and London, Balliere, 1843

39. Gautier JC: Cerebral ischemic in hypertension. *In* Vascular Diseases of the Central Nervous System, edited by Ross Russel, RW: London, Churchill-Livingston, 1983, p 235
40. Fisher CM: Lacunes: small, deep cerebral infarcts. Neurology (Minneapolis) **15**:774, 1965
41. Fisher CM: The arterial lesions underlying lacunes. Acta Neuropathol **12**:1, 1969
42. Donnan GA, Tress BM, Blandin PF: A prospective study of lacunar infarction using computerized tomography. Neurology **32**:49, 1982
43. Miller VT: Lacunar stroke. A reassessment. Arch Neurol **40**:129, 1983
44. Charcot JM, Bouchard C: Nouvelles recherches sur la pathogenie de l'hémorrhage cérébrale. Archives de physiologie normale et pathologique **1**:110, 643, 735, 1868
45. Ellis AG: The pathogenesis of spontaneous cerebral hemorrhage. Proc Pathol Soc Phil **12**:197, 1909
46. Green FHK: Miliary aneurysms in the brain. J Pathol Bacteriol **33**:71, 1930
47. Russell RWR: Observations on intracerebral aneurysms. Brain **86**:425, 1963
48. Jellinger K, Numayer E: Progressive subcorticale vasculare Encephalopathie Binswanger. Eine klinisch-neuropathologische Studie. Arch Psychiat Nervenkr **205**:523, 1964
49. Caplan LR, Schoene WC: Clinical features of subcortical arteriosclerotic encephalopathy (Binswanger's disease). Neurology (Minneapolis) **28**:1206, 1978
50. Binswanger O: Die Begrenzung der allgemeinen progressiven Paralysie. Berlin Klin Wochenschr **31**:1103, 1137, 1180, 1894
51. Loizou LA, Jefferson JM, Schmidt WT: Subcortical arteriosclerotic encephalopathy (Binswanger's type) and cortical infarcts in a young normotensive patient. J Neurol Neurosurg Psychiat **45**:409, 1982
52. Okeda R: Correlative morphometric studies of cerebral arteries in Binswanger's encephalopathy and hypertensive encephalopathy. Acta Neuropathol (Berlin) **26**:23, 1973
53. Feigin I, Poppoff N: Neuropathological changes late in cerebral edema: The relationship to trauma, hypertensive disease and Binswanger's encephalopathy. J Neuropathol Exp Neurol **22**:500, 1963
54. Feigin I, Budzilovich G, Weinberg G, Ogata J: Degeneration of white matter in hypoxia, acidosis, and edema. J Neuropathol Exp Neurol **32**:125, 1973
55. Hachinski D: Multi-infarct dementia. *In* Neurologic Clinics, Vol. 1, No. 1. Symposium on Cerebrovascular Diseases, edited by Barnett HJM, Philadelphia, Saunders, 1983, p 29
56. Terry RD, Katzman R: Senile dementia of the Alzheimer type. Ann Neurol **14**:497, 1983
57. Boller F, Vrtunski B, Mack JL, Kim Y: Neuropsychologic correlates of hypertension. Arch Neurol **34**:701, 1977
58. Wilkie F, Eisdorfer C: Intelligence and blood pressure in the aged. Science **172**:959, 1971
59. Ladurner G, Iliff LD, Lechner H: Clinical factors associated with dementia in stroke. J Neurol Psychiat **45**:97, 1982
60. Frackowiack RSJ, Pozzilli C, Legg NJ: Regional cerebral oxygen supply and utilization in dementia: A clinical and physiological study with oxygen $^{15}O_2$ and positron tomography. Brain **104**:753, 1981

61. Roth M: The natural history of mental disorder in old age. J Ment Sci **101**:281, 1955
62. Akesson HO: A population study of senile and arteriosclerotic psychoses. Hum Hered **19**:546, 1969
63. Hachinski VC, Lassen NA, Marshall J: Multi-infarct dementia. A cause of mental deterioration in the elderly. Lancet **2**:207, 1974
64. Ladurner G, Sager WP: Morphologische Bedingungskonstellation der vaskularen (Multiinfarkt) Demenz. Fortschr Neurol Psychiatr **49**:53, 1981
65. Marsden CO, Harrison MJG: Outcome of investigation of patients with presenile dementia. Brit Med J **1**:249, 1972

Chapter 11

Epidemiologic Appraisal of Hypertension and Stroke Risk

Philip A. Wolf, William B. Kannel,
and Joel Verter

Introduction

Stroke is the most common disabling and life-threatening neurological disease of adult life and the most devastating clinical manifestation of hypertension and atherosclerosis. It is not a chance or random occurrence, as the term cerebrovascular *accident* implies, but is the consequence of a course of events starting many years before. Elevated blood pressure is the major determinant of stroke occurrence. The evolution of hypertension and other host and environmental precursors into clinical manifestations of cerebrovascular disease have been delineated by prospective epidemiologic study of the general population. Prevention, not improved medical and surgical treatment of the stroke patient, is more likely to reduce the morbidity and mortality from stroke. Prevention requires correction of the precursors of stroke in susceptible individuals, notably vigorous and sustained control of hypertension. Evidence that such an approach is fruitful is emerging from controlled clinical trials in stroke and cardiovascular-disease-prone persons and mortality data that suggest an accelerating decline in death rates from stroke.

Identification of the precursors of stroke, their frequency, and relative impact has been accomplished in the prospective study of free-living popu-

Supported in part by grants numbers NIH-IPO-INS-16367 and 1-RO1-NS-17950-01 with Contract NO1-NS-2-2398 (Philip A. Wolf, M.D., National Institute of Neurological Communicative Disorders and Stroke); and Contracts numbers NIH-NO1-HV-92922 and NIH-NO1-HV-52971 (William B. Kannel, M.D., National Heart, Lung and Blood Institute).

lations such as the Heart-Disease Epidemiology Study at Framingham, Massachusetts. These studies provide data on the way clinical manifestations of cerebrovascular disease evolve and how stroke is related to the other cardiovascular consequences of atherosclerotic and hypertensive disease, particularly coronary heart disease (CHD) and congestive heart failure (CHF). The manifestations and precursors of stroke and CHD differ in men and women, at different ages, and in different racial groups. Assessment of these differences may disclose important clues to pathogenesis and thereby provide strategies for prevention.

Incidence

It is estimated that about 400,000 stroke patients are discharged annually from acute-care hospitals in the United States, three-fourths after an initial stroke and the remainder after a recurrence.[1] The reported incidence of stroke varies widely, depending on the source of the sample (hospitalized cases or general population), its age composition, and whether initial and recurrent strokes are included.[2] Stroke incidence is strikingly related to age, with incidence rates more than doubling in each successive decade above age 55. Clearly, the increasing numbers of elderly persons in the population makes stroke prevention a public health necessity.

Analagous manifestations of CHD and cerebrovascular disease may be compared by examining age and sex-specific incidence rates (per 1000) of myocardial infarction (MI) and atherothrombotic brain infarction (ABI) (Figure 11-1). These Framingham Study data represent 24 years of follow-up of approximately 5184 men and women 30 to 63 years old and free of stroke at entry to the study in 1950. They represent a sample of the general population of adults resident in the town of Framingham, MA.

Follow-up has been satisfactory, with 85% taking each exam and only 3% completely lost to follow-up. In men, the age-adjusted average annual incidence rate for MI is 8.5 per 1000 persons, three times the 2.7 per 1000 rate for ABI. For women, age-adjusted average annual incidence rates of MI and ABI are nearly identical at 2.4 and 2.1 per 1000 respectively. In both sexes, rates rise with age, but the 20-year lag in MI incidence experienced by women does not occur for ABI, where age-specific rates are similar. Overall, the incidence rate of ABI is about 30% greater in men than women, and this sex differential is slightly greater below age 65. Although stroke generally and ABI specifically occurs most frequently in old age, 20% of ABI's occur in persons below age 65.

Frequency of Stroke by Type

Estimates of the prevalence of the different clinical varieties of cerebrovascular disease vary widely depending upon the source of the data.

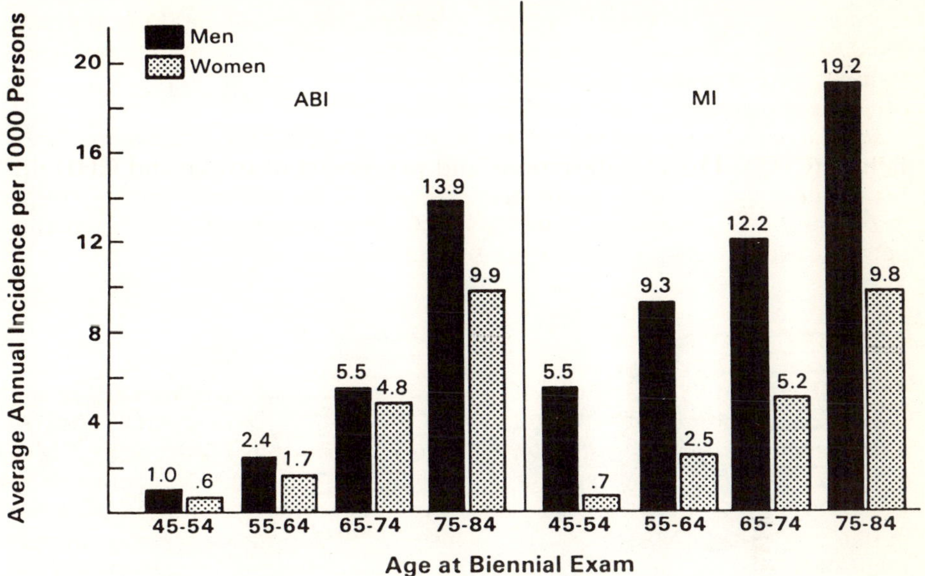

Figure 11-1. Incidence of myocardial infarction (MI) and atherothrombotic brain infarction (ABI) by age in each sex, 24-year follow-up. The Framingham Study.

Hospital data containing patients admitted to neurological services are subject to selective biases and are likely to over-represent younger, more severe, and diagnostically difficult stroke cases. Since it is frequently lethal, intraparenchymatous hemorrhage is over-represented in postmortem series. General population survey data, while more representative, often suffer from small numbers of cases, and lack the uniform and sophisticated clinical and laboratory evaluations needed to distinguish between stroke types.[3]

Distinctions by type of stroke—ABI due to occlusive disease of large arteries, lacunar infarction, cerebral embolism (CE), intraparenchymatous hemorrhage (IH), and subarachnoid hemorrhage (SH)—are clearly necessary for an understanding of the epidemiology of the various manifestations of cerebrovascular disease, since these manifestations may have different pathogenetic mechanisms.

In the Framingham cohort, at the end of 24 years of follow-up, 344 initial cases of stroke occurred (Figure 11-2). ABI is the most common type, accounting for 60%, with transient ischemic attacks (TIA's) unaccompanied by stroke representing an additional 10% of total stroke cases. Thus two-thirds of stroke cases are due to ischemia and infarction secondary to occlusive disease of the small and medium-sized arteries. Stroke due to CE, with a recognized embolic source, accounts for 14% of cases. Together, IH and SH comprise 14% of the total. SH, usually due to pathologically con-

FREQUENCY OF STROKE BY TYPE

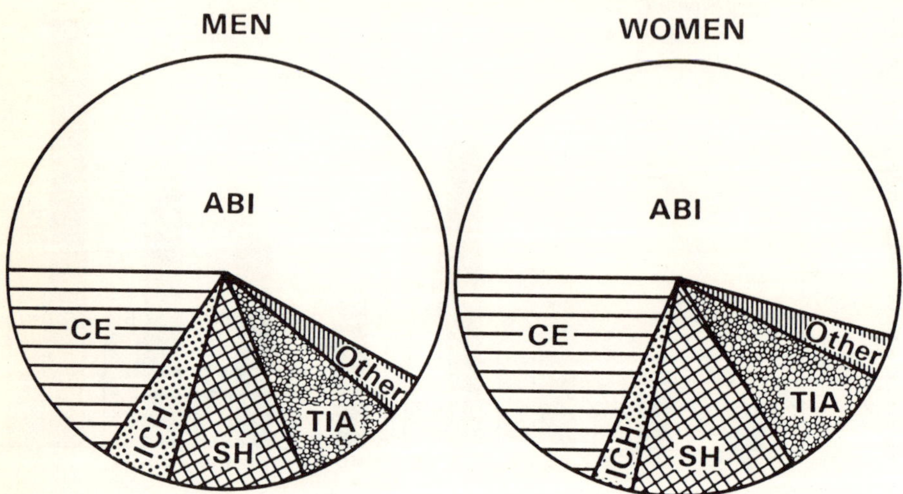

Figure 11-2. The relative frequency of clinical manifestations of stroke in men and women, ages 65–74, 24-year follow-up. The Framingham Study. ABT = atherothrombotic brain infarction; CE = cerebral embolus; ICH = intracerebral hemorrhage; SH = subarachnoid hemorrhage; TIA = transient ischemic attack.

firmed ruptured berry aneurysm of the circle of Willis, is about twice as frequent as spontaneous IH. The frequency of each stroke type is similar in the two sexes (Figure 11-2), in contrast to the frequency of the various clinical manifestations of CHD. A marked excess of MI and sudden death is seen in men, and an excess of angina pectoris in women (Figure 11-3).

Risk Factors

Major reduction in disability and death from stroke is more likely to come from prevention than from more effective medical or surgical treatment. Identification of the major risk factors for stroke and of the stroke-prone individual should facilitate preventive efforts. A universal finding in epidemiologic studies is that the most important risk factor for stroke, infarction as well as hemorrhage, is hypertension. Impaired cardiac function, with evidence of CHF, prior CHD, or electrocardiographic abnormalities, are also powerful contributors to stroke incidence. Elevated blood lipids, cigarette smoking, diabetes, and obesity are less potent precursors for stroke than for CHD or peripheral vascular disease.

FREQUENCY OF CORONARY HEART DISEASE BY TYPE

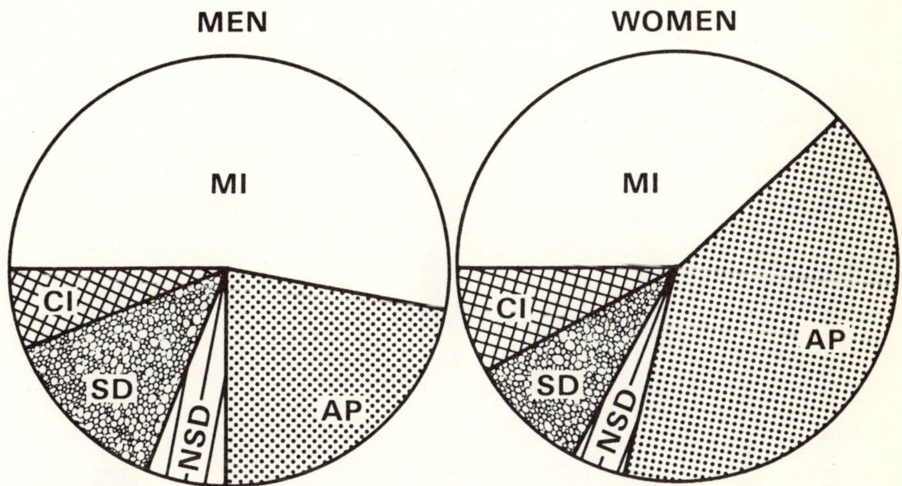

Figure 11-3. The relative frequency of clinical manifestation of coronary heart disease in men and women, ages 65-74, 24-year follow-up. The Framingham Study. MI = myocardial infarction; AP = angina pectoris; SD = sudden death; CI = coronary insufficiency; NSD = non-sudden death.

Cerebral embolism is chiefly a consequence of cardiac and valvular disease, MI, and irregular cardiac rhythm (notably atrial fibrillation), or complications of arteriography, carotid, and cardiac surgery.

Intraparenchymatous hemorrhage is chiefly due to rupture of a hypertension-induced Charcot-Bouchard microaneurysm, or as a complication of anticoagulant therapy. Spontaneous subarachnoid hemorrhage is chiefly secondary to rupture of a congenital aneurysm of the circle of Willis and may be associated with pre-existing hypertension.

Hypertension

Hypertension is the preeminent precursor of stroke generally and is strongly related to ABI and each of the other stroke types (Figure 11-4). Hypertension is not only the most powerful contributor to stroke incidence, it is also a highly prevalent abnormality having an adverse impact on a large portion of the population.[4] Risk of stroke is related to the height of the blood pressure throughout its range.[5] For ABI, incidence rises as pressure rises, with an adverse impact among mild, moderate, and severe hy-

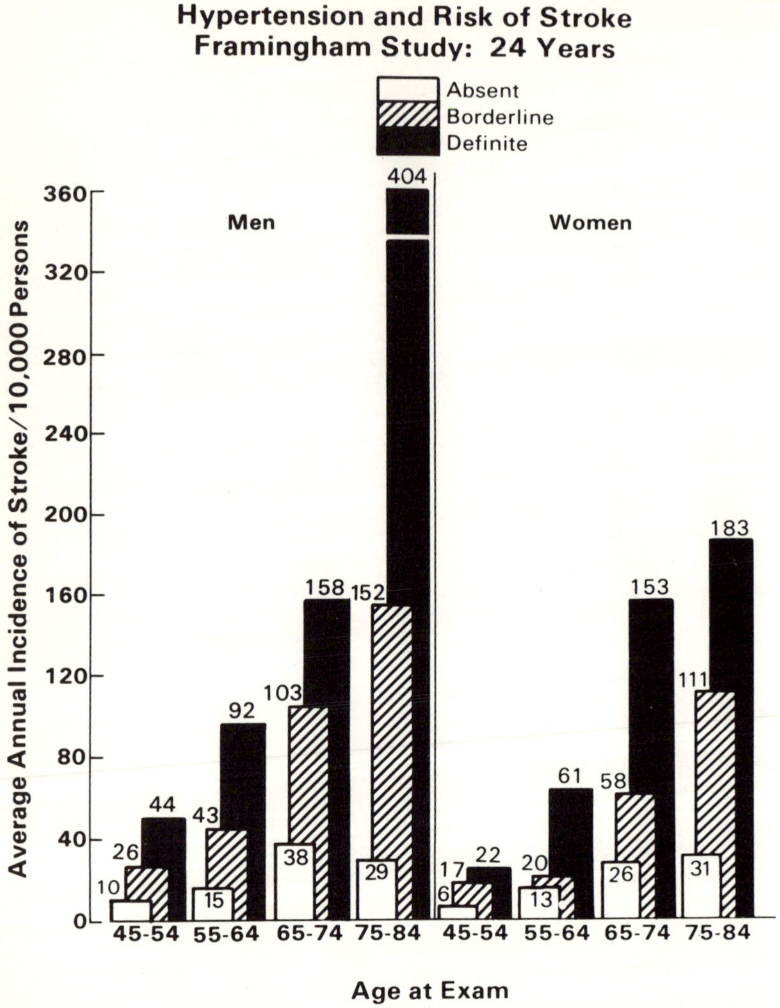

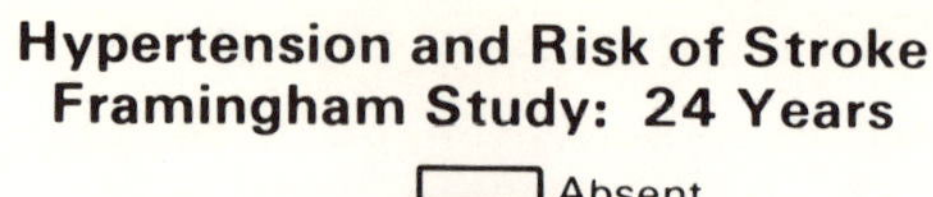

Figure 11-4. The relationship of hypertension to incidence of stroke in men and women, 24-year follow-up. The Framingham Study.

pertensives. There is no critical value of pressure level, systolic or diastolic, below which stroke or ABI does not occur. For stroke generally, and for ABI specifically, there is no evidence that women tolerate hypertension better than men, nor is there a waning of impact of hypertension in the elderly, where most cases occur (Table 11-1). These data strongly suggest that control of hypertension is no less important for stroke prevention in the eighth and ninth decades than it is at younger ages.

Table 11-1
Impact of Hypertension on Brain Infarction.
Incidence by Age and Sex.
Framingham Study, 24-Year Follow-up

Age	Risk Ratio Hypertension/ Normotension		Regression Coefficients*	
	Men	Women	Men	Women
45–54	5.0	7.0	0.850	1.022
55–64	22.0	14.3	1.389	1.371
65–74	3.7	10.8	0.597	1.176
75–84	12.7	— [a]	1.396	1.138
All Ages (Direct Adj.)	7.8	11.8	0.946	1.195

[a]No events in 75–84-year-old normotensive women.
Hypertension > 160/95
*All regression coefficients $p < 0.01$
The regression coefficients are based on the univariate logistic regression of brain infarction on hypertension status. The coefficients are tested against the null hypothesis that they are zero. This is similar to a test that the relative odds are one.

Components of Blood Pressure

An examination of various components of blood pressure in relation to incidence of brain infarction gives no indication that any feature of blood pressure is more closely linked than systolic pressure (Table 11-2). In order to place these components of blood pressure on equal footing for the different ranges of values, standardized regression coefficients are given for each; the larger the coefficient, the greater the impact on ABI incidence. Clearly, each component of blood pressure exerts a powerful effect; none is more powerful than systolic pressure, although there is no significant difference between the various components of blood pressure.

Compared with diastolic pressure, systolic pressure exerts no less impact on ABI incidence; this is true for the entire 45–84 year age group (Table 11-3). There is no substantial lessening of this impact with increasing age, for systolic pressure particularly. This contradicts the notion that the effect of blood pressure wanes with advancing age and that systolic elevations are innocuous, particularly in the elderly. With respect to stroke incidence generally, and ABI incidence particularly, systolic pressure exerts a greater influence than diastolic and does so through the mid and late adult years (Table 11-4).

Table 11-2
Comparison of Impact of Components of Blood Pressure
on Incidence of Brain Infarction. Subjects 45–84.
Framingham Study, 24-Year Follow-up

Component of Blood Pressure	Logistic Regression Coefficients Brain Infarction	
	Men	Women
Systolic Pressure	.031	.031
Diastolic Pressure	.032	.051
Mean Arterial Pressure	.042	.049
Pulse Pressure	.040	.037

$p < .0001$ for all coefficients

Other measures or components of the blood pressure include lability of systolic blood pressure and the tension-time index (the product of the systolic blood pressure and the heart rate). Both measures are highly correlated to the level of systolic blood pressure and neither makes any additional independent contribution to risk when systolic blood pressure is taken into account.

Table 11-3
Regression of ABI Incidence on Systolic vs. Diastolic
Blood Pressure, by Age. 24-Year Follow-up

Age	Regression Coefficients			
	Systolic BP		Diastolic BP	
	Men	Women	Men	Women
45–54	.029**	.025***	.036**	.053***
55–64	.036***	.033***	.070***	.069***
65–74	.018**	.026***	.008	.047***
75–84	.024**	.026***	.014	.036*
Bivariate Coefficient[1]	.026***	.028***	.038***	.054***

$*p < 0.05$
$**p < 0.01$
$***p < 0.001$
[1]Bivariate = age and blood pressure.

Table 11-4
Two-Year Incidence of Stroke According to Level of Systolic and Diastolic Blood Pressure, Men and Women, Age 50–79. Framingham Study, 24-Year Follow-up

		Systolic Blood Pressure					
	Diastolic Blood Pressure	<140 at Rate/1000		140–159 at Rate/1000		160+ at Rate/1000	
		Risk	Age Adj.	Risk	Age Adj.	Risk	Age Adj.
Men	<90	6735	5.3	1816	7.4	544	21.0
	90–94	478	6.5	911	12.1	499	10.8
	95+	137	13.1	761	12.3	1372	24.8
Women	<90	7827	3.8	2894	6.6	1295	9.6
	90–94	344	0.0	1195	8.3	1009	11.9
	95+	91	0.0	684	18.6	2192	16.8

Isolated Systolic Hypertension

With the disproportionate rise in systolic pressure that occurs with advancing age, isolated systolic hypertension becomes highly prevalent. Above age 75, 18% of men and 30% of women have this condition. However, it is far from innocuous. Not only is systolic blood pressure as powerful a predictor of brain infarction as the diastolic component, but isolated elevations of systolic pressure are also important. Even in the elderly (ages 65 to 84) there is at least a two-fold increased risk of brain infarction among those with systolic pressures exceeding 160 mm Hg accompanied by diastolic pressures consistently below 95 mm Hg (Table 11-5).

Because hypertension is the predominant contributor to stroke incidence, the importance of isolated systolic hypertension in the development of strokes was studied in the Framingham cohort, taking into account the degree of associated arterial rigidity. The arterial rigidity was estimated from pulse-wave recording using the degree of blunting of the pulse-wave diastolic notch as a measure of loss of arterial elastic recoil. Although this is an imperfect measure of arterial rigidity, risk of cardiovascular disease was found to be related to the degree of blunting.[6] Also, the prevalence of isolated systolic hypertension and pulse pressure were found to be related. All three—pulse pressure, systolic hypertension, and pulse-wave changes and diastolic notch blunting—increased with age.

Based on prospective data relating future stroke incidence to systolic pressure, diastolic pressure, age and pulse-wave configuration, isolated systolic hypertension was found to be an independent risk factor for develop-

Table 11-5
Risk of Brain Infarction in the Elderly with Isolated Systolic
Hypertension, Systolic 160+ mm Hg, Diastolic <95 mm Hg.
Framingham Study, 24-Year Follow-up

Isolated Systolic Hypertension	Average Annual Incidence Per 1000			
	65–74		65–84	
	Men	Women	Men	Women
Absent	4.6	3.8	9.4	7.9
Present	11.0	8.3	30.7	12.0
Risk Ratio	2.4*	2.2*	3.3*	1.5

*$p < .05$

ment of stroke, taking associated arterial rigidity into account. Subjects with isolated systolic hypertension were found to experience two to four times as many strokes as normotensive persons.[6] Taken alone, diastolic pressure was related to stroke incidence; in the subject with systolic hypertension, the diastolic component adds little to risk assessment. In men in this systolic hypertension subgroup the diastolic pressure was actually misleading (Figure 11-5).

These findings strongly suggest that the increased risk of stroke associated with systolic hypertension is probably a direct result of the pressure and not merely a reflection of the underlying arterial rigidity. Treatment to lower the systolic pressure may therefore be efficacious in reducing the risk of stroke in systolic hypertension. A controlled trial to determine the indications, contraindications, best drugs, dosage, side effects, benefits, and hazards has recently been undertaken.[7]

Stroke and CHD Incidence According to Severity of Hypertension

It is often asserted that at borderline levels of hypertension coronary disease is the chief risk, while at more severe levels of hypertension, stroke is the chief risk. This was examined by determining the ratio of CHD to stroke incidence at different levels of hypertension in the Framingham cohort (Table 11-6). The ratio of MI to ABI in men diminishes from about 6:1 to 2:1 going from normotension to moderately severe and severe hypertension. At borderline values the ratio is intermediate at 4:1. In women the ratio is smaller for all blood pressure classes. It diminishes with increasing severity of hypertension, and in moderately severe and severe hypertension the incidence of stroke exceeds that of MI by 25%.

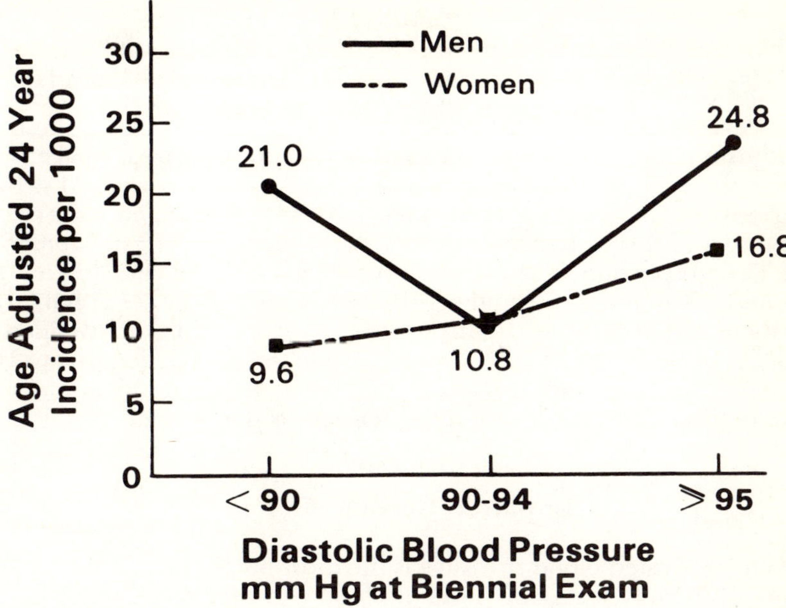

Figure 11-5. Risk of stroke according to diastolic blood pressure. Subjects with systolic pressures exceeding 160 mm Hg, men and women 50–79, 24-year follow-up. The Framingham Study.

Table 11-6
Ratio of Myocardial Infarction to Brain Infarction According to Blood Pressure Status

BP Status	Ratio of Age-Adjusted Average Annual Incidence	
	Men	Women
Normal BP	8.8	4.1
Borderline Hypertension	4.2	1.35
Hypertension	2.0	0.74

It is also alleged that at normal pressures or moderate elevations ABI's predominate, while at high pressures hemorrhage predominates. Actually, the proportion of strokes due to ABI increases as severity of hypertension increases, from 42% to 70% in men and from 37% to 77% in women (Table 11-7). Percentages were calculated after age adjustment using the ratio of age-adjusted annual incidence rates of ABI to those of total stroke. In normotensives, 42% of stroke in men and 37% in women were ABI's. In mild hypertensives, 54% of stroke in men and 54% in women were ABI. In moderate and severe hypertensives, 70% in men and 77% in women were ABI. The proportion of stroke due to IH was 3% in normotensives, 5% in mild, and 4% in moderate and severe hypertensives. Thus, with increasing severity of hypertension, the proportion of stroke due to ABI increased, usually at the expense of SAH and CE, while the proportion due to IH did not change. So the clinical dictum that IH is the predominant variety of stroke in moderate and severe hypertensives is not borne out.

Impaired Cardiac Function

While elevated blood pressure is the most potent risk factor for stroke, it is not uniformly so. At any level of blood pressure there are those whose risk of cardiovascular disease in general and stroke in particular is higher than others. This increased risk occurs in those with other risk factor abnormalities—notably, impaired cardiac function.

Cardiac impairment ranks third, following age and hypertension, as a risk factor for stroke in general and for ABI specifically. At any level of blood pressure, persons with cardiac disease, occult or overt, have more than twice the risk of stroke. Cardiac impairments include overt disease such as CHD and CHF, evidence of left ventricle hypertrophy (LVH) by ECG or x-ray, and rhythm abnormalities, particularly atrial fibrillation (AF).

Table 11-7
Ratio of ABI to All Strokes According to Blood Pressure Status

BP Status	Ratio of Age Adjusted Average Annual Incidence Rates	
	Men	Women
Normal BP	.42	.37
Borderline Hypertension	.54	.54
Hypertension	.70	.77

Overt evidence of impaired cardiac function, prior CHD, and CHF is significantly related to stroke and ABI incidence (Table 11-8). Risk of ABI is more than double in those men and women with CHD, and those with CHF have an even greater increase in risk.[8,9] LVH by ECG, probably reflecting the impact of prolonged or severe hypertension, increases in prevalence with age and blood pressure. Risk of brain infarction increases substantially, more than four-fold, in those who develop this ECG abnormality. This excess risk persists on adjustment for blood pressure and age. In contrast to ECG-LVH, generalized cardiac enlargement by x-ray is a less powerful predictor of ABI. Nonspecific ST and T wave abnormalities, intraventricular block, and atrioventricular block are also associated with an increased ABI incidence. Atrial fibrillation, even in the absence of rheumatic heart disease, is a powerful precursor of stroke—specifically of embolic stroke.[10,11] After adjusting for these variables, those with nonrheumatic atrial fibrillation develop strokes at more than five times the rate of those without this abnormality.[12,13,14,15]

Other Risk Factors

Unlike CHD, blood lipid abnormalities and cigarette smoking are not convincingly related to stroke or ABI. Diabetes does make a definite independent contribution to ABI incidence and is certainly strongly related to hypertension.

Assessment of the net effect of diabetes mellitus through multivariate analysis indicates an independent contribution in both sexes, but with more of the diabetic effect mediated through blood-pressure elevation for women than for men. While diabetes is a potent independent contributor

---

Table 11-8
Risk of Stroke with Pre-existing Evidence of Coronary Heart Disease and Heart Failure. Subjects 45–84. Framingham Study, 24-Year Follow-up

| | Average Annual Incidence per 10,000 Person Years (Age-Adjusted) | |
	Men	Women
No Pre-existing CHD	37	28
CHD without CHF	94	70
CHD and CHF	127	143

to ABI risk in both sexes in all age groups, the risk is strongly influenced by the frequently associated risk factors of elevated blood pressure and cardiac impairments. For stroke prevention, control of these associated risk factors would seem more important than vigorous treatment of the diabetes per se.

Obesity is clearly related to hypertension, and increase in weight is associated with an increase in systolic blood-pressure level. This direct relationship between weight change to change in blood pressure is significant and far more powerful than the relationship of blood pressure to basal weight level per se.[16]

An increase in relative weight of five units corresponds to an increase in systolic blood pressure of 3.3 mm Hg.[17] In addition to contributing to the development and worsening of hypertension, obesity adds a substantial burden of cardiac work. It does so in the form of expanded intravascular and circulating blood volumes to the heart already laboring under the high afterload induced by hypertension.[18]

Hemoglobin

Data from Framingham[19] have called attention to the relationship of high-normal blood hemoglobin concentration (or high-normal hematocrit level) to increased incidence of cerebral infarction. Confirmation of this relationship has come from a Japanese autopsy study[20] and from several clinical and radiologic studies of stroke patients.[21,22] While it had long been recognized that pathologically elevated hematocrits predisposed to stroke, the role of increased blood hemoglobin concentration in the upper-normal range in promoting cerebral infarction was not recognized.[20,22,23]

Elevated blood pressure and cigarette smoking are associated with high-normal blood hemoglobin concentrations. These associated variables account for much but not all of the relationship to ABI incidence.

Race

Substantial racial differences in stroke morbidity and mortality rates have been reported. Japanese (living in Japan) have high stroke death rates, higher than death rates from heart disease. Intracerebral hemorrhage as the chief type of stroke among Japanese has been declining relative to cerebral infarction. Autopsy studies derived from the prospective study of stroke in Hisayama, Japan where the rate of postmortem exam is high now show hemorrhage accounting for only 30% of all strokes.[24] Japanese migration to Hawaii and California is associated with correspondingly lower death rates from stroke.[25] These data suggest the presence of major environmental influences on racial and ethnic patterns of disease.

Mortality data consistently show higher death rates from stroke among blacks in the United States, undoubtedly related to the higher prevalence of hypertension among blacks.[26] Blacks in the southeastern part of the United States have especially high stroke death rates compared with whites at all ages in both men and women. The racial differences generally decrease with advancing age and have been diminishing over time.[27]

The Stroke Risk Profile

Risk factor information can be efficiently synthesized into a composite risk estimate using multiple logistic equations. These describe the conditional probability of a cerebrovascular event for any given set of risk variables from their known coefficients of regression on incidence and constants for the intercept.[28] This allows more logical selection of patients for preventive management and avoids underestimating the risk of persons with borderline levels of multiple risk factor according to categorical assessments of normal or abnormal. It also avoids over-reacting to those with only a single "abnormality."

Using such formulations, risk estimates can be obtained over a wide range, depending on the composite strength of the ingredients. Using a set of ingredients applicable to cardiovascular disease in general (systolic blood pressure, serum cholesterol, glucose tolerance, cigarette habit, and ECG-LVH), one-tenth of the asymptomatic population can be identified from which about one-third of the ABI's will emerge.[5]

Signs of Compromised Cerebral Circulation

The availability of medical treatment and effective surgery to restore flow through or around a narrowed or occluded carotid artery has stimulated interest in the detection of a compromised cerebral circulation prior to stroke occurrence. There are two clinical findings indicating that a compromised cerebral circulation may be present—asymptomatic carotid bruit and TIA—and both develop more frequently in hypertensives.

Asymptomatic Carotid Bruits

There is uncertainty about the prognostic importance and management of persons with asymptomatic carotid bruits. It is not clear what proportion of strokes are heralded by carotid bruits or whether, with bruits present, the stroke was actually caused by the obstructive disease in the vessel involved. Carotid bruits may be associated with a greater incidence of strokes either because they are directly related to critical narrowing of the internal carotid with resultant ipsilateral cerebral infarction, or indirectly as a nonspecific indicator of generalized atherosclerosis, which often includes the intracerebral vessels. It is also not clear how often asymptomatic carotid bruits lead to transient ischemic cerebral attacks or whether those that do are more specifically related to the subsequent occurrence of strokes.

In the Framingham Study, beginning with the ninth biennial examination in 1966 and in all subsequent examinations, carotid bruits were routinely sought out by auscultation. Over eight years, carotid bruits appeared in 171 subjects—66 in men and 105 in women—all of whom were initially asymptomatic and free of bruit. The incidence of bruits increased with age and was equal in men and women, rising from 3.5% at ages 45–54, to 7.0% at ages 67–79.[29] The incidence was greater in subjects with hypertension and in those with CHD and diabetes. TIA appeared in eight and strokes in 21 of the 171, a stroke rate over twice that expected for the age and sex groups. More often than not, however, the cerebral infarction occurred in a vascular territory different from that of the carotid bruit, and often in the posterior circulation.

Also, all strokes that occurred in these persons were not cerebral infarction due to large vessel atherosclerosis; ruptured aneurysm, embolism from the heart, or lacunar infarction was the mechanism of stroke in nearly half the cases. Interestingly, the incidence of myocardial infarction also increased two-fold in those with asymptomatic carotid bruit. General mortality also increased: 1.7-fold in men and 1.9-fold in women, with 79% of the deaths due to cardiovascular disease, including stroke.

Carotid bruit is clearly an indicator of increased stroke risk; however, in asymptomatic populations, the bruit is chiefly a nonfocal signal of advanced atherosclerotic disease and not necessarily an indicator of local arterial stenosis that will precede ipsilateral cerebral infarction in the territory of the carotid with the bruit.

Transient Ischemic Attacks (TIA)

Transient ischemic attacks are reversible focal neurologic deficits, lasting minutes to 24 hours. Based on retrospective clinical data from patients who have sustained a stroke, TIA's are believed to frequently precede development of brain infarction. However, best estimates indicate that only 10% of all strokes are actually preceded by TIA's.[3,30,31]

It is also estimated that atherothrombotic disease of the surgically accessible carotid artery accounts for less than 15% of strokes, and that atherothrombotic disease of the large extracranial arteries, including the carotid, altogether underlies about one-third of all strokes.[3]

The risk of TIA's and the risk of their evolving into brain infarctions is best discerned from prospective study of a general population sample. In the Framingham cohort, ABI was preceded by TIA's in 12% of the cases. The average annual incidence of TIA's was similar in men and women.

Incidence rose with age from four per 100,000 for those under age 40 at entry, to eight per 100,000 at age 40–49 at entry, to 14 per 100,000 at age 50–62 at entry. Of the persons with TIA, stroke developed in about 40%.

Precursors of TIA's are identical to precursors of ABI or stroke, with hypertension the major risk factor (Table 11-9). When compared with the prevalence by age and sex in the Framingham cohort, those with TIA had more hypertension and more cardiac disease, CHD, LVH by ECG, and CHF. Diabetes occurred more frequently among women but not men with TIA.

Although survival of TIA patients has been reported to be little different from the control population free of this condition,[30] in the Framingham cohort survival of those with TIA was intermediate between the cohort and stroke survivors. This is hardly surprising, since nearly half the TIA's develop ABI's.

Survival and Recurrence Following Stroke

Survival following stroke is clearly dependent on the type of stroke. In the Framingham cohort, 30-day case-fatality rates ranged from 15% for ABI and cerebral embolism to 46% and 83% for subarachnoid and intra-cerebral hemorrhage, respectively. Since ABI accounts for 60% of stroke cases, the overall immediate 30-day case-fatality rate is approximately 20%. As expected, mortality is clearly related to age at stroke, ranging for ABI from 8% below age 60 to 23% in men and women age 70 and older.

Long-term survival is strongly related to the presence of prestroke cardiac disease and to a lesser extent hypertension (Figure 11-6). In the absence of antecedent CHD, CHF, or hypertension, survival following stroke

Table 11-9
Frequency of Risk Factors (%) Among TIA's and in the Framingham Cohort of Age 65–74 Years

	Men		Women	
	TIA	Framingham Population (65–74 Years)	TIA	Framingham Population (65–74 Years)
Definite High Blood Pressure	50%	23%	69%	36%
Coronary Heart Disease	29%	19%	24%	15%
ECG-LVH	11%	5%	17%	5%
Congestive Heart Failure	5%	3%	7%	4%
Diabetes	5%	8%	17%	8%

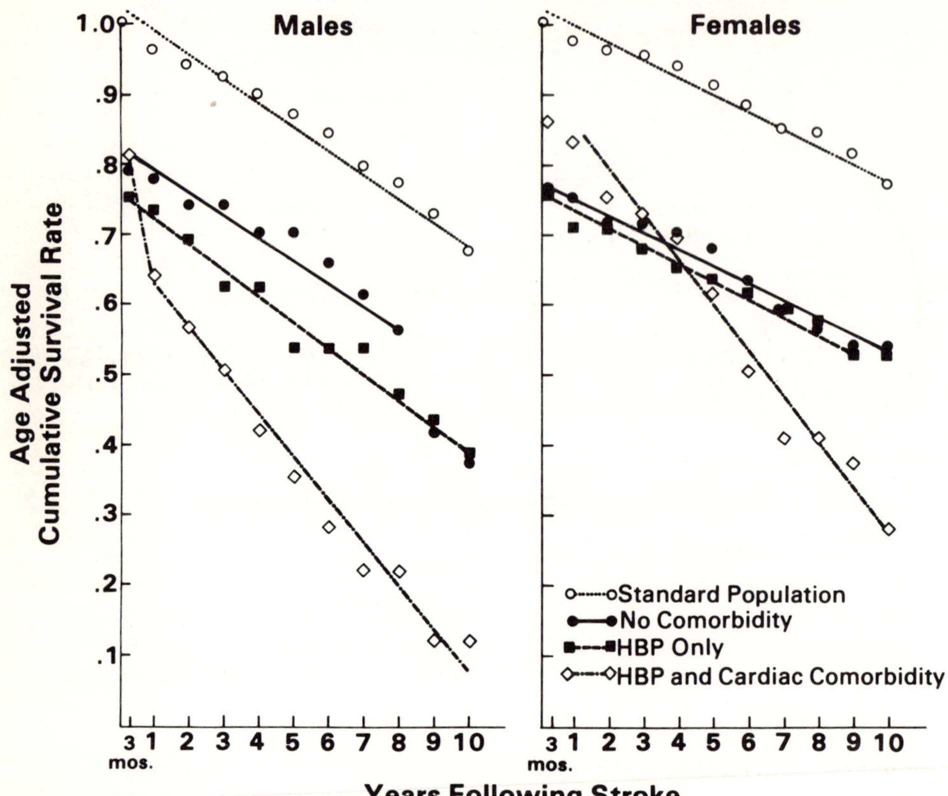

Figure 11-6. Survival following stroke. Effect of prior hypertension and cardiac comorbidity, 26-year follow-up. The Framingham Study.

or ABI closely approximates that of the rest of the cohort of the same age and sex. Cumulative age-adjusted fifth-year survival rates for brain infarction were reduced by prestroke cardiac disease (CHD and/or CHF) and hypertension prior to initial stroke from .85 to .35 in men and .70 to .56 in women. Hypertension alone reduced survival from .85 to .51 in men, but not in women. Not surprisingly, death following stroke is often due to cardiovascular disease in about 25% of cases and recurrent stroke in 45% (Figure 11-7). Survival was lower in men. Stroke of all types tends to recur, with five-year cumulative recurrence rates of 40% for men and 20% for women. Recurrences were frequently of the same type as the initial stroke. Recurrence was more common among persons with cardiac comorbidity and hypertension present prior to the initial stroke, and this impact was more substantial in men than women.

BRAIN INFARCTION

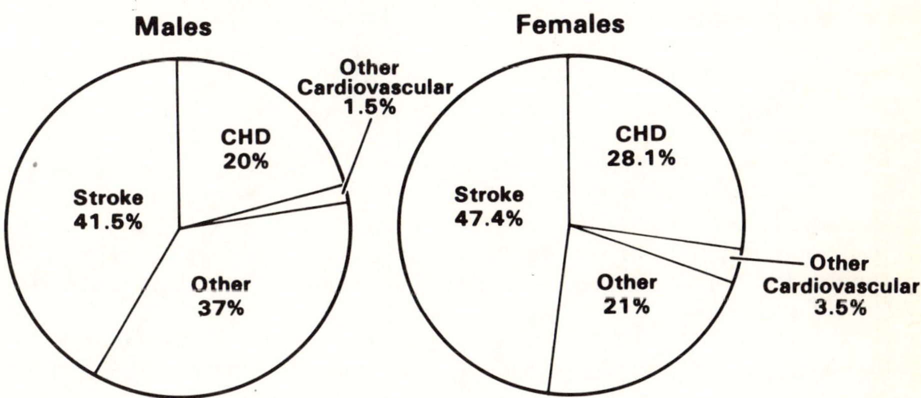

Figure 11-7. Proportionate mortality following stroke, 26-year follow-up. The Framingham Study.

The Declining Incidence of Stroke

Mortality trends in Western nations including the United States indicate a recent decline in stroke mortality.[32–38] This decline seems real despite recognized limitations imposed by fashions in death certification and inaccuracies in death diagnoses.[39,40] Morbidity statistics on the actual incidence of strokes are sparse, and the comparability of case ascertainment over time is questionable.[41–45] Study of secular trends in stroke incidence in the Framingham Study, where uniform criteria and case ascertainment has been maintained over three decades, confirm a decline in stroke incidence, but only in women.

Stroke is part of a larger problem of cardiovascular disease (CVD), and time trends must be examined from the perspective of overall mortality. Age-adjusted cardiovascular mortality rates in the United States have declined almost 32% over the past 30 years. This decrease has accelerated over the past decade, accounting for two-thirds of the 30-year decline. Despite an aging population of increasing size, the total number of deaths attributed to CVD recently fell below one million for the first time in almost a decade. The decline in cardiovascular mortality generally and stroke specifically has occurred in both sexes, in non-whites as well as whites and at all adult ages.

In the nine years following 1968, mortality rates from coronary heart disease, the leading cause of death in the United States, declined 25%. For stroke, the decline was 32%. This decline accelerated in the 1970's, with a rate of decrease about equal in men and women and in all age groups including ages 65 to 84 years. A downward trend in stroke mortality has been apparent for more than 50 years but has accelerated in recent years.[47] Death rates for stroke have fallen more rapidly than other components of cardiovascular disease. In the 1940's and 1950's, stroke mortality in the United States declined at a rate of 1% per year. Since 1972 the rate of decline has been 5% per year.[38]

The sizeable geographic differences in reported stroke death rates in the United States have narrowed, and stroke death rates from all regions have fallen over the past 15 years.[47,48] The decline has been especially notable in non-whites, and the 48.5% fall in stroke mortality for non-white females (1960–1975) represents a dramatic change in the racial patterns of stroke mortality.

It is not possible to determine at present whether the mortality is declining due to a fall in the incidence rate or because better treatment has lowered case fatality rates. It is not even clear whether the rates are declining for hospitalized or out of hospital deaths. It is likely, however, that the decline is real and not simply a result of changes in death certification practices. It is also likely that both primary prevention and better medical care have contributed to the decline.

Hypertension, a demonstrated contributor to stroke incidence and mortality, is being more effectively controlled; hence, the decline in stroke mortality is not unexpected.[38] The Veterans Administration Cooperative Study (1967, 1970) leaves little doubt that treatment of hypertension can prevent strokes.[49] However, effective hypertension control cannot be accepted unequivocally as the sole cause of the decline in stroke mortality since stroke mortality was declining for years before effective antihypertensive therapy became available. It is interesting that in the Framingham Study a decline in stroke incidence could be shown only for women, and women have had more effective blood pressure treatment and control than men.[12] It is difficult to escape the conclusion that hypertension control efforts have contributed to stroke death-rate declines. In the United States from 1972–1977, age-adjusted death rates for hypertension-related cardiovascular disease declined 20%, whereas unrelated cardiovascular disease declined only 9%.

Incidence of stroke, nonfatal as well as fatal, is difficult to determine accurately. Few defined populations are available where stroke has been studied over a sufficiently long time to draw conclusions about temporal trends. To discern changes in incidence of specific stroke types—i.e., thrombosis, embolism, intracerebral or subarachnoid hemorrhage—a degree of diagnostic sophistication is required. Studies in Rochester, Minnesota suggest a decline in thrombotic stroke occurrence during the period 1945 to 1974.

Clinicians have noted that hypertensive encephalopathy, a fairly commonly encountered condition prior to 1950, is now a rarity.[50,51] Massive hypertensive intracerebral hemorrhage also is less frequently seen in hospital emergency rooms and autopsy tables. In 1964, clinicians in Göteborg, Sweden noted a decline in the number of patients with hypertensive intra- cerebral hemorrhage, particularly below the age of 55.[52] Those with intra- cerebral hemorrhage proved to be untreated hypertensives with markedly elevated blood pressures. In a comparison of autopsy records representing 97% of all hospital deaths, cerebral hemorrhage rates were lower below age 65 than in prior years. Median age at hemorrhage was five years more in 1961 than it had been in 1948.

This decline in intracerebral hemorrhage was also noted in studies in Rochester, Minnesota, where incidence rates fell by 34% when the 15-year period from 1961 to 1976 was compared with the period from 1945 to 1960. Median age at onset of hemorrhage also increased—from 67 years in 1945–52 to 71 years in 1969–76.

This decrement in intracerebral hemorrhage rates predates the advent of the computerized tomographic (CT) scan of the head. The CT scan has demonstrated that many more restricted hemorrhages occur than had been suspected. These strokes were previously thought to be infarcts since the event was nonlethal, the deficit restricted, and the spinal fluid free of blood. Whether the rate of smaller hypertensive hemorrhage is also chang- ing may be determined in future years.

Control of Hypertension and Stroke Prevention

On the basis of clinical observation among groups of patients with treated and untreated severe hypertension, clinicians have noted com- parative improvement in outcome among the treated.[50,51] The Veterans Administration Cooperative Study demonstrated in a controlled clinical trial a highly significant benefit in stroke prevention and in survival among treated *severe* hypertensives whose pretreatment diastolic blood pressure levels were above 115 mm Hg. The degree of benefit correlated with levels of pre-randomization blood pressure and with the degree of blood pres- sure control.[53] In the moderately severe hypertensives with pretreatment diastolic blood pressure between 104 and 115 mm Hg, there were one- fourth the number of strokes among the group treated as in the placebo (control) group during the average 3.8-year follow-up period.

Control of moderately severe and severe hypertension has been re- peatedly shown to prevent or reduce stroke occurrence with few excep- tions.[54] In a recent community-based randomized controlled trial involving nearly 11,000 persons with high blood pressure including *mild* hyperten- sion, five-year mortality was significantly lower in the systematically treated and controlled antihypertensive treatment group than in those given stan- dard care.[55] In the group with mild hypertension (entry diastolic blood pressure 90 to 104), mortality was significantly reduced by 20% in the sys- tematic treatment group. This benefit was due to a reduction in death from cardiovascular disease, including a 45% reduction in stroke and a 46% decrease in acute MI. In the systematic treatment group, control of blood pressure was consistently better at all ages, in blacks and whites and in both sexes. This hypertension control was matched by a corresponding reduction in mortality in the older age groups, in white men and in black men and women.

These findings have potentially enormous significance for disease prevention, since about 70% of hypertensives in the United States fall in the mild hypertension category, with diastolic blood pressures averaging between 90 and 104 mm Hg. Sixty percent of the excess mortality attributable to hypertension occurs among persons in this blood pressure range.

The findings of a more conventional, treatment vs. placebo, controlled clinical trial—the Australian National Blood Pressure Study—confirm the efficacy of control of mild hypertension in prevention of cardiovascular morbidity and reduction of mortality.[56] As in the hypertension detection and follow-up program (HDFP), blood pressure control was most efficacious in prevention of cerebrovascular events, fatal and nonfatal.

Study of the effect of reduction of the blood pressure level in older persons with isolated systolic hypertension is being made in a controlled clinical trial, the Systolic Hypertension in the Elderly Program (SHEP). Acceleration in the decline in the incidence and mortality from cerebrovascular disease in recent years is a clear indication that stroke is not an inevitable consequence of aging or genetic constitution. Diminution of stroke mortality has occurred at all ages, including the eighth and ninth decades of life, providing evidence that control of hypertension and changes in environmental factors can effect changes in stroke occurrence.

Each physician can identify "prime" candidates for stroke among asymptomatic patients. Control of severe and moderately severe hypertension will definitely prevent stroke. Patients with these levels of blood pressure require vigorous and sustained therapy to maintain normotension. However, the greatest impact of elevated blood pressure on the public health is attributable to *mild* elevations of pressure because this abnormality is so common.

Medical treatment of the 40% of the adult population of the United States known to have mild hypertension, with diastolic pressure between 90 and 104 mm Hg, is an extraordinary therapeutic and financial endeavor. The rewards of such an effort—treatment of mild hypertension—may be correspondingly effective. Needed are hygienic measures that can be practiced by the individual to reduce the risk of cardiovascular disease including stroke. Weight loss, reduction of salt in the diet, and giving up cigarette smoking are measures that can be advocated for most people. In addition, the practicing physician, on the basis of a few historical, clinical, and laboratory tests, can identify 10% of the population in whom the majority of strokes will occur.

Utilizing a history of cigarette smoking, an ECG, a blood sugar, systolic blood pressure, and serum cholesterol, a cardiovascular risk profile can be determined for each person, and risk of subsequent stroke, CHD, or peripheral arterial disease determined. It is to the hypertensives among the 10% of the population whose cardiovascular or stroke risk profiles fall in the uppermost decile that vigorous antihypertensive therapy should be applied.

The appearance of impaired cardiac function—overt (CHD and CHF) or occult (enlarged heart on x-ray or LVH or intraventricular block by ECG)—heralds a definite increment in risk of stroke and marks the person as definitely stroke-prone. Initiation of antihypertensive therapy, including a diuretic, prior to the appearance of frank cardiac failure might help prevent stroke. Overt signs of a compromised cerebral circulation (the appearance of a carotid bruit or TIA) should alert the physician to the extreme hazard the patient faces. Forty percent of patients with TIA's develop stroke, half within three months of TIA onset. Ten percent of persons developing carotid bruit have a stroke within eight years of bruit appearance. These persons desperately need all the risk-reduction measures at the physician's disposal, particularly control of elevated blood pressure. Physicians have been loath to lower the blood pressure of patients following stroke or TIA for fear of precipitating a stroke. Reduction in blood pressure among hypertensives with prior stroke or TIA has been shown in fact to increase cerebral blood flow.[57]

Recurrence of stroke is common and occurs more frequently in stroke patients with higher blood pressures and in the presence of cardiac comorbidity. When antihypertensive treatment has been given to stroke survivors, the recurrence-rate of stroke has been closely related to the adequacy of control of hypertension.[58–60]

In the sole clinical trial where stroke recurrence was not *uniformly* reduced by antihypertensive therapy, no more strokes occurred among the treated group.[61] Overall, treatment reduced the occurrence of congestive heart failure and, specifically, reduced stroke recurrence among whites who comprised 20% of the study group.

There are no data to support the view, expressed more frequently in past years, that blood pressure reduction in stroke survivors is hazardous. It can be clearly stated that the benefits outweigh the hazards. *Control of blood pressure elevation is the single most effective means of stroke prevention.*

References

1. Robins M, Baum HM: Incidence, the national survey of stroke, edited by Weinfeld ED. Stroke **12**:supplement 1, I45–57, 1981
2. Kurtzke JF: Epidemiology of cerebrovascular disease. *In* Cerebrovascular Survey Report for Joint Council Subcommittee on Cerebrovascular Disease, National Institute of Neurological and Communicative Disorders and Stroke and National Heart and Lung Institute. Rochester, Minnesota. Whiting Press Inc., 1976, 213
3. Mohr JP, Caplan LR, Melski JW, et al: The Harvard Cooperative Stroke Registry: a prospective registry. Neurology **28**:754, 1978

4. Wolf PA: Hypertension as a Risk Factor for Stroke. *In* Cerebral Vascular Diseases, edited by Whisnant JP, Sandok B. New York, Grune and Stratton, 1975, pp 105–112

5. Kannel WB, Wolf PA, Verter J, et al: Epidemiologic assessment of the role of blood pressure in stroke: The Framingham Study. JAMA **214**:301, 1970

6. Kannel WB, Wolf PA, McGee DL, et al: Systolic blood pressure, arterial rigidity and risk of stroke: The Framingham Study. JAMA **245**(14):1442–1445, 1981

7. Smith M, Kuller L, Hulley S, et al: Systolic hypertension in the elderly program (SHEP), personal communication

8. Sacco RL, Wolf PA, Kannel WB, McNamara PM: Survival and recurrence following stroke, The Framingham Study. Stroke **13**:3, 1982

9. Toole JF, Janeway R, Choe K, et al: Transient ischemic attacks due to atherosclerosis, a prospective study of 160 patients. Arch Neur **32**:5, 1975

10. Friedman, GD, Loveland DB, Ehrlich SP: Relationship of stroke to other cardiovascular disease. Circulation **38**:533–541, 1968

11. Kannel WB, Abbott RD, Savage DD, et al: Epidemiologic features of chronic atrial fibrillation, The Framingham Study. N Engl J Med **306**:1018–22, 1982

12. Wolf PA, Dawber TR, Thomas HE, et al: Epidemiologic assessment of chronic atrial fibrillation and risk of stroke, The Framingham Study. Neurology **28**:973–977, 1978

13. Bharucha NE, Wolf PA, Kannel WB, McNamara PM: Epidemiological study of cerebral embolism, The Framingham Study. Annals of Neurology (Abstract), 1981

14. Hinton RC, Kistler JP, Fallon JT, et al: Influence of etiology of atrial fibrillation on incidence of systemic embolism. Am J Card **40**:509, 1977

15. Fairfax AJ, Lambert CD, Leatham A: Systemic embolism in chronic sinoatrial disorder. N Engl J Med **295**:190–192, 1976

16. Kannel WB, Sorlie P: Hypertension in Framingham. *In* Epidemiology and Control of Hypertension, edited by Oglesby, P. Miami, Symposia Specialists, 1975, pp 553–592

17. Kannel WB, Brand N, Skinner JJ, et al: The relation of adiposity to blood pressure and development of hypertension, The Framingham Study. Annals of Internal Medicine **67**:48–59, 1967

18. Masserli FH: Cardiovascular effects of obesity and hypertension. Lancet 1165–1168, 1982

19. Kannel WB, Gordon T, Wolf PA, et al: Hemoglobin and the risk of cerebral infarction. The Framingham Study. Stroke **3**:409–419, 1972

20. Tohgi H, Yamanouchi H, Murakami M, et al: Importance of the haematocrit as a risk factor in cerebral infarction. Stroke **9**:369–374, 1978

21. Pearson TC, Thomas DJ: Physiological and pharmacological factors influencing blood viscosity and cerebral blood flow. *In* Drug Treatment and Prevention in Cerebrovascular Disorders, edited by Tognomi G, Geratini S. Amsterdam, Elsevier/North-Holland, 1979, p 33

22. Harrison MJG, Mitchell JRA: The influence of red blood cells on platelet adhesiveness. Lancet **ii**:1163–64, 1966

23. Thomas DJ, Marshal J, Ross Russell RW, et al: Effect of haematocrit on cerebral blood-flow in man. Lancet **2**:941, 1977

24. Omae T, Takeshita M, Hirota Y: The Hisayama study and joint study on cerebrovascular disease in Japan. *In* Cerebrovascular Diseases, edited by Scheinberg P. New York, Raven Press, 1976, p 255

25. Worth RM, Kato H, Rhoads GG: Am J Epidemiol **102**:481–490, 1975
26. Heyden S, Heyman A, Camplong L: Mortality patterns among parents of patients with atherosclerotic cerebrovascular disease. J Chron Dis **22**:105, 1969
27. Miller GD, Kuller LH: Am J Epidemiol, **98**:233–242, 1973
28. Gordon T, Sorlie P, Kannel WB: An epidemiological investigation of cardiovascular disease. Coronary heart disease, atherothrombotic brain infarction, intermittent claudication. A multivariate analysis of some factors related to their incidence. *In* The Framingham Study, 16-Year Follow-up. Washington DC, United States Government Printing Office, 1971
29. Wolf PA, Kannel WB, Sorlie P: Asymptomatic carotid bruit and risk of stroke: The Framingham Study. JAMA **245**(14):1442–1445, 1981
30. Whisnant JP: Epidemiology of stroke: emphasis on transient cerebral ischemia attacks and hypertension. Stroke **5**:68, 1974
31. Hass WK: Aspirin for the limping brain: editorial. Stroke **8**:299, 1977
32. Acheson RM: Mortality from cerebrovascular accident and hypertension in the Republic of Ireland. Br J Prev Soc Med **14**:139–147, 1960
33. Wylie CM: Cerebrovascular accident deaths in the United States and in England and Wales. J Chron Dis **15**:85, 1962
34. Borhani NO: Changes in geographic distribution of mortality from cerebrovascular disease. Am J Public Health **55**:673–681, 1965
35. Prineas RJ: Cerebrovascular disease occurrence in Australia. Med J Australia **2**:509–515, 1971
36. Metropolitan Life Insurance Company. Recent trends in mortality from cerebrovascular disease. Statistical Bulletin **56**:2–4, 1975
37. Harborman S, Capildeo R, Rose FC: The changing mortality of cerebrovascular disease. Quart J Med **47**:71–88, 1978
38. Levy RI: Stroke decline: Implications and prospects. N Engl J Med **300**:490–491, 1979
39. Florey CDV, Senter MG, Acheson RM: A study of the validity of the diagnosis of stroke in mortality data. I. Certificate Analysis. Yale J Biol Med **40**:148–163, 1967
40. Israel RA, Klobba AJ: A preliminary report on the effect of eighth revision ICDA on cause of death statistics, 1969
41. Eisenberg H, Morrison JT, Sullivan A, et al: CVA's: incidence and survival rates in a defined population, Middlesex Country, Connecticut. JAMA **189**:883–888, 1964
42. Aho K, Fogelheim R: Incidence and early prognosis of stroke in Espoo-Kaunianen area, Finland. Stroke **5**:658–661, 1972
43. Abu-Zeid HAH, Choi NW, Nelson NA: Epidemiologic features of cerebrovascular disease in Manitoba: incidence by age, sex and residence, with etiologic implications. Can Med Assoc J **113**:379–384, 1975
44. Christie I: Stroke in Melbourne: a study of relationship between a teaching hospital and the community. Med J Australia **1**:565–568, 1976
45. Hansen BS, Marquardson J: Incidence of stroke in Frederiksberg, Denmark. Stroke **8**:663–665, 1977
47. Soltero I, Kiu K, Cooper R, et al: Trends in mortality from cerebrovascular diseases in the United States, 1960 to 1975. Stroke **9**:549, 1978
48. Moriyama IM, Krueger DE, Stamer F: Cerebrovascular diseases in the United States. Cambridge, Harvard University Press, 1971
49. Veteran's Administration Cooperative Study Group on Antihypertensive

NOTE: Reference #46 was deleted from the text.

Agents: effects of treatment on morbidity in hypertension. I. Results in patients with diastolic blood pressures averaging 115 through 129 mm Hg. JAMA **202:**116–122, 1967
50. Wolff FW, Lindeman RD: Effects of treatment in hypertension results of a controlled study. J Chron Dis **19:**227, 1966
51. Carter A, Barham A: Hypertensive therapy in stroke survivors. Lancet **1:**485, 1970
52. Aurell M, Hood B: Cerebral hemorrhage in a population after a decade of active anti-hypertensive treatment. Acta Med Scand **176:**377–383, 1964
53. Taguchi J, Freis ED: Partial reduction of blood pressure and prevention of complications in hypertension. New Engl J Med **291:**329, 1974
54. Beevers DG, Johnson J, Devine BL, et al: Relation between prognosis and the blood pressures before and during treatment of hypertensive patients. Clin Sci Mol Med **55**(supplement):333–336, 1978
55. Hypertension detection and follow-up program cooperative group. Five-year findings of the hypertension detection and follow-up programs. I. Reduction in mortality of persons with high blood pressure, including mild hypertension. JAMA **242:**2562–2571, 1979
56. Management Committee. The Australian therapeutic trial in mild hypertension. Lancet **i:**1261–67, 1980
57. Meyer JS, Sawada T, Kitamura A, et al: Cerebral blood flow after control of hypertension in stroke. Neurology **18:**772–781, 1968
58. Leonberg SC, Elliott FA: Prevention of Recurrent Stroke. Stroke **12:**731-735, 1981
59. Beevers DG, Fairman MJ, Hamilton M, et al: Antihypertensive treatment and the course of established cerebral vascular disease. Lancet 1407–1409, 1973
60. Rabkin SW, Mathewson FAL, Tate RB: The relation of blood pressure to stroke prognosis. Ann Intern Med **89:**15–20, 1978
61. Hypertension-Stroke Cooperative Study Group. Effect of antihypertensive treatment on stroke recurrence. JAMA **229:**409–418, 1974

Chapter 12

Acute Management of Stroke

Jeffrey E. Pearce, James I. Ausman,
and Fernando G. Diaz

Medical and surgical management of the stroke syndrome remains a controversial issue despite voluminous clinical and basic science research. Medical therapy has been described in a number of excellent recent articles.[1–5] We have attempted to outline current therapy of carotid distribution ischemia from a surgical viewpoint. The recent literature has been reviewed for indications and results of surgical therapy, medical adjuncts, and areas of active investigation in the therapy of thromboembolic cerebral ischemia.

Definitions

A classification of cerebral vascular diseases with standardization of the nomenclature has been established by the NINBB committee.[6] Clinical syndromes that will be addressed include transient ischemic attacks (TIA's), reversible neurologic deficits, actively changing neurologic status (stroke in evolution), and completed stroke.

TIA's of the anterior circulation are episodes of focal cerebral dysfunction with rapid onset, variable duration, and rapid resolution. TIA's most frequently last between two and 15 minutes; however, by definition they may extend to 24 hours. Anterior circulation TIA's include the following symptoms, alone or in combination: 1) motor deficits—unilateral motor impairment ranging from mild clumsiness to dense paresis; 2) sensory deficit—unilateral numbness with loss of sensation or paresthesias [a march of sensory deficit is not included as a TIA]; 3) aphasia—language disturbance that can involve abnormal expression, comprehension, reading, writing or calculation; 4) complete or partial loss of vision in one eye only; and 5) homonymous hemianopsia or dysarthria alone, which may be a manifestation of either anterior or posterior circulation ischemia.

Patients with actively changing neurologic deficits in the anterior circulation demonstrate a change in the severity or recruitment of new deficits (listed in the preceding paragraph) while under observation. This is frequently referred to as stroke in evolution or progressing stroke. Many authors include patients who present with carotid distribution deficits of less than 24 hours duration in this category.

Completed stroke includes deficits that are relatively stable for more than 24 hours. This category is further subdivided into reversible ischemic neurologic deficits (RIND)—deficits of 24 hours to three weeks duration, and completed stroke, greater than 3 weeks duration.

Cerebral Vascular Supply

Under physiologic conditions, blood flow to the gray matter is 75 ml/100 g-min, white matter 25 ml/100 g-min, and brain as a whole on an average 55 ml/100 g-min.[7,8] Experiments in animals and also in humans undergoing carotid endarterectomy indicate that blood flow between 15 and 20 ml/100 g/min results in decreased cortical evoked potentials and EEG changes, responses generally being abolished below 15 ml/100 g/min. Sodium-potassium pump failure does not occur until flow values have decreased to a level below 10 ml/100 g/min.[9,10] This suggests that for at least a limited period of time there is a significant discrepancy in the cerebral blood flow necessary for neuronal function and that necessary to maintain viability. The minimum cerebral blood flow compatible with cell survival and the duration of relative ischemia that can be tolerated have been investigated but are yet to be rigorously defined.[11]

Each carotid artery supplies 300–400 ml/min[12] and the vertebral arteries together supply approximately 100–150 ml/min[13] to the circle of Willis. From this point the distribution pool of arteries extends to the level of the penetrating arteries. A schematic of the normal cerebral circulation is presented in Figure 12-1. Very little resistance or drop in pressure occurs to the level of the arterioles. The arteriolar bed with a diameter of 70 μm at the cortical surface and 50 μm at the base of the brain, together with the capillary bed, is the primary source of cerebral vascular resistance and control of cerebral blood flow.[14] Since there is little resistance to flow in the distribution pool, augmentation of pressure or flow anywhere proximal to the arterioles may affect flow in remote areas of focal ischemia.

A joint study of extracranial occlusion described the distribution of vascular lesions by angiography in 4748 patients.[15] Because of the methodology involved and the failure to visualize all vessels uniformly, this study cannot be taken as an absolute index of atherosclerotic lesions. However, these findings are representative of the lesions visualized when treating symptomatic patients (Table 12-1).

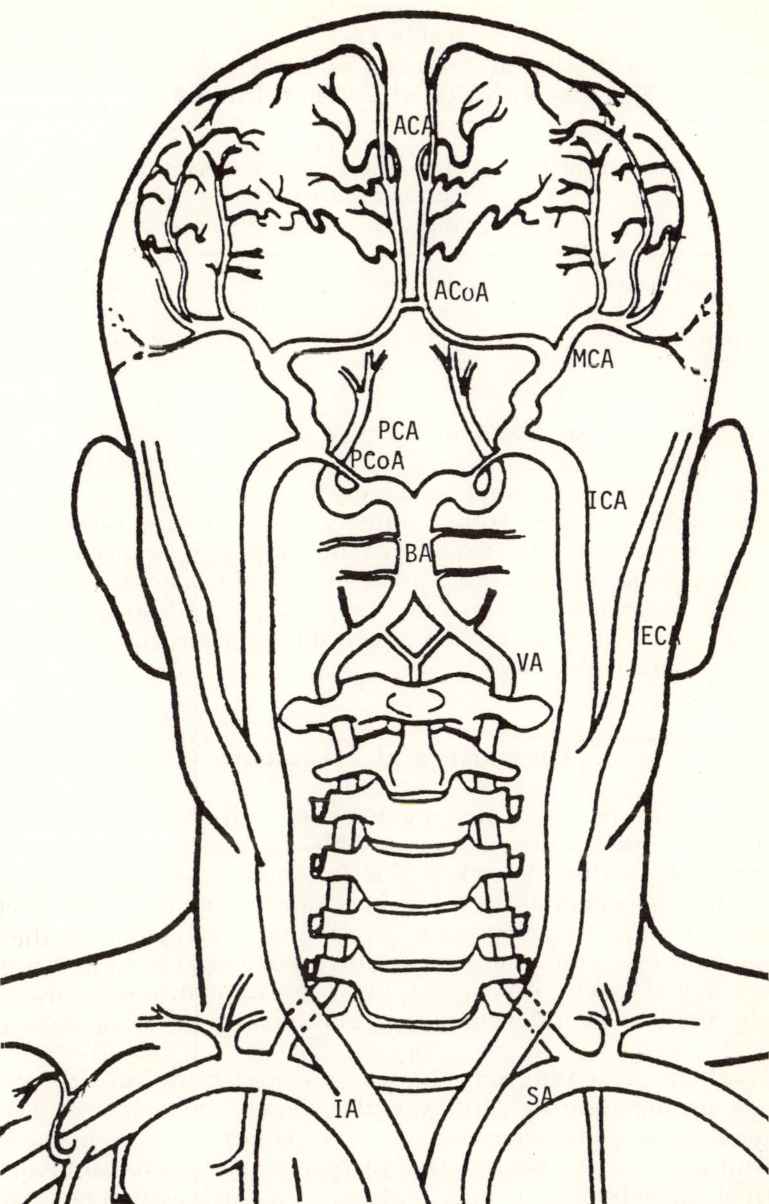

Figure 12-1. Schematic of the normal cerebral circulation. Abbreviations: IA = innominate artery; SA = subclavian artery; ICA = internal carotid artery; ECA = external carotid artery; ACA = anterior cerebral artery; MCA = middle cerebral artery; PCA = posterior cerebral artery; ACoA = anterior communicating artery; PCoA = posterior communicating artery.

Table 12-1
Frequency Distribution of Arterial Lesions (Cooperative Study[15] in Patients with TIA or Cerebral Infarction

	Greater Than 30% Stenosis		Occlusion	
	Right	Left	Right	Left
Cervical carotid artery	33.8	34.1	8.5	8.5
Intracranial carotid artery	5.5	6.0	1.5	1.7
Middle cerebral artery	3.5	4.1	2.2	2.1

General autopsy studies demonstrated an anatomically normal circle of Willis in only 50% of specimens,[16] however less than 25% have one or more posterior communicating arteries of less than 1 mm in diameter.[17] Collateral supply may arise from a number of sources and is conveniently grouped by territories. This would include external to internal, right carotid to left carotid, or vertebral basilar to carotid collateral channels. An angiographic study has demonstrated an average of 5.9 sources of collateral filling in patients with unilateral carotid occlusion and 11.0 in those with bilateral carotid occlusions.[18]

Diagnosis and Treatment

The first priority in managing patients with the stroke syndrome should be establishing a firm diagnosis. Although a myriad of systemic and vascular pathologies have been linked to stroke,[6] a reasonably comprehensive evaluation can generally be carried out rapidly with little morbidity. An accurate and complete history and neurovascular examination are the most important features in the evaluation of this syndrome. They will determine the direction and extent of proposed invasive and noninvasive studies and should be used in considering the significance of any abnormality uncovered.

All patients presenting with the stroke syndrome deserve a screening laboratory examination of cardiovascular, renal, and metabolic activity. This should include a baseline chest x-ray, EKG, urinalysis, complete blood count with differential, electrolytes, BUN, creatinine, prothrombin time and partial thromboplastin time, platelet count, sedimentation rate, and fasting glucose. Further testing must be tailored to specific findings and clinical judgment.

Therapeutic objectives in the management of cerebral ischemia will vary with the patient's clinical presentation. For those with TIA's, prevention of cerebral infarction is the first priority, followed by treatment of associated disease states and the amelioration of risk factors. The patients with a progressing stroke present the most complex and challenging problem. Goals include prevention of infarct progression, reversal of relative ischemia in the boundary zone, and prevention of secondary complications that can lead to increased injury. Patients with completed stroke require a risk assessment and treatment plan for prevention of recurrent infarction, alteration of risk factors, and rehabilitation.

Transient Ischemic Attacks

All proposed treatment modalities should be compared with each other and the natural course of the disease before they can be generally recommended. Numerous studies have followed the natural history of TIA patients.[19-26] Milliken[27] has recently reviewed these studies and found the incidence of cerebral infarction to vary between 20 and 40% over five years. The results of the Mayo Clinic study are frequently quoted.[28] They found a TIA incidence of 31 per 100,000 population, with subsequent infarction in 36%. Of those developing infarction, 21% occurred within one month and 52% within one year.

The management of patients who meet the criteria for TIA's as previously outlined will vary with the chronicity of the complaints. Patients with TIA's are at high risk for developing cerebral infarction early in their course. Almost all TIA patients without major contraindications to surgery will need eventual cerebral angiography. Since angiography is the most informative test and will to a large extent determine the course of subsequent therapy, it should be performed early in the course of evaluation rather than as a last resort. In our opinion, patients with recurrent TIA's within the past two months or a recent increase in frequency should undergo immediate CT scanning followed by cerebral angiography. If any delay in their evaluation is anticipated, anticoagulation with intravenous heparin is instituted.

The complication rate for angiography in patients with cerebral vascular disease varies widely in different series. This is most probably related to the criteria used in determining complications. The joint study reported a serious complication rate of 1.2%.[15] They failed to find an increased risk in patients with recent or severe deficits. Faught[34] and others also failed to show any increased angiographic risk in patients with acute or severe deficits.

In patients with well defined but more chronic TIA's who are acceptable surgical risks, we feel that noninvasive testing should not be the original procedure of choice. Significant surgical pathology can be missed using the best noninvasive methods, making angiography necessary in TIA patients with negative studies. If noninvasive testing does suggest significant pathology, angiography is needed for evaluation of surgical accessibility, intracranial pathology, tandem lesions, and collateral circulation.

A wide choice of noninvasive techniques are available and may be helpful under other circumstances.[29] They can be divided into direct, image-forming, or indirect nonimaging systems. High resolution B mode ultrasound gives a direct reconstruction of the carotid bifurcation based on differences in acoustical reflection by various tissues.[30] Imaging can also be obtained with Doppler scanning, which looks at frequency shifts related to velocity of blood flow.[31] Indirect methods include bruit analysis by phonoangiography or evaluation of secondary hemodynamic effects by oculoplethysmography, ophthalmodynamometry, and facial thermography.[32,33] Noninvasive tests could be valuable for patients with equivocal symptoms, significant angiographic risks, or asymptomatic bruits. They can also be used to follow atheromatous plaques that are not symptomatic or hemodynamically significant.

Carotid Endarterectomy for TIA

The role of carotid endarterectomy in the management of TIA's is well established, but its therapeutic efficacy remains poorly documented. Both medical and surgical series of various treatment modalities have failed to find significant improvement in mortality over untreated patients. This is not unexpected since the majority of patients with untreated TIA's die of a cardiac cause rather than cerebral infarction.[19] Prevention of morbidity from cerebral infarction must be used in addition to mortality as criteria for comparison of treatment modalities. Many large series have recorded morbidity and mortality statistics for carotid endarterectomy.[35–61] Morbidity and mortality rates vary by a factor of 10 among series, and a definite trend toward improvement in results over time is also seen (Table 12-2).

Before firm indications for surgical intervention can be made for an individual patient, classification of risk based on both the neurological status and the general medical condition must be established. Sundt et al.[47] devised a system for analyzing risk assessment on the basis of neurologic status and medical and angiographically determined risk factors. Their

Table 12-2
Combined Results of Published Studies on Carotid Endarterectomy for All Indications[35–61]

Year	Number	Transient Deficits	Permanent Deficits	Mortality
68–77	3820	2.1%	5.7%	3.0%
78–81	4149	1.8%	1.6%	1.5%

Group I and II patients with stable neurologic status and no major medical complicating factors had less than 2% total morbidity and mortality. Patients with significant medical risks had a 7% incidence of serious morbidity and mortality.

Although most studies of morbidity and mortality following carotid endarterectomy have not separated patients by their preoperative neurologic status, Thompson,[39] DeWeese,[36] and Sundt[47] have all shown a significant difference in operative morbidity and mortality between patients in the different diagnostic categories of stroke. Reviewing those series, which did classify patients by neurologic status, several difficulties are encountered. Strict criteria for inclusion were seldom employed, the operated lesions could not be classified as being directly related to the symptomatology in all cases, and in some cases patients were not classified as to the type of surgery performed. Table 12-3 groups data from a representative sample of more recent studies in patients with carotid endarterectomy for TIA's alone. When averaged they demonstrate a 2.5% significant morbidity and 1.7% mortality. If the excellent results of the largest reported series is excluded, however, average morbidity and mortality is 4.5% and 1.7% respectively.

Long-term follow up of TIA patients who have successfully undergone endarterectomy generally show decreased morbidity and mortality. Thompson[39] was the first to report decreased morbidity following successful carotid endarterectomy in 293 patients. Eighty-one percent were asymptomatic and 15.7% improved with long term follow-up. The joint study group of TIA patients demonstrated initial hospitalization morbidity and mortality figures of 11.2% in surgically treated patients versus 12.4% in medically treated patients.[38] However, in those successfully treated surgically, there were significantly more asymptomatic patients and fewer completed infarctions after the acute period. Overall significant infarct or mortality at 42 months in the two groups was about equal—26.6% in those treated surgically and 25.9% in those managed medically.

Several questions must be raised about the population in the study, however. The medically treated group demonstrated a 12.9% stroke rate over the average 42 month follow-up as opposed to the more commonly expected 30% with current medical therapy. The surgical morbidity of 11.2% is also, as previously noted, representative of the high morbidity in

Table 12-3
Combined Results of Carotid Endarterectomy for TIA[38,41,49,52,53,55,57,62]

Year	Number	Transient Deficits	Permanent Deficits	Mortality
68–80	2792	1.9%	2.5%	1.7%

the earlier experience with endarterectomy. A possible explanation is that 43% of medically treated patients had symptoms unrelated to carotid distribution disease and, in addition, 30% stenosis was considered a significant lesion.

Hass[63] used a best-case hypothesis chi-square analysis of the joint study to compare surgical and medical management for TIA's. He found that a permanent neurologic morbidity or mortality rate less than 2.9% is necessary to demonstrate significant superiority in surgically over medically managed patients. However, as previously mentioned, the patient population of the study on which these findings are based can be criticized as they evidence fewer completed infarctions than would be expected. Finally, it would appear that postoperative treatment with aspirin in patients undergoing carotid endarterectomy is of value in decreasing postoperative mortality and stroke.[64]

Recent statistics indicate that carotid endarterectomy can lower the stroke rate in patients experiencing TIA's, with moderate medical risk, and appropriate bifurcation lesions. Most authors would agree that a 50% stenosis and/or significant ulceration constitutes an operative lesion in a symptomatic patient. In addition, at least one study[65] has documented a great risk of infarction in highly stenotic lesions. Surgical therapy may still be considered on an individual basis in patients with heightened medical risks if they demonstrate severe stenoses.

Superficial Temporal Artery to Middle Cerebral Artery Anastomoses for TIA

The joint study of arteriography[15] in patients with the stroke syndrome demonstrated solitary intracranial lesions in 6.1% of cases and combined cervical and intracranial lesions in 33.3%. This included 6.6% stenosis and 8.5% occlusion of the internal carotid artery intracranially, together with 4% stenosis and 2% occlusion of the middle cerebral artery.

Surgical treatment of carotid bifurcation disease is generally aimed at removing a thromboembolic focus, whereas bypass surgery is most often performed to increase perfusion in areas of marginal supply. A number of studies have addressed the issue of what constitutes a flow limiting or critical stenosis.[66,67] Recently, Archie and Feldtman[68] demonstrated that lesions in the carotid artery begin to limit flow at the 60% diameter or 90% area-level of stenosis. In order to decrease flow in the carotid system by 40%, a 75% diameter or 96% area of stenosis is required.

The role of hemodynamic factors in the genesis of TIA is not as well documented as microemboli. Hypotension and arrhythmia are rarely associated with focal cerebral symptoms. Indirect evidence provided by changes in the EEG, and regional cerebral blood flow have been demonstrated in patients with TIA's.[69] Austin[70] also demonstrated abnormal autoregulation in approximately 50% of patients with TIA's or minimal infarction and diminished cerebral blood flow.

Because of hydrostatic effects, cerebral perfusion in patients with cerebral ischemia will vary with the patient position. Caplan[71] studied four patients with positional TIA's and found occlusive disease of the major vessels. In general, the distal territory of supply of an artery will be more sensitive to hemodynamic factors.[72] The watershed zone in man over the motor strip occurs in the region controlling the arm. The retina should also be sensitive to hemodynamic factors since the intraocular pressure is normally 16 mm Hg, more than twice that of intracranial pressure.

Barnett's literature search[73] for patients with complete occlusion of a proximal vessel and ongoing transient ischemic episodes also lends support to a hemodynamic etiology in selected TIA's. He documented 25 cases from a population of 500 with delayed transient ischemic episodes in the territory of a previously occluded vessel.

In selected patients, superficial temporal artery–middle cerebral artery anastomoses (STA-MCA) have been shown to increase cerebral blood flow in ischemic regions at statistically significant levels.[74–75] It is difficult to evaluate the results of bypass surgery for TIA's (Table 12-4). Most studies suffer from poorly defined criteria for TIA and short follow-up. An attempt to quantify flow through bypass grafts using angiographic criteria indicates that significant collateral flow can be provided by STA-MCA bypass procedures, at times approaching that of an intact carotid.[81] As noted in Table 12-4, surgical morbidity and mortality in patients undergoing STA-MCA bypass for TIA's is low. Reviewing major series reporting statistics for all indications combined, serious morbidity and mortality rates range from 2 to 5% with patency rates greater than 90%.[77–82]

It has been established that STA-MCA bypass can be performed with high patency and low morbidity and mortality. Patients with TIA's and appropriate lesions would appear to benefit from surgical therapy; however, the results are not conclusive. Long term follow up results are awaited.

Medical Management of TIA

A significant number of patients with classic TIA symptoms have a definite contraindication to surgery or no appropriate surgical lesion on angiography. Marshall and Wilkinson[83] followed 68 patients with classic TIA's and normal angiograms for an average of 5.4 years. They found several points of interest. Patients with fewer than six previous TIA's at the time of evaluation had fewer TIA's on follow-up but more cerebral infarctions and death. Twenty percent of patients had subsequent TIA's, 16% cerebral infarction, and 17% serious cardiovascular episodes.

Cardiac emboli related to myocardial infarction, valvular pathology, and prosthetic valves are a frequent cause of cerebral ischemia.[84] Unfortunately, these patients usually develop an acute infarction without antecedent TIA's. Rheumatic heart disease associated with atrial fibrillation or

Table 12-4
**Superficial Temporal Artery to Middle Cerebral Artery Bypass
for TIA[77-80]**

Year	Number	Persistent TIA	Permanent Deficit (Late)	Mortality	Relief TIA
76–80	206	5.8%	4.9%	2.4%	91.3%

mitral valvular pathology is a frequent source of embolism. Carter[85] found a recurrent stroke rate of 50% in the first year, which was significantly reduced with anticoagulation. Others have documented anticoagulant therapy as the treatment of choice in this condition.[86-91]

Cardiac dysrhythmia is rarely related to focal transient cerebral ischemia without underlying atherosclerotic flow-limiting lesions. Reed et al.[92] followed 290 patients undergoing pacemaker insertion. Four patients had focal symptoms but only two could be temporally related to a cardiac event. Diffuse cerebral ischemic symptoms, on the other hand, were very common among these patients. Because of the low incidence of TIA in patients with cardiac dysrhythmia or embolization and the high incidence of atherosclerosis in this patient population, angiography is probably indicated in the majority of older patients with transient focal cerebral ischemic events despite cardiovascular disease unless definite evidence of embolization is documented.

Transient ischemic symptoms have been attributed to polycythemia,[93] anemia,[94] hypoglycemia,[95] and a variety of other causes. Once again, atheromatous disease should be ruled out in patients with systemic disease but with focal symptoms. A sound diagnosis of migraine variants or hypertensive crises with focal ischemia can sometimes be established by history and examination. Mass lesions and focal seizures may be difficult to identify on a clinical basis; however, CT scanning and EEG may be helpful in the evolution of these disorders. The medical management of patients who are not surgical candidates includes anticoagulants, antiplatelet agents, control of hypertension, and manipulation of other risk factors.

Anticoagulant Therapy of TIA's

Fletcher et al.,[96] Milliken,[97] Sandok et al.,[4] and Byron and Easton[2] have all recently reviewed antiplatelet and anticoagulant therapy for TIA. The number of patients reported in most series of anticoagulant treatment has been quite small. In general, all studies failed to demonstrate differences in mortality between treated and untreated groups, randomized studies failed to show significant benefits, and nonrandomized studies tended to favor anticoagulant therapy. Because of the small number of patients and methodological problems, no indisputable evidence exists favoring anticoagulants. A more recent reassessment of the Mayo Clinic patients with TIA's does, however, demonstrate significant decreases in stroke rate over the first six months, which were then maintained over the following five years.[28] This was statistically significant only in patients with vertebrobasilar symptoms. The group studied was relatively small, however, and angiography was not performed. Little additional benefit of anticoagulation accrued after six months, and the risk of therapy greatly increased after one year of treatment.

Larger series have been completed on the use of antiplatelet agents for TIA. Four prospective randomized studies have been reported. They have shown statistically significant efficacy for aspirin but at a marginal level. A retrospective review of the data by Fletcher and Alkjaersig[96] pointed out that the primary benefit was seen in males in the Canadian study,[98] patients with multiple TIA's and an appropriate lesion in the US study,[99,100] and in carotid distribution TIA's in the final study from Germany.[101] All were undertaken with what is likely to be other than optimal dosing or combination of agents. Recent work has demonstrated antagonistic effects of aspirin on platelets and the endothelial cell, which are dose-dependent.[102,103] Combinations of aspirin and dipyridimole are also frequently employed clinically at present, and a marked dose and dose interval dependency has been shown for combinations.[104] The optimal dosing schedules and trial with these agents have not yet been documented.

In summary, anticoagulant therapy has documented efficacy in cases of embolization from a central source. It may be of value in nonsurgical candidates with TIA's early in the course of their disease. Antiplatelet therapy does have documented efficacy in at least some patients with TIA's, but the effects are not dramatic.

Stroke in Evolution

Patients in the category of stroke in evolution present with the highest potential for salvage and disaster. As previously defined, these patients present with an acute increase in the severity or recruitment of additional symptoms and signs of focal cerebral ischemia. The natural history of these patients is quite variable and less well-defined than patients with TIA. Several studies have followed patients with progressive stroke as controls for various medical therapies.[105–108] Cumulatively, there were 214 patients followed for 6 to 15 months. Of these, 49 patients (23%) died from cerebral infarction and 55 patients (26%) developed a progressive deficit that was permanent. The remainder improved or remained the same. Of all patients, therefore, 49% developed an increase in symptomatology. These results are comparable to a large early series of Milliken,[109] who followed

204 patients. At two weeks, 74% had developed moderate or severe deficits, 14% died and 12% improved.

General Medical Management

The patient in the early phase of an acute or progressive infarct is in a precarious position. Cerebral infarction is frequently a progressive process when secondary to a major vessel occlusion. The degree of ischemia seen with occlusion of a major vessel will vary with collateral supply and is almost never complete. This attested to by the variable course following carotid or middle cerebral occlusion in man.[110,111]

A number of factors, both local and systemic, can alter blood flow and metabolism in the region of an acute infarction.[112,113] Autoregulation is lost and local cerebral blood flow becomes dependent on perfusion pressure. Microcirculatory impairment secondary to intravascular sludging, together with endothelial and perivascular swelling, can add further injury. Intracellular calcium uptake secondary to ischemia of the arterioles may precipitate smooth muscle contraction and further increase cerebrovascular resistance.[114,115] Cerebral edema may cause significant mass effect and herniation with large infarcts, but also probably plays a role in the development of microcirculatory changes.

In addition to a progressive loss of perfusion after an ischemic insult, cellular metabolic damage appears to be an ongoing process. The role of Ca^{++} flux across membranes in relation to cytotoxicity is just beginning to be appreciated. Brief summaries have been presented by Siesjo,[116] Hass,[117] and Schanne.[118] The intracellular build up of Ca^{++} following anoxia has been implicated in energy failure due to blockade of ATP synthesis in the mitochondria. Ca^{++} is also instrumental in generating cytoplasmic free fatty acids initiating the synthesis of a number of toxins. These include thromboxanes, leukotrienes, and endobroxides.

Attention should be directed toward maintenance of normal homeostasis in acute stroke patients. Rapid correction of congestive heart failure or arrhythmias that compromise cardiac output is necessary. Pulmonary function must be watched closely to provide adequate oxygenation, ventilation, and prevention of secondary infectious complications. Normal renal function and fluid states must be established to maintain acid base balance and prevent electrolyte abnormalities, which can aggravate cerebral ischemia and edema. In addition, adequate nutritional support can be initiated once the acute insult has stabilized. Optimization of the patient's general organ function through strict attention to standard medical therapy can minimize secondary insults to the ischemic brain.

Manipulation of systemic arterial pressure may provide one means of affecting acute cerebral ischemia. Experimental[119] and clinical[120] studies have demonstrated loss of cerebrovascular autoregulation in areas of focal ischemia. Perfusion is therefore directly proportional to changes in systemic arterial pressure or resistance in the surrounding vascular bed. Induced hypertension has improved cerebral blood flow and cortical evoked potentials in animal models of middle cerebral occlusion.[121] Cerebral ischemia from vasospasm after subarachnoid hemorrhage can also improve with hypertensive therapy. In clinical situations this is generally accomplished with a combination of volume expansion and peripherally acting vasopressors.[122] Under these conditions, both improved viscosity from hemodilution and elevation of perfusion pressure may affect flow.

Spontaneous hypertension frequently accompanies acute cerebral infarction. Patients with hypertension are known to have an elevation of the range of pressures over which blood flow can be autoregulated. They may be unable to maintain flow at systemic pressures that are well tolerated by a normotensive individual.[123]

Unfortunately, there are detrimental effects in addition to benefits from systemic hypertension in acute cerebral ischemia. Vasogenic cerebral edema accumulates more rapidly and to a greater degree with elevation of arterial pressure.[124] High perfusion pressure in areas where vascular integrity is compromised and autoregulation lost could also precipitate hemorrhage.

There are no adequate clinical studies of blood pressure modification and clinical outcome in patients with focal ischemia. For the reasons outlined above it is likely that an abrupt fall in perfusion pressure would be detrimental in patients with acute infarcts. We attempt to gradually reduce arterial pressures if they are significantly elevated to levels that are mildly hypertensive for the age group to reduce complications of edema and hemorrhage. We have also seen patients with unusually low perfusion pressure benefit from volume expansion and elevation of arterial pressure. Neither approach has been studied and shown to be efficacious in a therapeutic trial, however.

Carotid Endarterectomy

In the past, carotid endarterectomy has played a limited role in the management of stoke in evolution. Early attempts at revascularization were generally unsuccessful. Wyle et al.,[126] Hunter et al.,[127] and Rob[128] have advocated conservative management. The joint study[129] reported a 42% mortality rate with surgical treatment and favored medical therapy. Hemorrhagic infarction has been a significant problem following thromboendarterectomy for acute occlusion. Occlusion of the carotid may develop secondary to obstruction at either the bifurcation or the intracranial segment of the carotid artery. Acute occlusion due to disease at the bifurcation will generally show occlusion of the entire internal carotid artery on angiography, whereas occlusion intracranially will usually be associated with a significant stump remaining at the origin of the internal carotid artery.

Attempts at cervical thromboendarterectomy for intracranial carotid occlusion are obviously bound to fail.

Several recent studies have reported excellent results in patients demonstrating acute deficits treated surgically.[130–133] Almost all patients who responded well to surgery demonstrated a fluctuating course with mild to moderate neurologic deficit. Ojemann treated patients with crescendo TIA's, stroke in evolution, sudden partial deficits, sudden severe deficits, or post-angiographic deficits.

If the patients with sudden severe deficits are excluded, there are 27 patients in the remaining categories. Of these, 63% showed marked improvement and 19% some improvement, with a mortality rate of 4% after acute carotid surgery. Those with sudden severe deficits, however, had a 44% mortality rate, and only one patient demonstrated marked improvement following surgery. Further, this one patient had flow restored in less than four hours. More recent data on patients operated for stroke in evolution are compiled in Table 12-5. Of 45 patients, 80% demonstrated marked improvement following surgery, with a mortality rate of 4.4%. This compares favorably with the natural history of the disease.

These results are clearly in contrast to those reported in the earlier studies. Patients with severe deficits were not operated on in the later surgical series. Although there are scattered case reports of dramatic recovery following surgery for acute dense neurologic deficits, the majority of these patients to date have done poorly with acute revascularization. Experimental evidence indicates that without adjunctive therapy to inhibit progressive cytotoxic and ischemic insults revascularization following severe ischemia is deleterious after two to four hours.[134–135] Until a method of selection based on cerebral blood flow, metabolic parameters, or as yet unspecified criteria can be established or an effective adjunct to prolong ischemic viability is documented, patients with severe deficits are best managed conservatively.

Hypertension is also clearly linked to the development of hemorrhagic infarction, intracerebral hematoma and complications following revascularization.[136,137] Diapedesis of red cells into an area of severe ischemia following revascularization with the formation of a hemorrhagic infarct is seen clinically[138] and experimentally.[139,140] Loss of autoregulation in ische-

Table 12-5
Carotid Endarterectomy for Stroke in Evolution

Author	Number	Improved	Worse or Unchanged	Mortality
Mentzer[132]	17	12	0	1
Goldstone[130]	18	18	0	0
Ojemann[131]	10	8	1	1
Totals	45	38	1	2

mic areas is well documented in animal models[141-143] and humans.[144,145] After reperfusion, even moderate levels of hypertension would be uncompensated, increasing the propensity to hemorrhagic infarction and hematoma formation. All studies reporting good results following acute revascularization included strict control of blood pressure in their postoperative protocol. It appears that acute endarterectomy can be of value in selected patients with stroke in progress. Results should improve as more explicit criteria for patient selection are developed.

Superficial Temporal Artery–Middle Cerebral Artery Bypass

Some patients with stroke in evolution have an established carotid or middle cerebral occlusion. A number of animal models have been devised to evaluate reperfusion after various intervals of ischemia.[146,147] Three have studied the efficacy of superficial temporal artery–middle cerebral artery anastomosis in the revascularization of lesions known to cause infarction. Levinthal[148] demonstrated a decrease in infarct size in dogs where superficial temporal artery–middle cerebral artery anastomosis was performed prior to middle cerebral artery embolization; however, animals treated five hours after occlusion did worse after bypass. Crowell and Olson[149] demonstrated improvement following bypass within two hours after occlusion in a dog model. Diaz,[150] however, looked at the effects of bypass at four hours and 24 hours post occlusion of the middle cerebral and internal carotid artery in dogs. Revascularization at both intervals was associated with increased infarct size and the development of hemorrhagic infarction. These three studies, together with the previously mentioned studies on the middle cerebral artery revascularization, suggest that a short but definite period of time exists between the onset of an ischemic event and irreversible injury. The natural duration of this interval and means of extending it are currently under study.

Early attempts at superficial temporal artery–middle cerebral artery anastomosis for progressing ischemia were disappointing.[77,78,80,82] Several factors no doubt contributed to these results. Initial mean flow rates through the anastomosis have been reported as 28/ml/min,[151] which may be inadequate to compensate for a major vessel occlusion with minimal collaterals. Probably more important, however, bypass operations were generally completed after a significant delay. This was presumably after cytotoxic and vascular injury had been irreversibly initiated.

Spetzler[152] has reported experimental and clinical efficacy with acute bypasses. Clinical results have also been recently reported by Suzuki[153] and Diaz.[154] All three reports suggest that acute revascularization could be performed with relative safety in select cases. All three also used medical adjuncts known to retard cytotoxic and vascular damage. The patient population that can benefit from these procedures and the most efficacious medical adjuncts have yet to be determined.

Acute middle cerebral artery embolectomy has also been reported by several authors.[155–160] Results are varied, and the number of cases remains too small for a rational judgment on the merits of the procedure. Animal studies have suggested that embolectomy can be successfully performed up to five hours after occlusion; however, occlusion of the perforating branches of the M1 segment frequently led to deep infarction.[161–163]

Ito[164] has attempted to identify a subgroup of acute ischemic lesions that would respond to acute revascularization. The EEG and somatosensory evoked potentials were followed with induced changes in perfusion pressure and diuretic agents. Based on these findings, Ito and Suzuki (164) selected a group of patients they felt would benefit from reperfusion. However, results of clinical trials were not presented. Future work toward refinement of patient selection and prolongation of the grace period prior to revascularization will undoubtedly improve results in acutely operated patients.

Medical Management of Acute and Progressive Stroke

Anticoagulants

The use of anticoagulants in acute or progressive stroke has both theoretical and experimental support. Elevated concentrations of fibrinogen complexes that can be identified chromatographically are indicative of increased fibrinogen to fibrin conversion. In the clinical setting this is most frequently seen with intravascular thrombus formation.[165] Significant elevation of circulating fibrinogen complexes have been documented for several days following acute cerebral infarction.[166] The same study also demonstrated increased levels of fibrinogen complexes in patients at high risk for stroke.

Several recent literature reviews support anticoagulant therapy in progressing strokes.[1,106,167] Factors such as decreased cardiac perfusion, cerebral edema, hypoxia, or metabolic insults must also be identified as they can lead to progressive neurologic deficit and would not be responsive to anticoagulant therapy. Lacunar infarcts in hypertensives frequently present as a slowly progressive lesion. They can sometimes be identified clinically by the specific focal nature of the deficit and should not be anticoagulated.[161,168] Finally, patients with severe deficits have near maximal ischemia and are unlikely to benefit from anticoagulation.

Thrombolytic Agents

Streptokinase and urokinase are the only thrombolytic agents that have undergone clinical trials for acute cerebral infarction in man. Two controlled studies have been completed with streptokinase.[169,170] In the first, a subtherapeutic dose was employed, and no effects were demonstrated. Patients receiving therapy in the second series did worse than those without therapy but a number of problems with this trial have been enumerated.[97] Urokinase, which has a number of advantages over streptokinase, has had relatively little therapeutic use. A single pilot study[171] demonstrated intracerebral hemorrhage in four of 31 cases treated. These modalities need further experimental investigation before widespread clinical use can be contemplated.

Antiplatelet Agents

No studies have been completed to date on the efficacy of aspirin or dipyridamole for acute or progressive cerebral infarction. Low molecular weight dextran decreases platelet adhesiveness and blood viscosity. Animal studies of dextran have suggested that it may prolong the interval of ischemia that can be tolerated prior to revascularization.[172] Clinical trials, however, have been disappointing. Gilroy et al.[173] found that dextran in patients with acute cerebral infarction decreased mortality. However, follow up was limited to 10 days. Matthews[174] demonstrated decreased mortality but persistence of severe deficits in patients with massive infarct. He could show no improvement in those with moderate deficits. Spudis et al.[175] found no significant difference in dextran-treated patients versus controls in a randomized study.

Future work in this area should be of interest and some clinical value. However, the routine use of dextran in acute or progressive cerebral ischemia cannot be strongly supported at present.

Glycerol

O'Brien[176] and Fugimoto[177] presented recent reviews of ischemic cerebral edema. With some simplification it can be considered to be initially cytotoxic with later aggravation by vasogenic changes that can then become dominant. Five clinical trials have been reported on glycerol therapy.[178–182] Four demonstrated improvement with therapy, which was generally seen in patients with moderate deficits after early observation. Glycerol tended to delay or prevent acute herniation in massive infarcts but had no efficacy in preventing severe deficits in patients with major infarctions. A significant or uncontestably beneficial effect of glycerol has not been documented to date although the therapy appears to have some promise.

Several clinical studies have concluded that mannitol has not been effective in cases of acute ischemia.[183,184] More recent work has reported beneficial effects when mannitol was used alone and in combination with perfluorochemicals as adjuncts for revascularization.[153,185,186]

Massive brain edema with herniation accounts for approximately 30%

of mortalities in the acute phase after cerebral infarction, frequently in young patients.[187] The mean survival in cases of herniation was 3.7 days. Selected patients with good rehabilitation potential and nondominant hemispheric lesions could benefit from decompressive surgical procedures if they were performed before secondary brainstem injury had occurred.[188]

Steroids

Conflicting results have obscured the evaluation of steroid therapy in acute or progressing stroke. Five controlled studies reported in the 70's failed to show significant benefit in steroid treated patients.[183,184,189–191] In order to demonstrate significant effects it is likely a selected population should be identified in whom significant mass effect in the infarcted area and spreading white matter edema are present. If this subgroup of patients was selectively treated with steroids, some benefit might accrue.

Barbiturates

Interest in barbiturate therapy for focal cerebral ischemia has grown as protective effects in animal models become increasingly well documented. Protection in global ischemia is not as well supported. These studies have been recently reviewed by Smith,[192] Belopavlovic and Buchthal,[193] and critiqued by Snyder.[194] Barbiturates cannot be expected to offer any protective effect in cerebral ischemia if local blood flow remains below that necessary for tissue survival. Possible benefits of therapy can only accrue if barbiturates either improve secondary local factors aggravating the ischemic process, thereby limiting infarct size, or provide a period of protection for ischemic tissues during which spontaneous hemodynamic changes or surgical intervention augmented cerebral blood flow.

The mechanism of barbiturate protection has not been conclusively demonstrated. Reduction of cerebral metabolic rate, decreased intracranial pressure, Ca^{++} channel blocking, inverse steal phenomenon, suppression of catechol-mediated hypermetabolism, and free-radical scavenging have all been offered as possible contributing factors.

High-dose barbiturate therapy does entail significant risk[195] and cannot be recommended routinely for the patient with an acute focal ischemic insult until indications and the efficacy of treatment are better established. Its use does appear to be justified in selected patients at present. They would include candidates for acute revascularization and patients where iatrogenic temporary ischemic insults are necessary, as seen with intracranial aneurysm surgery.

Animal studies have provided useful guidelines for managing barbiturates in these patients. The beneficial effects of barbiturate therapy are dependent on collateral circulation to the ischemic area so that maintenance of optimal cardiopulmonary function is essential.[196,197] The response to barbiturates is time-dependent, with good results more consistently seen if therapy is initiated less than one hour after the original insult.[152,195,198,199] The result is dose-dependent; however, toxicity probably outweighs any further advantages at very high dose levels.[200,201]

A number of other agents or treatments have had advocates. Recently, a report detailing transient reversibility of neurologic deficits after intravenous naloxone was presented.[202] Further follow up is awaited. A number of authors reported transient improvement after theophylline injections in acute ischemia, but recent reports have failed to document a difference in final outcome.[203] Hyperbaric oxygenation has also received trials, and some beneficial effects have been reported.[204,205]

In summary, patients with progressing stroke have a very poor prognosis without therapy. A diagnosis should be established on the basis of clinical presentation, CT, and angiography. Anticoagulation is probably of value in patients with reasonable control of hypertension and no major contraindications. This is generally instituted with intravenous heparin and maintained with coumadin after seven days. The optimal duration of therapy is not well defined but is probably from three to six months. Should an appropriate surgical lesion be found, both carotid endarterectomy and superficial temporal artery–middle cerebral artery bypass may be of value in select cases.

Completed Stroke

Patients who demonstrate a focal neurologic deficit of greater than 24 hours duration can be considered to have a completed infarction. Once such a completed infarct has occurred, treatment options are limited. Several studies of anticoagulant therapy for completed infarction had large control series, which reflect the natural history of this disorder.[206–208] Ninety-nine control patients in McDowell and McDevitt's[208] study had long-term follow-up. The recurrent rate of infarction was 22%, 7% of which were fatal. Total mortality was 57% at three years and primarily related to cardiac disease.

All patients with some rehabilitation potential should undergo a complete medical evaluation and treatment of associated disease processes. Currently, efforts are under way to select patients from this group who might benefit from more aggressive therapy.

The Framingham Study has shown that cerebral infarction is seven times more prevalent in hypertensive than normotensive individuals.[209,210] Reports on antihypertensive treatment in patients with chronic established cerebral infarction are conflicting. Some clinicians have been reluctant to treat hypertension in these patients for fear of precipitating further ischemia. Meyer et al[211] looked at cerebral blood flow in patients with chronic strokes treated for hypertension. Although they used a method that measured global rather than focal blood flow, perfusion appeared to improve after treatment.

Early studies by Adams[212] and Merrett[213] suggested that control of hypertension was not beneficial in patients with established cerebral infarction. A later study by Carter[214] found that patients under 65 years of age, but not those over, did benefit from treatment. Soon after, Beevors[215] also reported benefits with antihypertensive treatment but made no attempt to correlate the results with age. A large cooperative study of 452 hypertensive stroke patients found no improvement in the subsequent rate of cerebral infarction but fewer cardiac complications in patients treated for hypertension.[216]

It appears that the history of a previous remote cerebral infarction does not influence the indications for antihypertensive therapy. If transient ischemic symptoms appear after institution of therapy, flow-limiting cerebrovascular disease should be suspected. In any case, caution should be used in instituting therapy and drugs with significant orthostatic effects should be avoided.[125]

Surgical Treatment of Completed Stroke

Although reversal of longstanding ischemic neurologic deficits with EC-IC bypass has been reported,[217,218] revascularization procedures in patients with completed infarction are primarily performed for prophylaxis. The patient with a mild or moderate deficit but significant functional recovery in the appropriate hemisphere should be evaluated in a similar manner to TIA's. Indications for endarterectomy would remain the same. Although not well documented, most surgeons feel operation should be delayed four to six weeks to allow restoration of vascular integrity in the infarcted area. Complete occlusion of a proximal vessel in patients with a fixed neurologic deficit makes surgical selection more difficult. Ideally, patients at risk for a progressive or recurrent infarction on a hemodynamic basis need to be identified.

Two methods have been reported for selection of patients with these conditions. The first involves determination of regional cerebral blood flow and alterations in regional cerebral blood flow and somatosensory evoked potentials with induced hypertension.[219] Subjective selective value was demonstrated in 19 patients. The second used improvement following hyperbaric oxygenation on clinical and EEG criteria.[220] This also showed selective ability in detecting patients who would improve after surgery. Neither study was statistically significant because of the small number of cases. Although both methods show promise, further work on selection criteria is necessary before widespread evaluation and treatment of patients with completed infarctions and major vessel occlusions can be advocated.

Anticoagulants

Gentin et al[167] have reviewed anticoagulant therapy in completed stroke. Three studies were well designed with large numbers of patients.[221–223] All demonstrated no therapeutic benefit with anticoagulants, and one[224] suggested that they were actually contraindicated. This finding can be criticized, however, as slightly high levels of anticoagulation were used as endpoints in that study. Two nonrandomized studies were also reviewed and no definite advantage to anticoagulant therapy was demonstrable.

References

1. Millikan CH, McDowell FH: Treatment of progressing stroke. Stroke **12**:(4)397–409, 1981
2. Byer JA, Easton DJ: Therapy of ischemic cerebrovascular disease. Ann Int Med **93**:742–756, 1980
3. Toole JF: Management of TIA's and acute infarction. Adv Neurol **16**:71–80, 1977
4. Sandok BA, Furlan AJ, Whisnant JP, Sundt TM: Guidelines for the management of transient ischemic attacks. Mayo Clin Proc **53**:665–674, 1978
5. Whisnant JP: Indications for medical and surgical therapy for ischemic stroke. Adv Neurol **16**:133–144, 1977
6. Millikan CH, chairman NINCDS ad hoc committee on cerebrovascular diseases, et al: A classification and outline of cerebrovascular diseases. II. Stroke **6**:565–616, 1975
7. Austin G, Laftin D, Vasudevan R, Lichter E, Haywood W: Cerebral Blood Flow in Stroke Type Patients. *In* Microvascular Anastomosis for Cerebral Ischemia, edited by Fein JM, Reichman HO. New York, Springer Verlag, 1978, pp 241–265
8. Pasztor E, Symon L, Dorsch WWC, Branston WM: The hydrogen clearance method in assessment of blood flow in cortex white matter and deep nuclei of baboons. Stroke **4**:556–567, 1973
9. Sharbrough FW, Messick JM, Sundt TM: Correlation of continuous electroencephalograms with cerebral blood flow measurements during carotid endarterectomy. Stroke **4**:674–683, 1973
10. Astrup J, Symon L, Branston WM, Lassen WA: Thresholds of cerebral ischemia. *In* Microsurgery for Stroke, edited by Schmiedek P. New York, Springer Verlag, 1977, pp 16–21
11. Simon L: The relationship between CBF, evoked potentials and the clinical features in cerebral ischemia. ACTA Neurol Scand Suppl **78**:175–190, 1980
12. Hardesty WH, Roberts B, Toole JF, Royster HP: Studies of carotid-artery blood flow in man. New Engl J Med **263**:944–946, 1960
13. Hardesty WH, Whitacre WB, Toole JF, et al: Studies on vertebral artery blood flow in man. Surg Gyn Obst **116**:662–664, 1963
14. Kanzow E, Dieckhoff D: On the location of vascular resistance in the cerebral

circulation. *In* Cerebral Blood Flow, edited by Brock M, Feschi C, Inguan DH, et al. Berlin, Springer, 1969, pp 96–97

15. Hass WK, Fields WS, North RR, Kricheff RI, Chase WE, Bauer RB: Joint study of extracranial arterial occlusion. II. Arteriography techniques, sites and complications. JAMA **203**(11):159–166, 1968

16. Fawcett E, Blanchford JU: The circle of Willis: an examination of 700 specimens. J Anat (Lond) **40**:63–70, 1906

17. Alpers BJ, Berry RG, Paddison RM: Anatomical study of the circle of Willis in normal brain. Arch Neurol Psych **81**:409–418, 1959

18. Thompson JR, Rouhe SA, Austin GM, Simmons CR: Angiographic cerebral blood flow patterns in STA-MCA anastomosis candidates. *In* Microvascular Anastomoses for Cerebral Ischemia, edited by Fein J, Reichmann OH. New York, Springer Verlag, 1978, pp 145–157

19. Whisnant JP, Mastsumoto N, Elveback LR: Transient cerebral attacks in a community. Mayo Clin Proc **48**:194–198, 1973

20. Acheson J, Hutchinson EC: Observations on the natural history of transient cerebral ischemia. Lancet **2**:871–874, 1964

21. Friedman GP, Wilson JM, Colandrea MA, Wichaman MZ: Transient ischemic attacks in a community. JAMA **210**(8):1428–1434, 1969

22. Goldner JC, Whisnant JP, Taylor WF: Long term prognosis of transient cerebral ischemic attacks. Stroke **2**:160–167, 1971

23. Baker RN, Ramseyer JC, Schwartz WS: Prognosis in patients with transient cerebral ischemic attacks. Neurology **18**:1157–1165, 1968

24. Pearce JMS, Gubbay SS, Walton JM: Long term anticoagulant therapy in transient ischemic attacks. Lancet **1**:6–9, 1965

25. Ollson JE, Muller R, Berneli S: Long term anticoagulant therapy for TIA's and minor stroke with minimum residuum. Stroke **7**:444–451, 1976

26. Ziegler DK, Hassanein R: Prognosis in patients with transient ischemic attacks. Stroke **4**:666–673, 1973

27. Millikan CH: Treatment of occlusive cerebrovascular disease. *In* Cerebrovascular Survey. Report for Joint Council Subcommittee on Cerebrovascular Disease. National Institute of Neurological and Communicative Disorders and Stroke and the National Heart and Lung Institute, edited by Siekert RG. Washington DC, 1980

28. Whisnant JP, Cartlidge WEF, Elvebach LR: Carotid and vertebrobasilar transient ischemic attacks: effect of anticoagulants, hypertension and cardiac disorders on survival and stroke occurrence. Ann Neurol **3**:107–115, 1978

29. Ackerman R: Noninvasive carotid evaluation. Stroke **11**:675–678, 1980

30. Meredith J, Franklin E, Forbes G, et al: High resolution dynamic ultrasound imaging of the carotid bifurcations: a prospective evaluation. Radiol **144**:853–858, 1982

31. Spencer M, Reid J, Davis D, et al: Cervical carotid imaging with a continuous wave Doppler flow meter. Stroke **5**:145–154, 1974

32. Ginsberg M, Greenwood S, Goldberg H: Noninvasive diagnosis of extracranial cerebrovascular disease: oculoplethysmography, phonoangiography and directional Doppler ultrasonography. Neurol **29**:623–631, 1979

33. Ackerman R: A perspective on noninvasive diagnosis of carotid disease. Neurol **29**:615–622, 1979

34. Faught E, Trader SO, Hanna GP: Cerebral complications of angiography for transient ischemia and stroke. Neurology (Minneapolis) **29**:4–15, 1979

35. Rainer WG, Guillen J, Bloomquist CD, et al: Carotid artery surgery: morbidity and mortality in 257 operations. Am J Surg **116:**678–681, 1968

36. Deweese JA, Rob CG, Satran R, et al: Surgical treatment for occlusive disease of the carotid artery. Ann Surg **168:**85–94, 1968

37. Galbraith JG, McDowell HA: Stroke and occlusive cerebrovascular disease review and surgical results in 265 cases. J Med Assoc Alabama **38:**1107–1111, 1969

38. Fields WS, Maslenikov V, Meyer JS, et al: Joint study of extracranial occlusion, V: progress report of prognosis following surgery or nonsurgical treatment for transient cerebral ischemic attacks and cervical carotid artery lesions. JAMA **211:**1993–2002, 1970

39. Thompson JE, Austin DJ, Patman RD: Carotid endarterectomy for cerebrovascular insufficiency; long term results in 592 patients followed up to thirteen years. Ann Surg **172:**663–667, 1970

40. Tytus JS, Maclean JB, Hill HD: Prognosis in patients with transient ischemic attacks after endarterectomy. Am Surg **36:**623–626, 1973

41. Deweese JA, Rob DG, Satran R, et al: Results of carotid endarterectomy for transient ischemic attacks five years later. Ann Surg **178:**258–264, 1973

42. Howe JR, Kindt DW: Cerebral protection during carotid endarterectomy. Stroke **5:**340–343, 1974

43. Toole JF, Janeway R, Choi K, et al: Transient ischemic attack due to atherosclerosis: a prospective study of 160 patients. Arch Neurol **32:**5–12, 1975

44. Baker WH, Dorner DB, Barnes RW: Carotid endarterectomy: is an indwelling shunt necessary? Surg **82:**321–326, 1977

45. Matsumoto GH, Cossman D, Callow AD: Hazards and safeguards during carotid endarterectomy: technical considerations. Am J Surg **133:**458–462, 1977

46. Prioleau WH, Aiken AF, Hairston P: Carotid endarterectomy neurologic complications as related to surgical techniques. Ann Surg **185:**678–683, 1977

47. Sundt TM, Sandok BA, Whisnant JP: Carotid endarterectomy complications and pre-operative assessment of risk. Mayo Clin Proc **50:**301–306, 1975

48. Fleming JFR, Griesdale DE, Shutz H, et al: Carotid endarterectomy: Changing morbidity and mortality. Stroke **8:**14, 1977

49. Easton JD, Sherman DG: Stroke and mortality rate in carotid endarterectomy: 228 consecutive operations. Stroke **8:**565–568, 1977

50. West H, Burton R, Roon AJ, et al: Comparative risk of operation and expectant management for carotid artery disease. Stroke **10**(2):117–121, 1979

51. Hayes CD, Dempsey RL: Carotid endarterectomy. Review of 276 cases in a community hospital. Ann Surg **189:**758–762, 1979

52. Hertzer WR, Beven EG, Greenstreet RC, et al: Internal carotid artery back pressure, intraoperative shunting ulcerated atheromata, and the incidence of stroke during carotid endarterectomy. Surgery **83:**306–312, 1978

53. Duke LJ, Slaymaker EE, Lambeith JWC, et al: Carotid arterial reconstruction: a ten year experience. Am Surg **45:**281–288, 1979

54. Thompson JE: Complications of carotid endarterectomy and their prevention. World J Surg **3:**155–165, 1979

55. Boucher-Hayes D, DeCosta A, McGowan WAL: The morbidity and mortality of carotid endarterectomy. Br J Surg **66:**433–437, 1979

56. Towne JB, Bernhard VM: The relationship of postoperative hypertension to complications following carotid endarterectomy. Surg **88**(4):575–580, 1980

57. Whitney DG, Kahn EM, Estes JW, Jones CE: Carotid artery surgery without a temporary indwelling shunt. Arch Surg **115**:1393–1399, 1980
58. Carmichael JP: Carotid surgery in a community hospital. Arch Surg **115**:937–939, 1980
59. Ott DA, Cooley DA, Chapa L, Coelho A: Carotid endarterectomy without temporary intraluminal shunt. Ann Surg **191**(6):708–714, 1980
60. Lye CR, Downs AR: Carotid endarterectomy early and late results in 161 patients. Canadian J Surg **23**(6):536–540, 1980
61. White JS, Sirinek KR, Root D, Waid R: Morbidity and mortality of carotid endarterectomy: rates of occurrence in asymptomatic and symptomatic patients. Arch Surg **116**(4):409–412, 1981
62. DeWeese JA, Rob CG, Satran R, et al: Surgical treatment for occlusive disease of the carotid artery. Ann Surg **168**(1):85–94, 1968
63. Hass JS: An approach to the maximal acceptable stroke complication rate after surgery for transient cerebral ischemia (TIA). Stroke **10**(1):104, 1979
64. Fields WS, Lemak NA, Frankowski RF, Hardy RJ: Controlled trial of aspirin in cerebral ischemia. Part II. Surgical group. Stroke **9**(4):309–317, 1978
65. Ziegler DK, Hassanein RS: Prognosis in patients with transient ischemic attacks. Stroke **4**(7-8):666–672, 1973
66. DeWeese JA, May AG, Lipchik DO, Rob CG: Anatomic and hemodynamic correlations in carotid artery stenosis. Stroke **1**:149–157, 1970
67. Kartchner MM, McRae LP, Morrison FO: Non-invasive detection and evaluation of carotid occlusive disease. Arch Surg **106**:528–535, 1973
68. Archie JP, Feldtman RW: Critical stenosis of the internal carotid artery. Surg **89**(1):67–72, 1981
69. Naritomi H, Sakai F, Meyer JS: Pathogenesis of transient ischemic attacks within the vertebro-basilar arterial system. Arch Neurol **36**:121–128, 1979
70. Austin G, Zinke D, Lichter E, Hayward W: Changes in autoregulation in patients undergoing microanastomosis. *In* Microsurgry for Cerebral Ischemia, edited by Peerless SJ, McCormick CW. New York, Springer Verlag, 1980, pp 15–17
71. Caplan LR, Sergay S: Positional cerebral ischemia. J Neurol Neurosurg Psych **39**:385–391, 1976
72. Mohr JP: Distal field infarction. Neurology **19**:279, 1969
73. Barnett HJM: Delayed cerebral ischemic episodes distal to occlusion of major cerebral arteries. Neurology **28**:769–774, 1978
74. Austin G, Laffin D, Hayward W: Physiologic factors in the selection of patients for superficial temporal artery to middle cerebral artery anastomosis. Surg **75**(6):861–868, 1974
75. Little JR, Yamamoto YL, Feindel W, et al: Cerebral blood flow in superficial temporal artery to middle cerebral artery anastomosis. *In* Microsurgery for Cerebral Ischemia, edited by Peerless SJ, McCormick CW. New York, Springer Verlag, 1980, pp 59–69
76. Heilbrun MP, Reichman OH, Anderson RE, Roberts TS: Regional cerebral blood flow studies following superficial temporal-middle cerebral artery anastomosis. J Neurosurg **43**:706–716, 1975
77. Sundt TM, Seikert RG, Piepgras DG, et al: Bypass surgery for vascular disease of the carotid system. Mayo Clin Proc **51**(11):677–692, 1976
78. Gratzl O, Schmiedek H, Olteanu-Nerbe U: Long term clinical results following extracranial-intracranial arterial bypass surgery. *In* Microsurgery for

Stroke, edited by Schmiedek P. New York, Springer Verlag, 1977, pp 271–275

79. Sampson DS, Hodosh RM, Clark K: Microsurgical treatment of transient cerebral ischemia. JAMA **241**(4):376–378, 1979

80. Mehdorn H, Hoffman WF, Chater NL: Microneurosurgical arterial bypass for cerebral ischemia. The San Francisco experience. *In* Microsurgery for Cerebral Ischemia, edited by Peerless SJ, McCormick CW. New York, Springer Verlag, 1980, pp 350–356

81. Reichman OH: Estimation of flow through STA bypass graft. *In* Microvascular Anastomosis for Cerebral Ischemia, edited by Fein JM, Reichman OH. New York, Springer Verlag, 1978, pp 220–240

82. Crowell RM: STA MCA bypass for acute cerebral ischemia. *In* Microsurgery for Stroke, edited by Schmiedek P. New York, Springer Verlag, 1977, pp 244–250

83. Marshall J, Wilkinson IMS: The prognosis of carotid transient ischemic attacks in patients with normal angiograms. Brain **94**:395–402, 1971

84. Kane WC, Aronson SM: Cardiac disorders predisposing to embolic stroke. Stroke **1**:164–172, 1970

85. Carter AB: Strokes: natural history and progression. Proc R Soc Med **56**:483–486, 1963

86. Owren PA: Results of anticoagulant therapy in Norway. Arch Intern Med **111**:240–247, 1963

87. Easton JD, Sherman DG: Management of cerebral embolism of cardiac origin. Stroke **11**:433–442, 1980

88. Szekely P: Systemic embolism and anticoagulant prophylaxis in rheumatic heart disease. Br Med J **1**:1209–1212, 1964

89. McDevitt E: Treatment of cerebral embolism. Mod Treat **2**:52–63, 1965

90. Fleming HA, Bailey SM: Mitral valve disease, systemic embolism and anticoagulants. Postgrad Med J **47**:599–604, 1971

91. Adams GF, Merrett JD, Hutchinson W and Pollock AM: Cerebral embolism and initial stenosis: survival with and without anticoagulants. J Neurol Neurosurg Psych **37**:378–383, 1974

92. Reed RL, Siekert RG, Merideth J: Rarity of transient focal cerebral ischemia in cardiac dysrhythmia. JAMA **223**:893–895, 1973

93. Millikan CH, Siekert RG, Whisnant J: Intermittent carotid and vertebrobasilar insufficiency associated with polycythemia. Neurol (Minneapolis) **10**:188–196, 1960

94. Seikert RG, Whisnant JP, Millikan CH: Anemia and intermittent focal cerebral arterial insufficiency. Arch Neurol **3**:386–390, 1960

95. Portnoy HD: Transient ischemic attacks produced by carotid stenosis and hypoglycemia. Neurol (Minneapolis) **15**:830–832, 1965

96. Fletcher AP, Alkjaersig N: Prophylactic and therapeutic uses of antithrombotic drugs in cerebral vascular disease. *In* Cerebrovascular Survey Report for Joint Council Subcommittee on Cerebrovascular Disease. National Institutes of Neurological and Communicative Disorders and Stroke and the National Heart and Lung Institute, edited by Siekert RG. Rochester, MN, Whitney Press, 1980, pp 290–305

97. Millikan CH: Treatment of occlusive cerebrovascular disease. *In* Cerebrovascular Survey Report for Joint Council Subcommittee on Cerebrovascular Disease. National Institutes of Neurological and Communicative

Disorders and Stroke and the National Heart and Lung Institute, edited by Siekert RG. Rochester, MN, Whitney Press, 1980, pp 244–289

98. Canadian Cooperative Study Group: A randomized trial of aspirin and sulfanpyrazone in threatened stroke. New Engl J Med **299**:53–59, 1978

99. Fields WS, Lemak NA, Frankowski RF, Hardy RS: Controlled trial of aspirin in cerebral ischemia. Stroke **8**:301–315, 1977

100. Controlled trial of aspirin in cerebral ischemia. Part II. Surgical Group. Stroke **9**:309–319, 1978

101. Reuther R, Dorndorf W: Aspirin in patients with cerebral ischemia and normal angiograms or nonsurgical lesions. The results of a double blind trial. *In* Acetylsalicylic Acid in Cerebral Ischemia and Coronary Heart Disease, edited by Breddin K, Dorndorf W, Loen D, Marx R. New York, Schautter-Verlag, 1978, p 97

102. Jaffe EA, Weksler BB: Recovery of endothelial cell prostacyclin production after inhibition by low doses of aspirin. J Clin Invest **63**:532–535, 1979

103. Moncada S, Vane JR: Arachidonic acid metabolites and the interactions between platelets and blood vessel walls. New Engl J Med **300**:1142–1147, 1979

104. Moncada S, Korbut R: Dipyridamole and other phosphodiesterase inhibitors act as antithrombotic agents by potentiating endogenous prostacyclin. Lancet **1**:1286–1289, 1978

105. Fischer CM: Anticoagulant therapy in cerebral thrombosis and cerebral embolism. A national cooperative study interim report. Neurol (Minneapolis) **11**:119–131, 1961

106. Carter AB: Anticoagulant treatment in progressive stroke. Br Med J **2**:70–73, 1961

107. Baker RN, Broward JA, Fang HC, et al: Anticoagulant therapy in cerebral infarction. Neurol (Minneapolis) **12**:823–835, 1962

108. Millikan CH: Anticoagulant therapy in cerebrovascular disease. *In* Cerebrovascular Diseases. Fourth Princeton Conference, edited by Millikan CH, Siekert RG. New York, Grune & Stratton, 1965, p 183

109. Millikan CH: Evaluation of carbon dioxide inhalation for acute focal cerebral infarction. Arch Neurol Psych **73**:324–328, 1955

110. Jacobsen HH, Skinhoj E: Occlusion of the middle cerebral artery. An analysis of thirty-six arteriographic cases. Dan Med Bull **6**:9–12, 1959

111. Jacobsen HH, Skinhoj E: Thrombosis of the internal carotid artery verified by arteriography. Dan Med Bull **4**:240–248, 1957

112. Diaz FG, Ausman, JI: Experimental cerebral ischemia. Neurosurgery **6**(4):436–445, 1980

113. Paulson O: Cerebral apoplexy (stroke). Pathogenesis pathophysiology and therapy as illustrated by regional blood flow measurements in the brain. Stroke **2**:327–360, 1971

114. VanHoutte PM: Effects of anoxia and glucose depletion on isolated veins of the dog. Am J Physiol **230**(5):1261–1268, 1976

115. VanNueten JM, VanHoutte PM: Improvement of tissue perfusion with inhibitors of calcium ion flux. Biochem Pharm **29**:479–481, 1980

116. Siesjo BK: Cell damage in the brain: a speculative synthesis. J Cereb Blood Flow **1**:155, 1981

117. Hass WK: Beyond cerebral blood flow metabolism and ischemic thresholds: an examination of the role of Ca^{++} in the initiation of cerebral infarction. *In* Cerebral Vascular Disease. Vol. 3. Proceedings of the Salzburg Conference on Cerebral Vascular Disease. Amsterdam, Excerpta Medica, 1981, pp 3–17

118. Schanne, FA, Kane AB, Young EE: Calcium dependence of toxic cell death: a common pathway. Science **206**:700–702, 1979
119. Symon L, Branston N, Strong A: Autoregulation in acute focal ischemia, an experimental study. Stroke **7**:547–554, 1976
120. Hoedt-Rasmussen K, Skinhoj E, Paulson O, et al: Regional cerebral blood flow in acute apoplexy: the luxury perfusion syndrome of brain tissue. Arch Neurol **17**:271–281, 1967
121. Hope D, Branston N, Symon L: Restoration of neurological function with induced hypertension in acute experimental cerebral ischemia. Acta Neurol Scand **56**:506–507, 1977
122. Kassell N, Peerless S, Durward J, et al: Treatment of ischemic deficits from vasospasm with intravascular volume expansion and induced arterial hypertension. Neurosurg **11**:337–343, 1982
123. Standgaard S, Olesen J, Skinhoj E, Lassen N: Autoregulation of brain circulation in severe arterial hypertension. Br Med J **1**:507–510, 1973
124. Heiss W, Hayakawa T, Waltz A: Patterns of changes of blood flow and relationships to infarction in experimental cerebral ischemia. Stroke **7**:454–459, 1976
125. Breslin D, Swinton W: Hypertension and cerebrovascular disease. Primary Care **7**:49–59, 1980
126. Wylie EJ, Hein MF, Adams JE: Intracranial hemorrhage following surgical revascularization for the treatment of acute strokes. J Neurosurg **21**:212–215, 1964
127. Hunter JA, Julian OC, Dye WS, Javid H: Emergency operation for acute cerebral ischemia due to carotid artery obstruction: review of 26 cases. Ann Surg **162**:901–904, 1965
128. Rob CG: Operation for acute complete stroke due to thrombosis of the internal carotid artery. Surg **65**(5):862–865, 1969
129. Bauer RB, Meyer JS, Fields WS, et al: Joint study of extracranial arterial occlusion: 111 reports of controlled study of long term survival with and without operation. JAMA **208**:509–518, 1969
130. Goldstone J, Moore WS: A new look at emergency carotid artery operations for the treatment of cerebrovascular insufficiency. Stroke **9**(6):599–602, 1978
131. Ojemann RG, Crowell RM, Roberson GH, Fisher CM: Surgical treatment of extracranial carotid occlusive disease. Clinical Neurosurg **22**:214–263, 1975
132. Mentzer MD, Finkelmeier BA, Crosby IK, Wellons HA: Emergency carotid endarterectomy for fluctuating neurologic deficits. Surg **89**(1):60–66, 1981
133. Najafi H, Javid H, Dye WS et al: Emergency carotid thromboendarterectomy. Arch Surg **103**:610–613, 1971
134. Jones TH, Morawetz RB, Crowell RM, et al: Thresholds of focal cerebral ischemia in awake monkeys. J Neurosurg **54**:773–782, 1981
135. Selman WR, Spetzler RF, Roessmann VR, et al: Barbiturate-induced coma therapy for focal cerebral ischemia. J Neurosurg **55**:220–226, 1981
136. Satiani B, Vasko JS, Evans WE: Hypertension following carotid endarterectomy. Surg Neurol **11**:357–359, 1979
137. Caplan LR, Skillman J, Ojemann R, Fields WS: Intracerebral hemorrhage following carotid endarterectomy: a hypertensive complication. Stroke **9**:457–460, 1978
138. Fisher M, Adams RD: Observations on brain embolism with special reference to the mechanism of hemorrhagic infarction. J Neuropath Exp Neurol **10**:92–93, 1951

139. Fazio C, Sacchi U: Experimentally produced red softening at the brain. J Neuropath Exp Neurol **13**:476–481, 1954
140. Hain RF, Westhaysen PJ, Swank RL: Hemorrhagic cerebral infarction by arterial occlusion. J Neuropath Exp Neurol **11**:34–43, 1953
141. Kindt GW, Youmans JR, Albrand O: Factors influencing the autoregulation of cerebral blood flow during hypertension and hypotension. J Neurosurg **26**:299–305, 1967
142. Waltz AG: Effect of blood pressure on blood flow in ischemic and non ischemic cerebral cortex. The phenomenon of autoregulation and luxury perfusion. Neurol (Minneapolis) **18**:613–621, 1968
143. Waltz AG: Effect of $PaCO_2$ on blood flow and microvasculature of ischemic and nonischemic cerebral cortex. Stroke **1**:27–37, 1970
144. Fieschi C, Agnoli A, Battistini N, et al: Arrangement of regional cerebral blood flow and of its regulatory mechanisms in acute cerebrovascular lesions. Neurol (Minneapolis) **18**:1166–1179, 1968
145. Agnoli A, Fieschi C, Bozzao L, et al: Autoregulation of cerebral blood flow studies during drug induced hypertension in normal subjects and in patients with cerebral vascular diseases. Circ **38**:800–812, 1968
146. Sundt TM, Grant WC, Garcia JH: Restoration of middle cerebral artery flow in experimental infarction. J Neurosurg **31**:311–322, 1969
147. Laha RK, Dujovny M, Barrionuevo PJ, et al: Protective effects of methyl prednisolone and dimethyl sulfoxide in experimental middle cerebral artery embolectomy. J Neurosurg **49**:508–516, 1978
148. Levinthal R, Mosely J, Brown WJ, Stern WE: Effect of STA-MCA anastomosis on the course of experimental acute MCA embolic occlusion. Stroke **10**(4):371–375, 1979
149. Crowell RM, Olsson Y: Effect of extracranial intracranial bypass graft on experimental acute stroke in dogs. J Neurosurg **38**:26–31, 1973
150. Diaz F, Mastri A, Ausman J, Chou S: Acute cerebral revascularization after regional cerebral ischemia in the dog. J Neurosurg **51**:644–653, 1979
151. Spetzler RF, Chater NL: Microvascular bypass surgery. Part 2: Physiological studies. J Neurosurg **45**:508–513, 1976
152. Spetzler RF, Seleman WR, Rosk RA, Bonstelli C: Cerebral revascularization during barbiturate coma in primates and humans. Surg Neurol **17**(2): 111–115, 1982
153. Suzuki J, Takashi Y, Kodama W, et al: A new therapeutic method for acute brain infarctions: revascularization following the administration of mannitol and perfluosochemicals. A preliminary report. Surg Neurol **12**(5):325–332, 1982
154. Diaz FG, Ausman JI, de los Reyes RA, Dujovny M, Pearce J: Successful application of acute cerebral revascularization to stroke in evolution. *In* Microsurgical Anastomoses for Cerebral Ischemia, edited by Handa H, Kikuchi H. Kyoto, Japan, in Press
155. Weinstein P, Chater NL: Cerebral revascularization for stroke in evolution. *In* Microsurgery for Stroke, edited by Schmiedek P. New York, Springer Verlag, 1977, pp 240–243
156. Chou SN: Embolectomy of middle cerebral artery. Report of a case. J Neurosurg **20**:161–163, 1963
157. Jacobson HJ, Wallman LJ, Schumaker GA, et al: Microsurgery as an aid to middle cerebral artery endarterectomy. J Neurosurg **19**:108–115, 1962

158. Welch K: Excision of occlusive lesions of the middle cerebral artery. J Neurosurg **13**:73–80, 1956
159. Yasargil MG, Krayenbuhl HG, Jacobson JH: Microneurosurgical arterial reconstruction. Surgery **67**:221–233, 1970
160. Zlotnik EI: Thromboembolectomy of the middle cerebral artery. Case report. J Neurosurg **42**:723–725, 1975
161. Yonekawa Y, Handa H, Terano M, Tetsuaki T: Revascularization in the acute stage of MCA occlusion. *In* Microsurgery for Cerebral Ischemia, edited by Peerless SJ, McCormick CW. New York, Springer Verlag, 1980, pp 275–282
162. Dujovny M, Barrioneuvo PJ, Laha RK, et al: Experimental middle cerebral artery microsurgical embolectomy. *In* Microsurgery for Stroke, edited by Schmiedek P. New York, Springer Verlag, 1977, pp 91–97
163. Okada Y, Shima T, Yamamoto M, et al: Experimental middle cerebral artery embolization and embolectomy. Acta Neurochir Suppl **28**:222–225, 1979
164. Ito Z, Suzuki A: The emergency STA-MCA bypass evaluated by the induced functional EEG analysis in acute ischemic stroke. *In* Microsurgery for Cerebral Ischemia, edited by Peerless SJ, McCormick CW. New York, Springer Verlag, 1980, pp 117–121
165. Fletcher A, Alkjaersig N: The use and monitoring of antithrombotic drug therapy: the need for a new approach. Thromb Haemostas **38**:881–892, 1977
166. Fletcher A, Alkjaersig N, Brooks J, et al: Blood coagulation and plasma fibrinolytic enzyme system pathophysiology in stroke. Stroke **7**:337–348, 1976
167. Genton E, Barnett HJM, Fields WS, et al: XIV: Cerebral ischemia: the role of thrombosis and antithrombotic therapy. Stroke **8**(1):150–175, 1977
168. Mohr JP: Lacunes. Stroke **13**(1):3–11, 1982
169. Meyer J, Gilroy J, Barhart M, Johnson J: Therapeutic thrombolysis in cerebral thromboembolism: double blind evaluation of intravenous plasmin therapy in carotid and middle cerebral occlusion. Neurol (Minneapolis) **13**:927–937, 1963
170. Meyer J, Gilroy J, Barnhart M, Johnson J: Anticoagulants plus streptokinase therapy in progressive stroke. JAMA **189**:373, 1964
171. Hanaway J, Torack R, Fletcher A, Landau W: Intracranial bleeding associated with urokinase therapy for acute ischemic hemispheral stroke. Stroke **7**:143–147, 1976
172. Laha RK, Isroeli J, Dujovny M, et al: Low molecular weight dextran in experimental embolectomy. Stroke **11**(1):59–63, 1980
173. Gilroy JM, Barnhart M, Meyer JS: Treatment of acute stroke with dextran 40. JAMA **210**:293–302, 1969
174. Matthews WB, Moxbury J, Grainger KMR, et al: A blind controlled trial of dextran 40 in the treatment of ischemic stroke. Brain **99**:193–206, 1976
175. Spudis EV, de la Torre E, Pikula L: Management of completed strokes with dextran 40. A community hospital failure. Stroke **4**(6):895–897, 1973
176. O'Brien MD: Ischemic cerebral edema. A review. Stroke **10**(6):623–628, 1979
177. Fujimoto T, Walker JT, Spatz M, Klatzo I: Pathophysiologic aspects of ischemic edema. *In* Dynamics of Brain Edema, edited by Pappius HM, Feindel W. Berlin, Heidelberg, Springer Verlag, 1976, pp 171–180
178. Mathew NT, Rivera VM, Meyer JS, et al: Double blind evaluation of glycerol therapy in acute cerebral infarction. Lancet **2**:1327–1329, 1972
179. Gilsanz V, Rebollar JL, Buencuerpo J, Changues MT: Controlled trial of glycerol versus dexamethasone in the treatment of cerebral oedema in acute cerebral infarction. Lancet **1**:1049–1051, 1975

180. Fritz G, Werner I: The effect of glycerol infusion in acute cerebral infarction. Acta Med Scand **198**:287–289, 1975
181. Larsson O, Marinovich W, Barber K: Double blind trial of glycerol therapy in early stroke. Lancet **1**:832–834, 1976
182. Fawer R, Justafre JC, Berger JP, Schelling JL: Intravenous glycerol in cerebral infarction. A controlled 4 month trial. Stroke **9**(5):848–486, 1978
183. Candelise L, Colombo A, Spinnler H: Therapy against brain swelling in stroke patients. A retrospective clinical study on 227 patients. Stroke **6**:353–356, 1975
184. Santanbrogio S, Martinotti R, Sardella J, et al: Is there a real treatment for stroke? Clinical and statistical comparison of different treatments in 300 patients. Stroke **9**:130–132, 1978
185. Kagawa S, Keiji K, Yoshimoto T, Suzuki J: The protective effect of mannitol and perfluorochemicals on hemorrhagic infarction: An experimental study. Surg Neurol **17**(1):66–70, 1982
186. Little JR: Modification of acute focal ischemia by treatment with mannitol. Stroke **9**:5–9, 1978
187. Bounds JV, Okazaki H, Reagan TJ, Whisnant JP: Recent cerebral infarction in the distribution of the internal carotid artery. Stroke **8**:5, 1977
188. Rengachary SS, Batnitzky S, Morantz RA, et al: Hemicraniectomy for acute massive cerebral infarction. Neurosurgery **8**(3):321–328, 1981
189. Patten BM, Mendell J, Bruun B, et al: Double blind study of the effects of dexamethasone on acute stroke. Neurology (Minneapolis) **22**:377–383, 1972
190. Bauer RB, Tellez H: Dexamethasone as treatment in cerebral vascular disease. II. A controlled study in acute cerebral infarction. Stroke **4**:547–555, 1973
191. Norris JW: Steroid therapy in acute cerebral infarction. Arch Neurol **33**:69–71, 1976
192. Smith AL: Barbiturate protection in cerebral hypoxia. Anesthesiology **47**:285–293, 1977
193. Belopavlovic M, Buchthal A: Barbiturate therapy in cerebral ischemia. Anaesthesia **35**:235–245, 1980
194. Snyder BD: Barbiturate therapy in cerebral ischaemia. Anaesthesia **36**(1):77–78, 1981
195. Michenfelder JD, Milde HJ, Sundt TM: Cerebral protection by barbiturate anesthesia. Arch Neurol **33**:345–350, 1976
196. Mosely JI, Laurent JP, Molinari GF: Barbiturate attenuation of the clinical course and pathological lesions in the primate stroke model. Neurol **25**:870–874, 1975
197. Molinari GF, Lightfoote WE, Fein JM: Evidence for barbiturate protection in focal cerebral ischemia: a hypothesis for mechanism and clinical utility. *In* Microsurgical Anastomosis for Cerebral Ischemia, edited by Fein JM, Reichman OH. New York, Springer Verlag, 1978, pp 86–93
198. Corkill G, Chikovani OK, McLeisch R, et al: Timing of pentobarbital administration for brain protection in experimental stroke. Surg Neurol **3**:147–179, 1976
199. Selman WR, Spetzler RF, Roessmann U, et al: Barbiturate induced coma therapy for focal cerebral ischemia: effect after temporary and permanent MCA occlusion. J Neurosurg **55**:220–226, 1981
200. Corkill G, Sivalingam S, Reitan JA, et al: Dose dependency of the post insult protective effect of pentobarbital in the canine experimental stroke model. Stroke **9**:10–12, 1978

201. Hoff JT, Smith AL, Hankinson HL, et al: Barbiturate protection from cerebral infarction in primates. Stroke **6**:28–33, 1975
202. Baskin DS, Hosobuchi Y: Naloxone reversal of ischaemic neurologic deficits in man. Lancet, Aug. 8, pp 272–275, 1981
203. Britton M, Faire VD, Helmers C, et al: Lack of effect of theophylline on the outcome of acute cerebral infarction. Acta Neurol Scand **62**:116–123, 1980
204. Inguar DH, Lassen NA: Treatment of focal cerebral ischemia with hyperbaric oxygen. Report of four cases. Acta Neurol Scand **41**:92–95, 1965
205. Heyman A, Saltzman HA, Whalen RE: The use of hyperbaric oxygenation in the treatment of cerebral ischemia and infarction. Circ **33**:(Suppl II):20–27, 1966
206. Baker RN: An evaluation of anticoagulant therapy in the treatment of cerebrovascular disease: report of the Veterans Administration cooperative study of atherosclerosis, Neurology Section. Neurol (Minneapolis) **11**:132–138, 1961
207. Baker RN, Broward JA, Fang HC, Fisher CM, Giroch SN, Heyman A: Anticoagulant therapy in cerebral infarction. Neurology (Minneapolis) **12**:823–835, 1962
208. McDowell F, McDevitt E: Treatment of completed stroke with long term anticoagulant: Six and one half year experience. *In* Cerebral Vascular Diseases, Fourth Princeton Conference, edited by Kiekert RG, Vhisnant JP. New York, Grune & Stratton, 1965, pp 185–199
209. Kannel W, Wolf P, McGee D, et al: Systolic blood pressure, arterial rigidity, and risk of stroke. JAMA **245**:1225–1229, 1981
210. Kannel W, Dawber T, Sorlie P, Wolf P: Components of blood pressure and risk of atherothrombotic brain infarction: the Framingham study. Stroke **7**:327–331, 1976
211. Meyer S, Sawada T, Kitzmura A, Toyoda M: Cerebral blood flow after control of hypertension in stroke. Neurol **18**:772–781, 1968
212. Adams G: Prospects for patients with strokes, with special reference to hypertensive hemiplegics. Br Med J **2**:253–259, 1965
213. Merrett J, Adams G: Comparison of mortality rates in elderly normotensive and hypertensive hemiplegic patients. Br Med J **2**:802–805, 1966
214. Carter A: Hypotensive therapy in stroke survivors. Lancet **1**:485–489, 1970
215. Beevors D, Fairman M, Hamilton M, Harpur J: Antihypertension treatment and the course of established cerebral vascular disease. Lancet **II**:1407–1409, 1973
216. Hypertensive-Stroke Cooperative Study Group: Effect of antihypertension treatment on stroke recurrence. JAMA **229**:409–418, 1974
217. Roski R, Spetzler RF, Owen M, et al: Reversal of a seven-year-old visual field defect with extracranial intracranial arterial anastomosis. Surg Neurol **10**:267–268, 1978
218. Jacques S, Garner JT: Reversal of aphasia with superficial temporal artery to middle cerebral artery anastomosis. Surg Neurol **5**:143–145, 1976
219. Ito Z, Nakajima K, Suzuki A, Vemura K: Selection of completed stroke patients for STA-MCA anastomosis based on measurements of somatosensory evoked potential and CBF dynamics. *In* Microsurgery for Stroke, edited by Schmiedek P. New York, Springer Verlag, 1977, pp 177–184
220. Holbach KH, Wassmann H: Extra-intracranial anastomosis operation associated with hyperbaric oxygenation in the treatment of completed stroke. *In* Microsurgery for Cerebral Ischemia, edited by Peerless SJ, McCormick CW. New York, Springer Verlag, 1980, pp 286–291

221. Baker RN, Broward JA, Fang HC, et al: Anticoagulant therapy in cerebral infarction. Neurol (Minneapolis) **12:**823–835, 1962
222. Enger E, Boyesen S: Long term anticoagulant therapy in patients with cerebral infarction. A controlled clinical study. Acta Med Scand **178**(Suppl 438):1–61, 1965
223. Hill AB, Marshall J, Shaw DA: Cerebrovascular disease: trial of long term anticoagulant therapy. Br Med J **2:**1003–1006, 1962

Neurogenic Hypertension:
Pathogenesis and Therapy

Chapter 13

Experimental Neurogenic Hypertension

Robert M. Carey

Introduction

The sympathetic nervous system has been implicated as an initiating and potentially sustaining mechanism responsible for elevated blood pressure in essential hypertension. Increased blood pressure could occur through a direct effect of the neurotransmitter, norepinephrine, on vascular smooth muscle, or through norepinephrine-induced effects of salt and water retention on the circulation.

Recent focus on the relationship of the sympathetic nervous system to the initiation and maintenance of elevated blood pressure in essential hypertension has resulted from the following basic and clinical observations: 1) The circulatory changes of high cardiac output, tachycardia, increased dP/dT, and venoconstriction with normal peripheral resistance in early hypertension suggest excessive sympathetic nervous system activity.[1–3] 2) Concentrations of catecholamines in blood, cerebrospinal fluid, and certain tissues such as the vas deferens, in many patients with hypertension, indicate increased synthesis, storage, and release or impaired re-uptake of catecholamines at peripheral sympathetic or central adrenergic sites.[4–7] 3) Pharmacologic agents that lower blood pressure in hypertensive patients, particularly alpha-methyldopa or clonidine, act centrally and/or peripherally to reduce sympathetic neuronal activity.[8–11] 4) Psychosocial stress can contribute to or cause arterial hypertension in experimental animals and man.[12] 5) In hypertensive man, arterial blood pressure falls during sleep, suggesting that decreased sympathetic drive at least in part sustains the elevation of blood pressure during the wake period.[13] 6) Lesions of the brain, most notably the anteroventral third ventricle (AV3V) area of the anterior hypothalamus, can prevent or abolish elevated arterial pressure in animals with several forms of experimental hypertension.[14–16] 7) In a subgroup of patients with essential hypertension, plasma renin activity is elevated, and blood pressure and circulating renin can be reduced together with a beta-adrenergic blocking agent, suggesting that elevation of sympathetic nervous system activity contributes to the hypertension and hyperreninemia in these patients.[17] 8) Sympathetic nerve activity correlates with blood pressure as spontaneously hypertensive rats develop hypertension.[18]

Increased activity of the sympathetic nervous system may bring about chronic elevation of blood pressure by means of a variety of pathophysiologic mechanisms. 1) Sustained arteriolar vasoconstriction may be caused directly by release of norepinephrine in several peripheral vascular beds. Adaptive changes resulting in vascular smooth muscle hypertrophy may serve to maintain the hypertensive state.[19] 2) Sympathetic stimulation of the heart increases stroke volume, heart rate, and cardiac output. A high cardiac output may bring about a rise in arterial pressure, which may lead to arteriolar hypertrophy or autoregulatory vasoconstriction and increased peripheral vascular resistance.[20–22] Venous constriction may contribute to the high cardiac output by increasing central blood volume.[23] 3) Sympathetic stimulation to the kidney, perhaps in selective fashion, causes sodium and water retention as well as renin release, with associated elevation of angiotensin and aldosterone concentrations.[24–26] These factors result in enhanced peripheral resistance through arteriolar vasoconstriction, increased vascular wall stiffness, or increased vascular wall-to-lumen ratio, which augments the contractile response.[22,27,28] 4) Sympathetic neuronal stimulation may result directly in abnormal electrogenic ion transport and exaggerated vasoconstrictor responses by means of a membrane defect in arteriolar smooth muscle.[29] In addition, sympathetic neurons stimulate the rate of synthesis of contractile proteins in vascular smooth muscle, which may lead to enhanced vasoconstriction and a rise in peripheral resistance.[19,30]

A large body of evidence indicates that increased sympathetic nervous system activity, possibly modulated by the central nervous system, results in the development and/or maintenance of elevated arterial blood pressure in essential hypertension. Under normal circumstances, arterial blood pressure is maintained within the "normal" range by the activity of neuronal systems in the central nervous system.[31,32] These central neuronal systems provide preganglionic sympathetic stimulation to the spinal cord, creating a background vasoconstriction, which elevates peripheral resistance and maintains systemic arterial pressure. This vasopressor system is counterbalanced in turn by a central vasodepressor system inhibiting sympathetic activity and lowering blood pressure.[31,32] Normally, pressor and depressor systems are counterbalanced, maintaining a normal blood pressure. However, an imbalance of these central pressor and depressor systems may result in augmentation of peripheral sympathetic discharge, increasing peripheral vascular resistance and elevating arterial blood pressure.

Central sympathetic neuronal output is continuously modulated by afferent signals from various sensors through the body. The influence of efferent sympathetic activity is determined by factors operating at the level of the target organ, vascular smooth muscle. Thus, neurogenic hypertension may originate (1) within the central nervous system; (2) at the level of the efferent pathways, the adrenergic nerve terminals, or the target tissues; or (3) at the level of the afferent or sensory endings, where the input to the central nervous system originates. Any increase in excitation or reduction in the inhibition of the sympathetic vasomotor neurons at any of these levels may theoretically produce an elevation of arteriolar blood pressure, termed "neurogenic hypertension."

If neurogenic mechanisms are indeed involved in the pathophysiology of essential hypertension, it should be possible to demonstrate in animals that abnormalities of neurotransmission can elevate arterial blood pressure. Although such models cannot prove the pathogenesis of the human disease, they demonstrate that abnormalities of neuronal function are capable of producing a disorder comparable in many respects to that observed in humans.

Over many years, numerous investigators have performed animal experiments to produce hypertension by manipulation of normal neuronal function.[33] In most studies a direct increase in sympathetic excitation was obtained with a variety of methods, including chronic emotional or environmental stress, central nervous system ischemia, chronic ablation of specific sites in the central nervous system, or chronic electrical stimulation of the sympathetic nervous system. In addition, some investigators have sought to produce hypertension by withdrawing inhibition of sympathetic neuronal discharge—for example, by interrupting input from arterial baroreceptors to the central nervous system.

Most of the models of experimental neurogenic hypertension have produced a few of the features of human hypertensive disease. However, none of the models has been successful in producing chronic sustained hypertension. Thus, there is no uniformly accepted model of chronic experimental neurogenic hypertension, in which the elevation of blood pressure is clearly dependent upon enhanced sympathetic neuronal activity.

Attempts to validate any model of experimental neurogenic hypertension should demonstrate that manipulations of the sympathetic nervous system cause chronic sustained hypertension, that the hypertensive process exhibits many features of the human disease, and that the hypertension is responsive to antihypertensive agents. For example, the elevation of the mean arterial pressure should be associated with an increase in the variability of pressure from minute to minute; a phasic increase in blood pressure should occur in response to a defined stimulus or during a behavioral manipulation; and hormonal parameters, such as circulating catecholamines and plasma renin activity, should be similar to the human disease.

Up to now, attempts to establish an animal model of neurogenic hypertension with chronic sustained elevation of blood pressure have been difficult and generally unsuccessful. This chapter reviews critically the various animal models of experimental neurogenic hypertension reported to the present time. The review will be confined strictly to experimental manipulations producing hypertension acutely or chronically. No attempt will be made to cover the broader topics of neurogenic factors involved in experimental renal or renovascular hypertension, or in the spontaneously hypertensive rat, nor will there be any discussion of manipulations of the nervous system designed to inhibit or prevent elevation of blood pressure in these models of experimental hypertension.

The following animal models will be discussed in detail: (1) production of sustained hypertension by continuous stimulation of sympathetic ganglia; (2) production of sustained hypertension by continuous stimulation of the splanchnic and renal nerves; (3) production of sustained hypertension by chronic intrarenal norepinephrine infusion; (4) production of labile hypertension by sinoaortic denervation; (5) acute and chronic hypertension resulting from interruption of transmission through the nucleus tractus solitarii and its immediate connections; (6) production of acute hypertension by electrical stimulation of the nucleus locus coeruleus, and (7) production of acute hypertension by electrical stimulation of the anterior hypothalamus.

Stimulation of the Sympathetic Ganglia

Several studies have demonstrated that electrical stimulation of the cervical sympathetic ganglia produces an acute pressor response in experimental animals.[34–36] Most of these studies were performed in anesthetized dogs and demonstrated that electrical stimulation of either the right or the left stellate ganglion increases cardiac output and raises arterial pressor. The pressor response under certain conditions may be maintained for several hours in the anesthetized dog.[37]

More recently, Liard et al. electrically stimulated the left stellate ganglion of six conscious dogs continuously for a seven-day period while monitoring cardiac output and arterial blood pressure.[38] In all six dogs, stimulation elicited an abrupt rise in systemic arterial pressure related entirely to an increase in cardiac output lasting at least six hours. After 24 hours of continuous electrical stimulation, cardiac output returned to control values, but blood pressure remained elevated. After seven days of continuous stimulation, blood pressure was increased by an average of 25 mm Hg and peripheral resistance by 35%. Alterations of blood volume, plasma renin activity, circulating catecholating catecholamines, and sodium balance could not explain the development of sustained hypertension. Alpha-adrenergic blockade with phenoxybenzamine largely prevented the rise in blood pressure in the short-term stellate ganglion stimulations, while propranolol had no effect on the pressor response, although it nearly abolished the increase in cardiac output.

These experiments (38) demonstrated that sustained elevation of mean arterial blood pressure could be elicited by continuous stimulation of the left stellate ganglion in conscious dogs. Although the precise mechanism responsible for increase in blood pressure was not defined in these experiments, the authors felt that a pressor reflex might have been activated, through which stimulation of afferent fibers from the heart would increase sympathetic tone. Another possibility was that total body autoregulation occurred rapidly such that the initial increase in cardiac output (or high flow) led to an increase in peripheral vasoconstriction and structural changes in the vascular wall, returning flow to a level in accord with the metabolic needs of the tissues. In any case, these studies strongly suggest that continuous stimulation of the sympathetic nerves at the level of sympathetic ganglion can result in chronic experimental neurogenic hypertension. However, the degree of technical difficulty in producing this animal model render it impractical for extensive investigation.

Chronic Splanchnic and Renal Nerve Stimulation

As stated, studies have demonstrated that selective sympathetic stimulation to the kidney may be important in the control of systemic arterial pressure. Perhaps the earliest demonstration of this phenomenon was performed in 1945 by Kottke et al.,[24] who showed that chronic renal artery-nerve stimulation resulted in sustained elevation of blood pressure in dogs. However, the autopsy finding of renal hemorrhage and nearly complete occlusion of the renal arteries by thrombus formation in the region of the stimulating electrodes in one of the dogs rendered interpretation of these studies difficult. It was possible that renal ischemia may have contributed to the pathogenesis of the observed hypertension.

In 1953, Kubicek et al.[25] chronically stimulated splanchnic nerves of 19 conscious dogs. Stimulation produced an unequivocal elevation of arterial pressure for the duration of stimulation, which varied from 12 to 41 days. Pulse rate during hypertension was normal. Renal plasma flow, glomerular filtration rate, and filtration fraction were increased during the hypertension in some instances. None of the animals showed a distinct decrease in renal plasma flow and glomerular filtration rate. Although the contribution of possible renal ischemia was not assessed pathologically, the hypertension was probably produced by vasoconstriction of the splanchnic bed.

From these studies it is possible that selective sympathetic stimulation to the kidney may produce chronic experimental neurogenic hypertension, but these experiments are too laborious to provide a functional model for future study.

Chronic Intrarenal Norepinephrine Infusion

In 1977, studies from our laboratory demonstrated that selective sympathetic stimulation to the kidney could produce sustained arterial hypertension.[26] Dogs were infused with norepinephrine chronically into the renal artery and responses were compared with a similar norepinephrine infusion into the inferior vena cava in uninephrectomized conscious dogs. Intrarenal norepinephrine produced a sustained rise in mean arterial pressure of approximately 25 mm Hg associated with a 32 meq positive sodium balance. Inferior venacaval infusion of norepinephrine produced a transient rise in blood pressure accompanied by a pressure natriuresis of 54 meq of sodium. With renal artery infusion, peripheral renin activity rose from 1.1 $\pm$ 0.2 to 4.4 $\pm$ 0.8 ng/ml/hr at 1 hour and fell to control at 24 hours. Inferior venacaval infusion of norepinephrine produced a similar result. Saralasin ([Sar^1, Ala^8]-angiotensin II) produced no significant change in blood pressure, but phentolamine normalized blood pressure. Renal plasma flow was decreased chronically by 25%, but glomerular filtration rate was unchanged by intrarenal norepinephrine. The chronic sustained elevation of blood pressure with intrarenal norepinephrine was characterized by decreased cardiac output and elevated total peripheral resistance.

These data indicated that proportionally greater sympathetic stimulation to the kidney may be important to the pathogenesis of sustained arterial hypertension, and established this animal model of experimental neurogenic hypertension. Further, the model of chronic intrarenal norepinephrine infusion is technically straightforward, with a predictable dose-dependent sustained increase in mean arterial pressure in each animal. These results were subsequently confirmed by others.[39] Thus, the reproducibility of benign hypertension with this model affords an excellent practically feasible model of experimental neurogenic hypertension. It is possible that with higher doses of intrarenal norepinephrine severe intrarenal vasoconstriction could provide a model of accelerated or malignant hypertension as well.

The hypothesis resulting from these data is in agreement with the principles of Guyton, who has proposed that a generalized increase in total peripheral vascular resistance producing an increase in blood pressure would result in a pressure natriuresis and return of arterial pressure to normal levels.[40] However, with selective sympathetic stimulation to the kidneys, pressure natriuresis did not occur, and blood pressure was sustained at an elevated level.[26]

Sinoaortic Deafferentation

Baroreceptors of the carotid sinus and aortic arch respond to changes to arterial blood pressure by reflex vasomotor and cardiac responses, which tend to return pressure to normal. A reduction in impulses traveling from these receptors to the medullary cardiovascular control centers causes vasomotor and cardiac changes that raise arterial pressure. Conversely, an increase in impulses traveling via these pathways causes a decrease in arterial pressure.

The sensory terminals for systemic arterial baroreceptors are located in segments of the arterial circulation with highly elastic properties.[41] Baroreceptor endings are most densely concentrated in the medio-adventitial border of the carotid sinus, aortic arch, and right subclavian artery. Baroreceptor fibers transmitting information to the central nervous system are mostly medullated type A nerve fibers, but nonmedullated type C fibers have also been found in the aortic arch and carotid sinus of several species.[42] The importance of the baroreceptor C fibers in the tonic control of arterial blood pressure, however, is controversial.[42]

Precise knowledge of the anatomical location of afferent neurons conveying baroreceptor information to the central nervous system has been established recently by the development of new sensitive anatomical tracing techniques employing horseradish peroxidase histochemistry.[43,44] Afferent baroreceptor fibers originating in the carotid sinus, aortic arch, and right subclavian artery pass into the brain via the carotid sinus and aortic depressor nerves, the former being a branch of the glossopharyngeal nerve (IXth cranial nerve), and the latter a portion of the vagus nerve (Xth cranial nerve). Using the horseradish peroxidase technique, Kalia[44] has identified the termination of baroreceptor afferents in the region of the nucleus tractus solitarii (NTS). Fibers originating in the aortic-arch and traveling via the aortic nerve terminate in the dorso-lateral and medial subnuclei of the NTS. Afferent projections from the carotid sinus baroreceptor fibers terminate in a larger distribution along the rostro-caudal medulla, projecting not only to the ventro-lateral nuclei of the NTS, but also extending to the ventro-lateral medulla in the region of the nucleus ambiguus and the paramedian reticular nucleus. Furthermore, Kalia[44] and Chernicky et al.[45] have shown termination of horseradish peroxidase-labelled vagal fibers in both the ipsilateral and contralateral aspects of the area postrema, a circumventricular organ in the 4th ventricle contiguous with the NTS.

Baroreceptor nerve endings are mechanoreceptors that are stimulated by a stretch of the arterial wall as a result of change in pressure within the blood vessel. Baroreceptor nerve endings are quite sensitive to small changes in both static and pulsatile pressures, although they are more strongly stimulated by the latter.[46]

Increased baroreceptor activity resulting from a rise in intra-arterial pressure causes inhibition of vasomotor discharge in the sympathetic nervous system and simultaneously increases cardiac vagal activity.[47] The resultant vasodilation and reduction in heart rate thus oppose the rise in pressure, acting to return the pressure toward normal. A decrease in arterial pressure evokes the opposite series of events. The baroreceptor control system provides a powerful cardiovascular negative feedback system. Normally, baroreceptor reflexes serve their major purpose by preventing a fall in arterial pressure. In their absence, severe orthostatic hypotension would occur in an upright position, as a consequence of venous pooling.[47]

In 1927, Herring discovered that denervation of the sinoaortic areas caused an abrupt rise in arterial pressure.[47] In 1929, Koch and Mies demonstrated that ablation of these areas resulted in chronic hypertension, and this prompted interest in the possibility that baroreceptor dysfunction could account for the development of essential hypertension.[47]

A large number of studies have shown that excision of the sinoaortic nerves is associated with tachycardia and increased blood pressure lability, most apparent in the active animal.[33] The exaggerated lability of blood pressure may or may not be accompanied by a sustained rise in baseline mean arterial pressure. Although controversial, it is likely that the magnitude of the blood pressure rise is dependent upon the degree of alertness or stress associated with the procedure of recording the arterial pressure.[48,49]

In cats the normal fall in arterial pressure during sleep is remarkably exaggerated after sinoaortic denervation.[50] Severe hypotensive episodes may occur, associated with symptoms of cerebral ischemia. The hypotension during sleep in cats is related to removal of the chemoreceptor component carried by the carotid sinus nerve.

In dogs and rats the opposite effects occur. After sinoaortic denervation, arterial pressure rises rather than falls during sleep. In dogs, Ferrario et al.[48] found significant elevations in arterial pressure during slow wave sleep without changes in heart rate. Averill et al.[51] also found transient hypertensive episodes characteristic of deep sleep in dogs with neurogenic hypertension. Junqueira et al.[49] showed that blood pressure also rises during slow wave sleep in rats subjected to sinoaortic denervation. The mechanism of the hypertensive episodes during slow wave sleep in neurogenic hypertensive dogs and rats is unknown.

As early as 1932, Wright[52] recognized that the carotid sinus and aortic baroreceptors act to "buffer" abrupt changes in arterial blood pressure. During the 1930s and 40s, baroreceptor denervation as described by Nowak[53] and Thomas[54] became an accepted method to produce "neurogenic hypertension." The hypertension following chronic baroreceptor denervation was unquestioned, until it was observed by Cowley et al.[55] in 1973 that the mean level of arterial blood pressure generally was not elevated when averaged over long periods from continuously recorded denervated dogs. Thus, there was no significant difference in the average level of arterial pressure around which the daily fluctuations occurred.

Yet, immediately following baroreceptor denervation, these dogs exhibited marked increases in pressure as classically described. They showed no bradycardia in response to injections of various pressor agents or carotid occlusion, a finding related to the inability of the animals to stabilize rapidly fluctuating pressures. Excitement or arousal caused by visual, auditory, or olfactory stimuli, anticipation of feeding, grooming, pain, etc. were associated with dramatic elevations of arterial pressure. Postural movements, exercise, and other as yet unidentified events resulted in abrupt falls of arterial pressure. These observations indicate that arterial baroreceptors exert an important influence on the stabilization of blood pressure, but may not determine the long-term level of arterial pressure.

Observations by Ito and Scher,[56] also in the dog, support the concept that sinoaortic denervation is associated with sustained hypertension. The magnitude of the hypertension correlates roughly with the extent of denervation. For example, section of the carotid sinus nerves alone does not cause hypertension or increased blood pressure lability. On the other hand, extensive denervation of the aortic arch receptors alone or combined with cervical sinoaortic denervation results in elevation of the level of mean arterial pressure as well as its variability. Several other studies also support Ito and Scher's conclusions. Ferrario et al.[48] showed that sinoaortic denervation caused mild hypertension in dogs, but the predominant changes were persistent increases in lability of arterial pressure and heart rate. Laubie and Schmitt[57] also document a more severe form of hypertension present for several months after sinoaortic denervation. In the rat, Krieger and colleagues[58,59] and Fink et al.[60] report sustained hypertension from moderate or extensive baroreceptor denervation in rats. Many of these studies were performed with long-term continuous recordings. However, these findings have recently been challenged by Norman et al.,[61] who failed to observe hypertension after sinoaortic denervation.

From the preceding description of studies to date, it is apparent that controversy exists concerning the appropriateness of peripheral baroreceptor denervation as a model of experimental neurogenic hypertension. This debate concerning the relationship between baroreceptor denervation and hypertension will undoubtedly remain until definitive answers to several questions are provided.

First, does technically inadequate denervation of baroreceptors account for failure of some investigators to produce sustained elevation of blood pressure? The location of the aortic nerve in relationship to the vagal sympathetic trunk is variable among species. Also, baroreceptor fibers are present within the vagus nerve itself. Thus, there appears to be no certain way of interrupting all baroreceptor fibers, and it is possible that those remaining few may eventually assume the function of controlling bulbar cardiovascular neurons.

Second, what physiologic procedures should be used to evaluate the adequacy of the denervation process and the possible occurrence of reinnervation? Extensive studies to evaluate the completeness of denervation have not been carried out consistently and the methods used have not been entirely appropriate. The most commonly used method for evaluating baroreceptor denervation consists of measurement of bradycardia due to an intravenous bolus injection of an alpha-adrenergic agonist such as phenylephrine. This method does not test the sympathetic component of the baroreflex arc, but measures vagal activity to the heart, only one component of the afferent pathway. Other procedures should be developed to evaluate changes in sympathetic nerve activity in conscious experimental animals.

Lesions of the Nucleus Tractus Solitarius (NTS) and Its Immediate Connections

Experimental neurogenic hypertension has been produced in animals by surgical or chemical interventions in specific central nervous system sites, resulting in increased peripheral sympathetic activity. The most commonly studied site has been the nucleus of the tractus solitarii (NTS). The neurons of the NTS in the medulla are probably the most important in the integration of sensory input from various afferent pathways and in the modulation of reflex autonomic cardiovascular activity. The cells of the medial part of the NTS, at the level of the obex, are involved in blood pressure regulation. Impulses originating in arterial or cardiopulmonary baroreceptors travel by way of the glossopharyngeal (IXth cranial nerve) and vagal (Xth cranial nerve) afferent fibers with cell bodies in the petrosal and nodose ganglia, which have central process terminating in the NTS.[62–66] The NTS also receives input from the trigeminal, facial, and vestibular cranial nerves; from hypothalamic nuclei such as the paraventricular and supraoptic nuclei, which may contain vasopressin and neurophysin; and from noradrenergic neurons such as the A2 group of neurons and the nucleus of the locus coeruleus (NLC).[67,68]

NTS neurons are rich in catecholamines such as dopamine, norepinephrine, and epinephrine and receive, in addition to adrenergic terminals, other terminals containing substance P, enkephalin, and other peptides. The origin of these terminals is not yet known. The NTS may also be influenced by hormonal factors in blood and cerebrospinal fluid because of close vascular and neural connections with the area postrema, which is devoid of a blood brain barrier and is adjacent to the ventricular system.[67]

Efferent fibers from the NTS project to three groups of neurons: (1) vagal (nucleus ambiguus and dorsal motor vagal nucleus) and sympathetic preganglionic nuclei (intermediolateral nucleus in the spinal cord) to modulate autonomic control of the circulation; (2) the other brain-stem nuclei such as the locus coeruleus, the parabrachial nucleus, and the reticular formation; and (3) the higher centers of the forebrain including the hypothalamus and amygdala.[69]

Reis has proposed a role of central nervous system structural or biochemical abnormalities in causing acute as well as chronic hypertension.[70] He proposes that a central "neural imbalance" may cause hypertension either by causing excitation of sympathetic neurons or by suppressing inhibitory influences on sympathetic neurons. The NTS is used to study brain-blood pressure relationships because (1) the NTS is the principal site of termination of afferent fibers from arterial baroreceptors; (2) electrical stimulation of the NTS stimulates baroreflexes, whereas acute lesions abolish baroreflexes; (3) neurons from the NTS project into or receive inputs from other regions of the CNS important to cardiovascular control, and (4) the NTS is richly innervated by neurons containing a number of potential neurotransmitters and/or modulators.

In 1973, Doba and Reis[71] first sought to determine whether small bilateral lesions of the NTS would result in changes in arterial blood pressure in unanesthetized rats. These studies were performed in rats with indwelling arterial and venous catheters. After the instruments were placed, while the animals were awake and unrestrained, basal values of cardiovascular activity were obtained. The animals were then re-anesthetized, usually with halothane, and lesions were placed bilaterally in the NTS at the obex. After administration of the anesthetic was discontinued, cardiovascular variables were observed.

Lesions of the NTS in the rat invariably produced fulminating hypertension.[71] Within minutes after placement of bilateral lesions of the NTS and discontinuation of anesthesia, the arterial pressure of the lesioned rats began to rise, reaching systolic levels over 200 mm Hg. The elevation of arterial pressure was sustained until the animals invariably died with acute pulmonary edema three to five hours later. Reis showed that the acute hypertension in rats with NTS lesions was caused by marked increase of sympathetic nerve activity in association with vasoconstriction.[72] The responses were mediated by alpha-adrenergic receptors and could be blocked by alpha-adrenergic blocking drugs, ganglioplegic agents, and reserpine. The elevation of blood pressure also was substantially ameliorated by the alpha-adrenergic agonist, clonidine.[73]

The increase in peripheral vasoconstriction after NTS lesions was selective and representative of a differentiated activation of sympathetic nerves. The greatest sympathetic effects were observed in the skin and muscle, and to a lesser degree in the lower gastrointestinal tract.[74] Although there was evidence of augmented release of adrenal medullary catecholamines after NTS lesions, the adrenal hormones did not contribute substantially to the elevation of blood pressure.[72]

NTS hypertension in the rat is likely to be caused by central interruption of baroreflexes in the NTS. The electrolytic lesions resulted in the disappearance of baroreflexes, and the pattern of redistribution of blood flow is similar to that produced by sinoaortic denervation but different from that produced in other experimental forms of hypertension.[71]

According to Reis[71] the production of NTS hypertension requires bilateral lesions that are restricted to or near the intermediate zone of the NTS. Whether the changes result from destruction of surrounding neurons, destruction of incoming afferent fibers from arterial baroreceptors, or a combination of these effects is still not clear. However, Palkovitz et al.[75] demonstrated that small knife cuts at the level of the obex, presumably interrupting the entering baroreceptor afferents, also caused hypertension.

The precise regions of the brain stem necessary for expression of hypertension after NTS lesions remain to be established. The possible involvement of basal hypothalamic structures is supported by recent observations of Brody and associates[76,77] that electrolytic lesions in the anterior portions of the third ventricle (AV3V) abolish NTS hypertension. The efferent pathways required for maintenance of elevated blood pressure also are unknown. Intracisternal administration of 6-hydroxydopamine, which destroys noradrenergic neurons, blocks the development of NTS hypertension and selectively decreases norepinephrine content of the spinal cord.[72] These observations suggest that a descending noradrenergic pathway may be important in sustaining the pressor response.

In the hope of producing a more chronic form of hypertension, Nathan and Reis[78] have investigated the effects of placement of bilateral electric lesions in the NTS in the cat. Although cats develop a marked elevation of blood pressure within minutes of placement of the lesions, most animals survive to develop chronic abnormalities of blood pressure control. NTS hypertension in cats has been characterized by the following major features: (1) lability of arterial blood pressure; (2) sustained tachycardia; (3) exaggerated reactivity of arterial pressure; (4) absent or attenuated baroreceptor reflexes; (5) preservation of the hypotensive action of clonidine; and (6) facilitated conditioned pressor responses. The most striking feature of the abnormal arterial pressure in the cat is marked lability characterized by large fluctuations in arterial blood pressure sometimes as great as 100 mm Hg. These changes occurred while the animals were resting quietly and were unrelated to behavioral changes or to environmental stimulation.[79,80]

The average value of arterial blood pressure in cats with NTS lesions is significantly higher than that of controls at all times during the day. While the pressures of the normal cat are about 80 ± 1.5 mm Hg, the hypertensive animals averaged 114 ± 2 mm Hg, significantly different from controls. In control cats the heart rate was 154 ± 8.1 beats per minute after lesions, heart rate increased to 191 ± 5.6 beats per minute. However, there is no change in the variability of heart rate despite wide fluctuations of arterial pressure. The NTS lesions also greatly exaggerated the normal small fluctuations of pressure associated with various behaviors, or in response to controlled environmental stimuli. Cats with NTS lesions also have substantially larger elevations of arterial pressure in response to classic Pavlovian conditioning.[80]

Reis has emphasized that cats with NTS lesions have many features in common with the essential hypertension in man, including chronicity, lability, exaggerated reactivity to environmental stimuli, and intact responses to centrally acting hypotensive agents. However, these animals do not have chronic sustained hypertension characteristic of the human disorder.

Carey et al.[81] and Laubie and Schmitt[57] recently have shown that bilateral electrolytic lesions in the NTS of dogs produce sustained elevation of blood pressure. In studies from our laboratory,[81] 13 female American foxhounds had placement of bilateral electrical lesions in the NTS at the level of the obex. After recovery from anesthesia the dogs could be divided into two groups on the basis of their blood pressure responses. In the first group, comprised of six dogs, sustained hypertension with an increase of mean arterial pressure 25–35% above control values was observed for 10 days after placement of the lesions. In the second group, composed of the remaining seven dogs, a transient increase of blood pressure on postoperative day one was observed, but the animals became normotensive for the subsequent nine days of observation. All of the dogs in the first group with sustained hypertension were hypertensive at the time of sacrifice, and all of the animals in the second normotensive group were normotensive at sacrifice. The histologic sections from the first group showed complete cellular destuction of the nucleus and the tractus solitarius bilaterally at the level of the obex. In the second group, unilateral or incomplete cellular destruction of the NTS at the obex or bilateral NTS lesions caudal to the obex were observed.

Two studies,[81,57] published simultaneously in 1979, showed for the first time that central nervous system lesions can produce chronic sustained hypertension with many features similar to those of essential hypertension in man. Studies from our laboratory[81] characterized the hemodynamic and hormonal characteristics of the first group of dogs with sustained hypertension. These dogs had an increase in total peripheral resistance, a decrease in cardiac output, and a slight decrease in heart rate. All of these hemodynamic abnormalities were reversed to control levels after phentolamine treatment. Plasma renin activity, aldosterone concentration, and blood pressure responses to angiotensin-converting enzyme inhibitor (teprotide, SQ20881) were unaffected by NTS lesions. The hypertensive dogs in the first group had sodium retention on the first postoperative day, but no change in renal plasma flow or glomerular filtration rate was observed during the chronic hypertensive phase.

In the studies of Laubie and Schmitt,[57] the acute and chronic hemodynamic effects of bilateral lesions of the NTS were observed. Bilateral lesions of the NTS abolished baroreceptor reflexes, as quantified by absence of pressor responses to carotid occlusion and by bradycardic responses to carotid sinus nerve stimulation and norepinephrine administration. Immediate and marked hypertension and tachycardia were observed in the anesthetized dogs, without change in cardiac output. Left ventricular end diastolic pressure was elevated and *dP/dT* was increased. These hemodynamic effects resulted from increased sympathetic activity because blood pressure and heart rate were decreased by the central and peripheral sympatholytic agents.

On the basis of pharmacologic studies it was felt that destruction of the NTS interrupts cardiopulmonary as well as baroreceptor reflexes. During the chronic phase after NTS lesions in conscious animals, blood pressure remained elevated from baseline values for 12 months and baroreceptor reflexes remained abolished during this period. Again, clonidine decreased blood pressure and heart rate.

Talman and co-workers[82] have further investigated mechanisms of central neurogenic hypertension in the rat. In one set of studies, central catecholamine projections into the NTS were destroyed by local microinjection of the neurotoxin, 6-hydroxydopamine.[82] In the second set of experiments, the cells of origin of one portion of the noradrenergic innervation of the NTS, those arising from the so-called A2 group of neurons of the dorsal medulla, were electrolytically lesioned.[82] In both the six hydroxydopamine and A2-lesioned animals, chronic changes in blood pressure control were observed. Both lesions resulted in development of marked lability of arterial pressure without any change in mean blood pressure values. No change in the average value or lability of heart rate was found. Hydroxydopamine administration did not alter baroreceptor responses. A2 lesions interrupted the baroreceptor reflexes—cardiovagal responses were abolished, but vasodepressor responses remained intact.

Interestingly, the lability of arterial blood pressure caused by interference with noradrenergic innervation of the NTS produced by A2 lesions remained unchanged for up to one year. However, the animals did not develop increased arterial pressure nor any evidence of pathology of the blood vessels, kidneys, or heart. Thus, lability of arterial pressure per se may not evolve into hypertension.

Blessing and colleagues[83] have determined blood pressure and baroreceptor reflex responses to brainstem lesions coinciding with the A1 group of catecholaminergic neurons. In the rabbit, electrolytic lesions in this area attenuate baroreceptor reflexes and result in an immediate increase in arterial blood pressure and bradycardia. The increase in blood pressure is related to an increase in total peripheral vascular resistance. However, the hypertension is short lived, with return to control values four hours after lesioning. Interestingly, total peripheral vascular resistance remains elevated for two weeks despite the normalization of blood pressure at four hours. Since both the A1 and A2 neuron areas appear to innervate the NTS, and since both produce disturbances of blood pressure control, it is possible that both the A1 and A2 neurons areas act in concert to control arterial baroreceptor reflexes through their influence on the NTS.

In recent interesting experiments, Talman and colleagues[84] have demonstrated that glutamic acid may be the neurotransmitter of baroreceptor afferents terminating in the NTS. Microinjection of minute quantities of glutamic acid or glutamic acid analog into the NTS stimulate baroreceptor reflexes, producing a dose-dependent fall of arterial blood pressure, bradycardia and apnea. Bilateral injection of a relatively selective antagonist of glutamic acid on central neurons blocks baroreflexes and produces transient hypertension and tachycardia. Interestingly, glutamic acid microinjected into the rat NTS in doses greater than that required to produce hypotension elicits fulminating hypertension similar to that produced by bilateral electrolytic lesions. It is felt that larger doses of glutamic acid and its agonist produce hypertension by depolarization blockade of glutamatergic receptors in the NTS that mediate the baroreceptor reflexes. No investigations yet have indicated whether continual administration of glutamic acid antagonist can produce chronic sustained hypertension.

In further studies to delineate the site of neuronal destruction, it has been demonstrated that administration of kainic acid, a material that destroys cell bodies with minimal or no damage to nerve terminals or axons passing through the lesioned area, into both the NTS and the A1 group of catecholaminergic neurons increases blood pressure.[85,86] Similar experiments have not been conducted on the A2 group of catecholaminergic neurons.

Most recently, Ferrario and colleagues[87] have dissected the mechanisms of NTS hypertension, by comparing the cardiovascular effects of bilateral NTS lesions with those of bilateral NTS lesions *plus* subsequent sinoaortic denervation in the same dogs. Destruction of the lateral but not the medial component of the NTS between 0.5 and 3 mm anterior to the obex produced mild hypertension and tachycardia, not always sustained for more than two weeks. The increase in blood pressure was accompanied by increased lability, which was not present consistently in all dogs, but which correlated with the baseline level of arterial pressure. Sinoaortic denervation following lateral NTS lesions produced the first demonstration of fulminant hypertension in the dog, leading to death within hours, as previously demonstrated for the rat.

These data were interpreted as indicating that in the dog NTS lesions probably only partially interrupt the central baroreceptor pathways, but the addition of sinoaortic denervation completely disrupts baroreceptor inputs to the central nervous system, thus releasing central sympathetic outflow completely from baroreceptor inhibition.

Up to now, no studies of the effects of lesions of the NTS *plus* lesions of the area postrema have been reported. This is surprising in view of the baroreceptor and NTS neuroanatomical connections with the area postrema. Further studies of the NTS and its connections are necessary to produce a consistent model of sustained neurogenic hypertension.

Electrical Stimulation of the Nucleus Locus Coeruleus

Few studies are available in which manipulations have been performed on the nucleus of the locus coeruleus (NLC), a midbrain nucleus with the highest norepinephrine content in the brain and an important center influencing hypothalamic, cortical, cerebellar, medullary, and spinal function, as well as in the modulation of arterial pressure control.[88,89] Frohlich and co-workers[90] have stimulated the NLC in normotensive and spontaneously hypertensive rats. Electrical stimulation in normotensive rats results in a significant rise in mean arterial pressure during stimulation. However, in spontaneously hypertensive rats, this response is attenuated. The stimulatory pressor response is apparently the result of stimulation of an ascending fiber system of the posterior hypothalamus and of its descending fiber system, which projects to the ventrical and lateral reticular formation.

To date, no studies are available on chronic NLC stimulation.

Acute Hypothalamic Stimulation

In 1966, Folkow and Rubinstein[91] reported that chronic electrical stimulation of the "hypothalamic defense area" elevates blood pressure progressively in conscious rats. The elevation of blood pressure was not immediate, but was delayed for more than eight weeks. However, in more recent studies (1979) by Bunag and Riley,[92] these results were not confirmed. In this study, daily electrical stimulation of the posterior hypothalamus for twelve weeks in awake rats caused persistent cardioacceleration but no significant increase in systolic pressure. Chronic stimulation was then repeated following the exact stereotaxic coordinates originally employed by Folkow and Rubinstein. Systolic pressure rose, but the elevation was only significant at weeks eight and ten. The stimulated rats gained weight more rapidly than the unstimulated controls, and electrical current strengths had to be increased in stepwise fashion to maintain behavioral effects during the chronic stimulation period.

In further experiments, electrical thresholds were higher and pressor and sympathetic nerve responses were smaller in rats that had been stimulated chronically than those that had not. Thus, in these more recent experiments, blood pressure could not be elevated by hypothalamic stimulation alone. The reason for the inability of Bunag and Riley to produce sustained hypertension in the stimulated rats is not clear, but may have to do with the extensive fibrosis observed at the sites of electrode implantation, and associated brain damage.

Ciriello and Calaresu[93] recently investigated the role of paraventricular and supraoptic nuclei in the central cardiovascular regulation of the cat. These hypothalamic nuclei have traditionally been associated with production of posterior pituitary hormones. However, recent evidence has suggested that these nuclei may play an important role in the neural regulation of the cardiovascular system. Electrophysiological studies have demonstrated that single units in these nuclei alter their discharge rate during electrical stimulation of the buffer nerves[94] and during selective excitation of baroreceptors, chemoreceptors, and atrial stretch receptors.[95] Also, the paraventricular nucleus projects directly to sites involved in cardiovascular regulation in the medulla and thoracic spinal cord, and receives direct projections from the region of the NTS, the primary site of termination of the buffer nerves.[96,97]

Ciriello and Calaresu[93] stimulated histologically verified sites in the region of the paraventricular and supraoptic nuclei in 26 anesthetized cats. Electrical stimulation elicited increases in arterial blood pressure in bilaterally vagotomized animals and increased heart rate in both C_2 spinal animals and in animals bilaterally vagotomized. In addition, electrical stimulation of the paraventricular and supraoptic nuclei inhibited reflex vagal bradycardia elicited by stimulation of the carotid sinus nerve, and bilateral lesions in these areas increased the magnitude of this response. On the other hand, stimulation and lesions of these hypothalamic regions did not alter the magnitude of the cardiovascular responses to stimulation of the aortic depressor nerve.

Thus, this study demonstrated that acute electrical stimulation of the hypothalamus in the region of the paraventricular and supraoptic nuclei in anesthetized cats could elicit cardioacceleration and arterial hypertension. The pressor response was related to activation of vasoconstrictor neurons, and was not secondary to the changes in heart rate or cardiac output, as the arterial pressure response was not affected by the administration of beta-adrenergic blocking agents.

Nathan and Reis[98] have demonstrated that electrolytic lesions produced with anodal current and stainless steel electrodes placed in the anteromedial, anterolateral, or ventromedial hypothalamus cause acute arterial hypertension and tachycardia, leading rapidly to pulmonary edema in the rat. The hypertension was related to a marked increase in peripheral resistance. Similar lesions produced with platinum electrodes (noncorrosive) failed to elicit the cardiovascular syndrome.[99] The acute hypertension produced by stainless steel electrodes appears to mediate excitation of the hypothalamus, possibly due to the irritative action of metallic ions deposited at the lesion site. The hypertension and tachycardia were blocked by adrenalectomy, indicating a critical role of adrenal catecholamines in the production of the syndrome.

As indicated, various hypothalamic nuclei may be found to play a role in neurogenic hypertension. However, there are no established models of chronic neurogenic hypertension involving hypothalamic stimulation or destruction.

Summary and Conclusions

The sympathetic nervous system plays an important role in initiating and sustaining elevated blood pressure in essential hypertension. The increased activity of the sympathetic nervous system in essential hypertension undoubtedly is modulated by the central nervous system. However, despite attempts by many investigators, a suitable animal model of experimental neurogenic hypertension demonstrating chronic sustained elevation of blood pressure has not been defined.

Chronic intrarenal norepinephrine infusion in the dog perhaps best approximates human hypertension, as this model is characterized by chronic sustained hypertension, increased total peripheral vascular resistance, normal cardiac output, antinatriuresis, and a broad spectrum of plasma renin activity. Similar hormonal and hemodynamic features are found in dog NTS hypertension, but the hypertensive process does not persist chronically in the majority of animals. NTS lesions in other species have led either to acute fulminating hypertension or chronic blood pressure lability with little increase in mean arterial pressure. Experimental models involving chronic central or peripheral neuronal stimulation are technically difficult and the results are variable and unpredictable.

Clearly, one or more reliable models of experimental neurogenic hypertension would be valuable tools for assessment of the role of central and/or peripheral neural mechanisms in human essential hypertension. Further study of this important area should be timely and rewarding.

References

1. Eich RH, Peters RJ, Cuddy RP, Smulyan H, Lyons RH: The hemodynamics of labile hypertension. Am Heart J **63**:188, 1962
2. Eich RH, Cuddy RP, Smulyan H, Lyons RH: Hemodynamics in labile hypertension. Circulation **34**:299, 1966
3. Frolich ED, Tarazi RC, Dustan HP: Re-examination of the hemodynamics of hypertension. Am J Med Sci **257**:9, 1969
4. deChamplain J, Farley L, Cousineau D, vanAmeringen MR: Circulating catecholamine levels in human and experimental hypertension. Circ Res **38**:109, 1976
5. DeQuattro V, Campese V, Miura Y, Meijer D: Increased plasma catecholamines in high renin hypertension. Am J Cardiol **38**:801, 1976
6. Louis WJ, Doyle AE, Anavekar SN, Johnson CI, Geffen LB, Rash R: Plasma catecholamine, dopamine-beta-hydroxylase and renin levels in essential hypertension. Circ Res **34** and **35** (Suppl I):I–57, 1974
7. Goldstein DS: Plasma catecholamines and essential hypertension: an analytical review. Hypertension **5**:86, 1983
8. Antonoccio MJ: Neuropharmacology of central mechanisms governing the circulation. *In* Cardiovascular Pharmacology, edited by MJ Antonoccio. New York, Raven, 1977, p 131
9. DeJong W, Nijkamp FP: Hypertension action of noradrenaline and alpha-methylnoradrenaline in the area of the nucleus tractus solitarii in the rat brainstem. *In* Central Action of Drugs in Blood Pressure Regulation, edited by DS Davies and JL Reid. London, Pitman, 1975, p 179
10. Finch L, Buckingham RE, Moore RA, Bucker TJ: Evidence for a central-sympathetic action of clonidine in the rat. J Pharm Pharmacol **27**:181, 1975
11. Scriabine A: Methyldopa. *In* Pharmacology of Antihypertensive Drugs, edited by A Scriabine. New York, Raven, 1980, p 43
12. Henry JP, Meehan JP: Psychosocial stimuli, physiological specificity and cardiovascular disease. *In* Brain Behavior and Bodily Disease, edited by H Weiner, MA Hofer, AJ Stunkard. New York, Raven, 1981. p 305
13. Zanchetti A, Bartonelli C: Central nervous mechanisms in arterial hypertension: experimental and clinical evidence. *In* Hypertension, edited by J Genest, O Kuchel, E Koiw. New York, McGraw-Hill, 1977. p 59
14. Buggy J, Fink GD, Johnson AK, Brody MJ: Prevention of the development of renal hypertension by anteroventral third ventricular tissue lesions. Circ Res **40** (Suppl I):I–110, 1977
15. Johnson AK, Hoffman WE, Buggy J: Attenuated pressor responses to intracranially injected stimuli and altered antidiuretic activity following pre-optic hypothalamic periventricular ablation. Brain Res **157**:161, 1978

16. Brody MJ, Haywood JF, Touw KB: Neural mechanisms in hypertension. Ann Rev Physiol **42**:441, 1980
17. Buhler FR, Laragh JH, Baer L, Vaughan ED Jr, Brunner HR: Propranolol inhibition of renin secretion: a specific approach to diagnosis and treatment of renin-dependent hypertensive disease. New Engl J Med **287**:1209, 1972
18. Lais LT, Bhatnogar R, Brody MJ: Role of the sympathetic nervous system in development and maintenance of spontaneous hypertension. *In* The Nervous System in Arterial Hypertension, edited by S Julius and MD Esler. Springfield, Charles C Thomas, 1976, p 76
19. Bevan RD: Effect of sympathetic denervation on smooth muscle cell proliferation in the growing rabbit ear artery. Circ Res **37**:14, 1975
20. Ferrario C, Page I, McCubbin J: Increased cardiac output as a contributory factor in experimental renal hypertension in dogs. Circ Res **27**:799, 1970
21. Guyton AC, Coleman TG, Granger HJ: Circulation: overall regulation. Ann Rev Physiol **34**:13, 1972
22. Folkow B, Cardiovascular structural adaptation: its role in the initiation and maintenance of primary hypertension. The Fourth Volhard Lecture. Clin Sci Molec Med **55**:3, 1978
23. Takeshita A, Mark AL: Decreased vasodilator capacity of forearm resistance vessels in borderline hypertension. Hypertension **2**:610, 1980
24. Kottke FJ, Kubicek WG, Visscher MB: The production of arterial hypertension by chronic renal artery-stimulation. Am J Physiol **145**:38, 1945
25. Kubicek WG, Kottke FJ, Laker DJ, Visscher MB: Renal function during arterial hypertension produced by chronic splanchnic nerve stimulation in the dog. Am J Physiol **174**:397, 1953
26. Katholi RE, Carey RM, Ayers CR, Vaughan ED Jr, Yancey MR, Morton CL: Production of sustained hypertension by chronic intrarenal norepinephrine infusion in conscious dogs. Circ Res **40** (Suppl I):I–118, 1977
27. Tobian L Jr, Janecek J, Tomboulian A, Ferreira D: Sodium and potassium in the walls of arterioles in experimental renal hypertension. J Clin Invest **40**:1922, 1961
28. Abboud FM: Effects of sodium, angiotensin and steroids on vascular reactivity in man. Fed Proc **33**:143, 1974
29. Abel PW, Hermsmeyer K: Sympathetic cross-innervation of SHR and genetic controls suggest a trophic influence on vascular muscle membranes. Circ Res **49**:1311, 1981
30. Hart MM, Heistad DD, Brody MJ: Effect of chronic hypertension and sympathetic denervation on wall/lumen ratio of cerebral vessels. Hypertension **2**:419, 1980
31. Alexander RS: Tonic and reflex functions of medullary sympathetic cardiovascular centers. J Neurophysiol **9**:205, 1946
32. Dampney RAL: Functional organization of central cardiovascular pathways. Clin Exp Pharmacol Physiol **8**:241, 1981
33. Reis DJ, Doba N: The central nervous system and neurogenic hypertension. Prog Cardiovasc Dis **17**:51, 1974
34. Shipley RE, Gregg DE: Cardiac response to stimulation of the stellate ganglia and cardiac nerves. Am J Physiol **143**:396, 1945
35. Anzola J, Rushmer RF: Cardiac responses to sympathetic stimulation. Circ Res **4**:302, 1956
36. Sarnoff SJ, Brockman SK, Gilmore JP, Linden RJ, Mitchell JH: Regulation of

ventricular contraction: influence of cardiac sympathetic and vagal nerve stimulation on atrial and ventricular dynamics. Circ Res **8:**1108, 1960

37. Rohse WG, Kaye M, Randall WC: Prolonged pressor effects of selective stimulation of the stellate ganglion: Circ Res **5:**144, 1957

38. Liard JF, Tarazi RC, Ferrario CM, Manger WM: Hemodynamic and humoral characteristics of hypertension induced by prolonged stellate ganglion stimulation in conscious dogs. Circ Res **36:**455, 1975

39. Cowley AW Jr, Lohmeier TE: Changes in renal vascular sensitivity and arterial pressure associated with sodium intake during long-term intrarenal norepinephrine infusion in dogs. Hypertension **1:**549, 1979

40. Guyton AC, Hall JE, Lohmeier TE, Manning RD Jr, Jackson TE: Position paper: the concept of whole body autoregulation and the dominant role of the kidneys for long term blood pressure regulation. *In* Frontiers in Hypertension Research, edited by JH Laragh, FR Buhler, DW Seldin. New York, Springer-Verlag, p 125

41. Boss J, Green JH: The histology of the common carotid baroreceptor areas of the cat. Circ Res **4:**12, 1956

42. Sleight P, editor: Arterial Baroreceptors and Hypertension. Oxford, Oxford University Press, 1980

43. Mesulam MM: Tetramethyl benzidine for horseradish peroxidase neurohistochemistry: a non-carcinogenic blue reaction-product with superior sensitivity for visualizing neural afferents and efferents. J Histochem Cytochem **26:**106, 1978

44. Kalia MP: Localization of aortic and carotid baroreceptor and chemoreceptor primary afferents in the brain stem. *In* Central Nervous System Mechanisms in Hypertension. New York, Raven Press, 1981, p 9

45. Chernicky CL, Barnes KL, Conomy L, Ferrario CM: Distribution within the brainstem of vagal afferents in the dog. Neurosci Abstr **7:**115, 1981

46. Ead HW, Green JH, Neil E: A comparison of the effects of pulsatile and non-pulsatile flow through the carotid sinus on the reflexogenic activity of the sinus baroreceptors in the cat. J Physiol **118:**509, 1952

47. Kirchheim HR: Systemic arterial baroreceptor reflexes. Physiol Rev **56:**100, 1976

48. Ferrario CM, McCubbin JW, Page IH: Hemodynamic characteristics of chronic experimental neurogenic hypertension in unanesthetized dogs. Circ Res **24:**911, 1969

49. Junqueira LF Jr, Krieger EM: Blood pressure and sleep in the rat in normotension and in experimental hypertension. J Physiol **259:**725, 1976

50. Guazzi M, Zanchetti A: Blood pressure and heart rate during natural sleep of the cat and their regulation by carotid sinus and aortic reflexes. Arch Ital Biol **103:**789, 1965

51. Averill DB, Ferrario CM, McCubbin JW, Nadzam GR: Paradoxical hypertension during sleep in dogs with buffer nerve section. Physiologist **18:**215, 1975

52. Wright S: Recent work on the afferent control of the circulation in health and disease. Br Med J **1:**457, 1932

53. Nowak SJG: Chronic hypertension produced by carotid sinus and aortic-depressor nerve section. Am Surg **111:**102, 1940

54. Thomas CB: Experimental hypertension from section of moderator nerves. Johns Hopkins Hosp Bull **74:**335, 1944

55. Cowley AW Jr, Liard JF, Guyton AC: Role of the baroreceptor reflex in daily

control of arterial blood pressure and other variables in dogs. Circ Res **32**:564, 1973

56. Ito CS, Scher AM: Hypertension following denervation of aortic baroreceptors in unanesthetized dogs. Circ Res **45**:26, 1979

57. Laubie M, Schmitt H: Destruction of the nucleus tractus solitarii in the dog: comparison with sinoaortic denervation. Am J Physiol **236**:H736, 1979

58. Krieger EM: Neurogenic hypertension in the rat. Circ Res **15**:511, 1964

59. Vasquez EC, Krieger EM: Sequence of tachycardia following baroreceptor denervation in the rat. *In* Arterial Baroreceptors and Hypertension, edited by P Sleight. Oxford, Oxford University Press, 1980, p 413

60. Fink GD, Kennedy F, Bryan WJ, Werber A: Pathogenesis of hypertension in rats with chronic aortic baroreceptor deafferentation. Hypertension **2**:319, 1980

61. Norman RA Jr, Coleman TG, Dent AC: Continuous monitoring of arterial pressure indicates sinoaortic denervated rats are not hypertensive. Hypertension **3**:119, 1981

62. Cottle MK: Degeneration studies of primary afferents of IXth and Xth cranial nerves in the cat. J Comp Neurol **122**:329, 1964

63. Crill WE, Ries DJ: Distribution of carotid sinus and depressor nerves in the cat brainstem. Am J Physiol **214**:269, 1968

64. Humphrey DR: Neuronal activity in the medulla oblongata of cat evoked by stimulation of the carotid sinus nerve. *In* Baroreceptors and Hypertension, edited by P Kezdi. New York, Pergamon, 1967, p 131

65. Miura M, Reis DJ: The role of the solitary and paramedian reticular nuclei in mediating cardiovascular reflex responses from carotid baro- and chemoreceptors. J Physiol London **223**:525, 1972

66. Seller H, Illert M: The localization of the first synapse in the carotid sinus baroreceptor reflex pathway and its alteration of the afferent input. Pfluegers Arch **306**:1, 1969

67. Palkovits M: The anatomy of central cardiovascular neurons. *In* Central Adrenaline Neurons: Basic Aspects and their Role in Cardiovascular Functions, edited by Fuxe K, Goldstein M, Hökfelt B, Hökfelt T. Oxford, Pergamon, 1980

68. Sofroniew MV, Weindl A: Projections from the parvocellor vasopressin and neurophysin-containing neruons of the suprachiasmatic nucleus. Am J Anat **153**:391, 1978

69. Palkovitis M, Zaborski L: Neuroanatomy of central cardiovascular control. Nucleus tractus solitarii: afferent and efferent neuronal connections in relation to the baroreceptor reflex arc. Progr Brain Res **47**:9, 1977

70. Reis DJ: The brain and arterial hypertension: evidence for a neural-imbalance hypothesis. *In* Disturbances in Neurogenic Control of the Circulation, edited by Abboud FM, Fozzard HA, Gilmore JP, Reis DJ. American Physiological Society, Bethesda, 1981, p 87

71. Doba N, Reis DJ: Acute fulminating neurogenic hypertension produced by brainstem lesions in the rat. Circ Res **32**:584, 1973

72. Doba N, Reis DJ: Role of central and peripheral adrenergic mechanisms in neurogenic hypertension produced by brainstem lesions in the rat. Circ Res **34**:273, 1974

73. Rockhold RW, Caldwell RW: Effects of lesions of the nucleus tractus solitarii on the cardiovascular actions of clonidine in conscious rats. Neuropharmacol **18**:347, 1979

74. Snyder DW, Doba N, Reis DJ: Regional distribution of blood flow during arterial hypertension produced by lesions of the nucleus tractus solitarii in the rat. Circ Res **42**:87, 1978
75. Palkovitz M, DeJong W, Zandberg P, Versterg DHG, Van der Gugten J, Larenth C: Central hypertension and nucleus tractus solitarii catecholamines after surgical lesions in the medulla oblongata in the rat. Brain Res **127**:127, 1977
76. Brody MJ, Fink GD, Buggy J, Haywood JR, Gordon FJ, Knuepfer M, Mow M, Mahoney L, Johnson AK: Critical role of the anterior third ventricle (AV3V) region in the development and maintenance of experimental hypertension. *In* Nervous System and Hypertension, edited by Meyer P, Schmitt H. New York, Wiley, 1979, p 76
77. Hartle DK, Brody MJ: Hypothalamic vasomotor pathways mediating the development of hypertension in the rat. Hypertension **4** (Suppl III):III−68, 1982
78. Nathan MA, Reis DJ: Chronic labile hypertension produced by lesions of the nucleus tractus solitarii in the cat. Circ Res **40**:72, 1977
79. Nathan MA, Tucker LW, Severini WP, Reis DJ: Enhancement of conditioned arterial pressure responses in cats after brainstem lesions. Science **201**:71, 1978
80. Nathan MA, Severini WA, Tucker LW and Reis DJ: Effect of environment on labile arterial hypertension. Circulation Suppl III:242, 1977
81. Carey RM, Dacey RG, Jane TA, Winn HR, Ayers CR, Tyson GW: Production of sustained hypertension by lesions of the nucleus tractus solitarii of the American foxhound. Hypertension **1**:246, 1979
82. Talman WT, Snyder D, Reis DJ: Chronic lability of arterial pressure produced by destruction of A2 catecholamine neurons in rat brainstem. Circ Res **46**:842, 1980
83. Blessing WW, West MJ, Chalmers J: Hypertension, bradycardia and pulmonary edema in the conscious rabbit after brainstem lesions coinciding with the A1 group of catecholamine neurons. Circ Res **49**:949, 1981
84. Talman WT, Perrone MH, Reis DJ: Evidence for L-glutamate as the neurotransmitter of primary baroreceptor afferent nerve fibers. Science **209**:813, 1980
85. Talman WT, Perrone MH, Reis DJ: Acute hypertension after the local injection of kainic acid ito the nucleus tractus solitarii of rats. Circ Res **48**:292, 1981
86. Blessing WW, Sued AF, Reis DJ: Destruction of noradrenergic neurons in rabbit brainstem elevates plasma vasopressin, causing hypertension. Science **217**:661, 1982
87. Ferrario CM, Barnes KL, Bohonek S: Neurogenic hypertension produced by lesions of the nucleus tractus solitarii alone or with sinoaortic denervation in the dog. Hypertension **3** (Suppl II):II−112, 1981
88. Anden NE, Dahlstrom A, Fuxe K, Larsson K: Mapping out of catecholamine and 5-hydroxytryptamine neurons innervating the telencephalon and diencephalon. Life Sci **4**:1275, 1965
89. Saavedra JM, Grobecker H, Axelrod J: Adrenaline-forming enzyme in brain stem: elevation in genetic and experimental hypertension. Science **191**:483, 1976
90. Kawamura H, Gunn CG, Frohlich ED: Cardiovascular alteration by nucleus locus coeruleus in spontaneously hypertensive rat. Brain Res **140**:137, 1978
91. Folkow B, Rubinstein E: Cardiovascular effects of acute and chronic stimulations of the hypothalamic defense area in the rat. Acta Physiol Scand **68**:48, 1966

92. Bunag RD, Riley E: Chronic hypothalamic stimulation in awake rats fails to induce hypertension. Hypertension **1:**498, 1979
93. Ciriello J, Calaresu FR: Role of paraventricular and supraoptic nuclei in central cardiovascular regulation in the cat. Am J Physiol **239:**R137, 1980
94. Calaresu FR, Ciriello J: Electrophysiology of hypothalamus in relation to central regulation of the cardiovascular system. *In* Nervous System and Hypertension, edited by Meyer P, Schmitt H. New York, Wiley, 1979, p 129
95. Kannan H, Yagi K: Supraoptic neurosecretory neurons: evidence for the existence of converging inputs from carotid baroreceptors and osmoreceptors. Brain Res **145:**385, 1978
96. Saper CB, Loewy AD, Swanson LW, Cowan WH: Direct hypothalamic-autonomic connections. Brain Res **117:**305, 1976
97. Ricardo JA, Koh ET: Anatomical evidence of direct projections from the nucleus of the solitary tract to the hypothalamus, amygdala, and other forebrain structures in the rat. Brain Res **153:**1, 1978
98. Nathan MA, Reis DJ: Fulminating arterial hypertension with pulmonary edema from release of adrenomedullary catecholamines after lesions of the anterior hypothalamus in the rat. Circ Res **37:**226, 1975
99. Gauthier P, Reis DJ, Nathan MA: Arterial hypertension elicited either by lesions or by electrical stimulations of the rostral hypothalamus in the rat. Brain Res **211:**91, 1981

Chapter 14

Neural Mechanisms in Clinical Hypertension

Stevo Julius, M. Andrew Fitzpatrick,
Brent Egan, and Robert Schneider

The evidence for the role of the nervous system in the etiology of human hypertension is reviewed in this chapter. We will describe those aspects of neural mechanisms that are of clinical relevance and operative regardless of the etiology of hypertension.

Nervous System and Blood Pressure Variability in Hypertension

Naturally occurring blood pressure variability appears to depend on the average blood pressure level; patients whose blood pressure is higher will have higher excursions of their blood pressure.[1,2] When the oscillation is expressed as a percentage of the mean, there is no difference between various sub-groups of hypertensive patients. The important point is that one should not expect excessive blood pressure responses to exercise,[3] isometrics,[4,5] or cold pressor test[6,7] in any group of hypertensive patients.

Whereas the overall blood pressure variability in hypertension is not characteristically increased, there is no doubt that an occasional patient with hypertension shows excessive blood pressure oscillation. There are two subgroups of such patients, and in both of them the blood pressure oscillation has a neurogenic origin. Centrally acting antihypertensive compounds such as clonidine, methyldopa or reserpine may be particularly suitable for the treatment of such patients.

Office Hypertension

Occasionally, patients show high readings in the physician's office, but at home and in everyday situations tend to have much lower values. The patient does not necessarily look apprehensive nor is always aware of inner tension. Blood pressure values in such patients are reproducibly elevated over periods of years, even when the patient and not the physician takes the blood pressure reading. An example of such a patient followed for ten years in our clinic is given in Figure 14-1. It is impossible to chart all the drugs this patient received; however, we tried almost all known antihypertensive compounds as they became available and could not eliminate the home-to-office blood pressure difference. One should suspect such "office hypertension" if the optic fundi are benign but the blood pressure is resistant to treatment. Another clue in treated patients is the presence of symptoms compatible with hypotension at home. Postural dizziness and extreme lassitude call for caution. If the blood pressure is taken at the time when these symptoms occur, one frequently finds surprisingly low blood pressure values.

Thus, office hypertension is neurogenic. Since the pioneering description by Brod[8] of a permanent state of "defense reaction" in hypertension, it has repeatedly been demonstrated that hypertensives respond to laboratory-induced mental stresses by excessive blood pressure, heart rate, and plasma norepinephrine responses.[9–12] This peculiar tendency to respond to mental stressors, but not to other physical stresses, may be related to the patient's personality. In our own work, anxiety[13] is related to blood pressure fluctuations, but other personality traits (submissiveness, suppressed anger) may relate to elevated average blood pressure levels.

The clinical importance of this blood pressure variability in the physician's office remains unclear. The weight of evidence indicates that the average blood pressure, not the peaks or valleys, determines a patient's prognosis. This has been elegantly demonstrated by Sokolow et al.[14] Regardless of the relative prognostic importance of the average blood pressure vs. peak blood pressure oscillation, in practice the limiting value is that of the home blood pressure reading. Patients may develop symptoms of hypotension at home, while appearing hypertensive in the office. Further increase of dosage based on office readings may cause harm to the patients, particularly if compounds that interfere with blood pressure homeostasis in upright posture are used. Since the control of blood pressure by pharmacologic means may be rather difficult, these patients are prime candidates for various forms of behavorial therapy.

Cardiogenic Hypertension

Pressor reflexes originating in the heart have been well described.[15–17] The clinical counterpart of such cardiogenic hypertension is the sudden

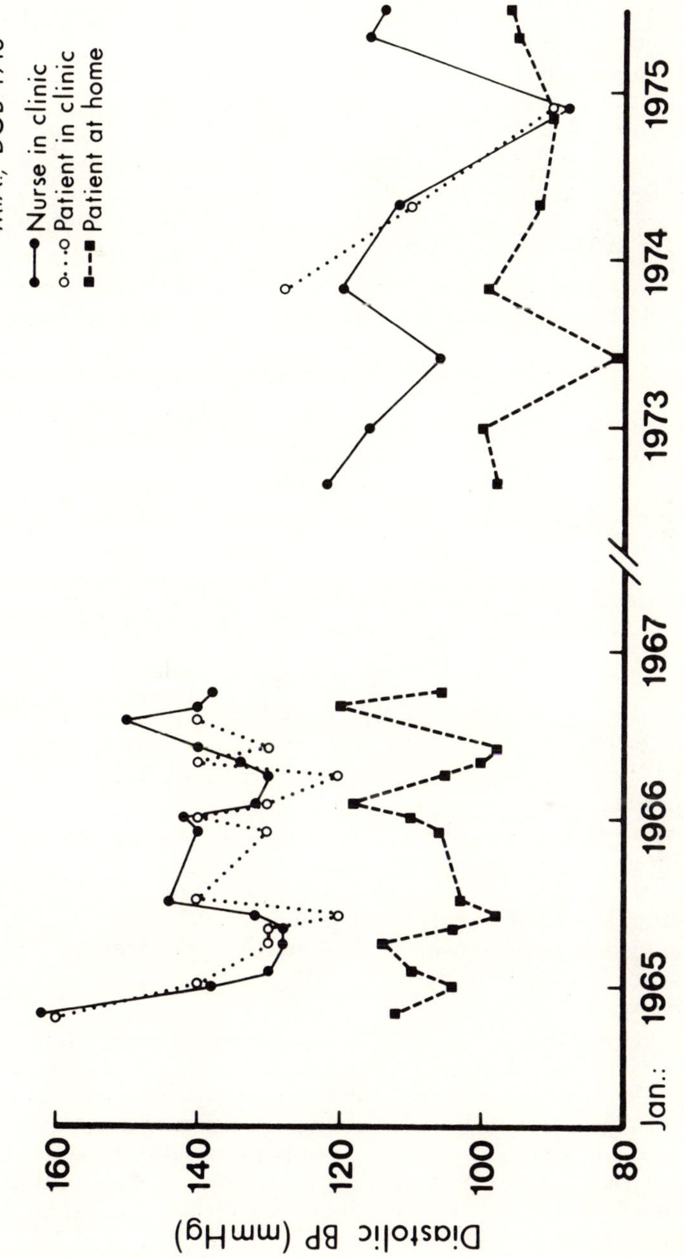

Figure 14-1. Sequential blood pressure measurements taken under measured conditions in a patient followed over 10 years.

increase of blood pressure after coronary revascularization,[18] which can be abolished by blocking afferent cardiac nerves.[19]

Less recognized and not well described is the "pseudopheochromocytoma" syndrome in patients with unstable angina[20] or fresh myocardial infarction.[21] Such patients have paroxysmal attacks of severe hypertension. Plasma catecholamines may well be in the pheochromocytoma range. Frequently it is assumed that the patient had an attack of pheochromocytoma, which in turn caused angina. Once the angina resolves, the blood pressure oscillation disappears. Analgesics do not necessarily decrease the hypertensive attack, and in protracted cases small doses of clonidine may be more effective than treatment with nitroprusside or other vasodilators.

Tachycardia in Hypertension

Clear signs for a neurogenic etiology of blood pressure elevation can be found only in a minority of patients with hypertension. Similarly, in animal experimental hypertension it is very difficult to find good evidence for a primary role of the nervous system. Animal experiments, however, point toward a permissive role of the nervous system in such non-neurogenic models as DOCA-induced, renovascular, and salt-dependent genetic hypertension.[22,23] In human hypertension a similar permissive role of the autonomic nervous system may be inferred. It has been shown that the arterial baroreceptors in human hypertension are reset to function at the hypertensive level,[24] e.g.—not to oppose the elevated blood pressure but in fact to maintain the higher readings. Whereas the mechanism of this resetting may be either peripheral or central, there is good evidence that a central resetting of the cardiovascular control occurs in a large proportion of patients with hypertension.

The argument is based on the prevalence of tachycardia in hypertension. Epidemiologic studies have confirmed the association between tachycardia and higher blood pressure levels.[25] Clinically, tachycardia is present not only in young, so-called hyperkinetic patients[26,27] but also in many patients with established hypertension.[28,29] A particularly dramatic form of such hyperkinetic circulation in patients with established hypertension has been described by the Cleveland group.[30]

One could argue that tachycardia in hypertension is secondary to the blood pressure elevation. A higher sympathetic discharge to the heart is noticeable in patients who are marginally decompensated. We and others have shown that patients with borderline hypertension whose cardiac output is normal and whose blood pressure is only minimally elevated already have a limited stroke volume and maintain a normal cardiac output by a higher heart rate.[28,31,32] Thus, even in mild hypertension the fast heart rate may be secondary to hypertension. However, the elevation of heart rate actually precedes hypertension, and this argues for an early involvement of the nervous system in the pathophysiology of hypertension.

When evaluated prospectively,[33–35] tachycardia is an independent predictor of the future development of hypertension. Particularly convincing is the work by Levy et al.,[35] who have shown that subjects with normal blood pressure and tachycardia after five years develop three times more hypertension than those who have normal blood pressure and normal heart rates. The predictive strength of isolated tachycardia was of a similar magnitude as borderline hypertension without tachycardia. When transient (borderline) hypertension and tachycardia were found together, the risk for future established hypertension was additive, and those individuals were at a five-times higher than normal risk for hypertension.

The tachycardia in hypertension is neurogenic. When the heart is isolated from autonomic influence by propranolol and atropine, the "intrinsic pacemaker" rate is not different than in normal subjects.[29,31] We have shown that in early phases of hypertension the autonomic abnormality is of central nervous origin.[36,37] First, there is no evidence for an increased beta-adrenergic responsiveness in patients with hypertension. Whereas such a hyper-responsiveness has been described in a small subgroup of normotensive or hypertensive individuals,[38] patients with hypertension in fact show a decreased responsiveness to beta-agonist infusion.[31,39,76] Second, the autonomic abnormality does not involve only sympathetic drive to the heart. After blockade with large doses of propranolol the heart rate is still elevated and becomes comparable to the normal controls only after an additional blockade of the parasympathetics with atropine.[26]

Consequently, the parasympathetic nervous system is also involved in the maintenance of tachycardia. Involvement of two branches of the autonomic system strongly suggests that a central mechanism is responsible for the resting tachycardia. Third, the direction of changes in sympathetic drive and parasympathetic inhibition helps to localize the central nervous system area responsible for the faster resting heart rate. Hypertensives with tachycardia have more sympathetic drive and less parasympathetic inhibition of the heart. Such a reciprocal change where activation of the sympathetics is coupled with deactivation of parasympathetics or vice versa is characteristic of functional organization in the cardiovascular centers, presumably in the medulla oblongata.

This picture changes in the course of the disease. Patients without signs of hyperkinetic circulation[31] and those with more severe established hypertension[28,29,32] continue to have tachycardia, but with pharmacologic blockade one can show only decreased vagal inhibition. This change from the combined sympathetic-parasympathetic to only parasympathetically mediated tachycardia is very likely due to the decreased cardiac chronotropic responsiveness to sympathetic stimulation. Heart rate response to isoproterenol is decreased in patients who have normal cardiac output along with slight, but significant, resting tachycardia.[31] We postulated,[31] and others have provided supporting evidence,[40] that this decreased responsiveness to isoproterenol may reflect a "down-regulation" of beta-adrenergic receptors secondary to a consistently increased cardiac sympathetic drive.

Norepinephrine in Hypertension

Clear elevation of plasma norepinephrine is found only in young patients with hypertension, but such patients show no correlation between blood pressure and plasma norepinephrine levels.[27] On the other hand, a correlation is found in patients with more severe forms of hypertension[41,42] who generally do not have high plasma norepinephrine levels. This discrepancy may in part be explained by the different sources of plasma norepinephrine. In those with high catecholamines, plasma norepinephrine may reflect the patient's emotional state at the time of blood drawing. Patients with high norepinephrine are characterized by an unusual personality pattern[43] that may render them overresponsive to mental stress.

An increased heart rate response is always associated with an increased blood pressure responsiveness to stress in such patients.[9,10] Plasma norepinephrine, while not correlated with the blood pressure, is correlated with the heart rate[27] and pre-ejection period.[44] It is conceivable that in these patients the plasma norepinephrine reflects the emotionally induced increased cardiac sympathetic drive. However, this increased drive is not responsible for the hypertension, since even when the heart rate and cardiac output are brought to normal range by autonomic blockade[29,31] the blood pressure remains elevated due to an increase of vascular resistance.

Although other instances of abnormal reflex response of vascular resistance can be demonstrated in such patients,[45,46] there is no relationship between plasma norepinephrine and vascular resistance in these patients.[44] However, as hypertension progresses, a correlation of norepinephrine with vascular resistance and blood pressure levels becomes more evident,[41,42] in spite of the fact that plasma norepinephrine levels are not elevated.[41,42]

How can one explain the better correlation between the blood pressure and norepinephrine in patients who have normal plasma norepinephrine levels? It is possible that patients with advanced hypertension develop increased vascular sensitivity to sympathetic stimuli. The evidence for such increased sensitivity is usually derived by comparing blood pressure and resistance responses to infused sympathetic agonists or antagonists. One of the earliest reports[49] indicated that patients with hypertension show an excessive blood pressure response to ganglionic blockade. In a more recent study, Louis et al.[41] reported that the decline in blood pressure during ganglionic blockade with pentolinium correlated with resting norepinephrine.

As receptor blocking agents become available, the experiments become more sophisticated but somewhat harder to explain. Agabiti-Rosei[47] found that phentolamine when given alone did not completely lower the blood pressure, due to compensatory tachycardia, but the fall in total peripheral resistance correlated with resting plasma norepinephrine levels. With a stepwise autonomic blockade in borderline[31] and mild established hypertension[27] we found that blood pressure was normalized in only a small number of patients. These responders to autonomic blockade did have high plasma norepinephrine levels.[27]

Overall, then, the picture is consistent with an increased blood pressure and/or vascular responsiveness to adrenergic antagonists in patients with established hypertension, and the degree of response correlates with the plasma norepinephrine levels. However, before this is taken as a sign of an involvement of the nervous system in the maintenance of blood pressure in hypertension, one has to consider methodological problems.

First is the question of the adequacy of the baroreceptor response in hypertension. Baroreceptor sensitivity is known to be reduced in hypertension.[50] The second problem lies in the structural changes of the arterioles. As the arteriolar wall becomes hypertrophic and encroaches upon the lumen, the blood vessel responds more than a normal vessel to all vasoconstricting and vasodilating agents.[51] The end result of both of these processes is that the blood pressure should fall more in all patients, that the response should be greater in those with a higher blood pressure, and that the response should be exaggerated to all vasoactive agents. If plasma norepinephrine increases in response to the rising blood pressure, as it may if more sympathetic tone is needed to maintain a normal flow against the higher afterload, one can explain the result of Louis et al.[41,52] in a "reverse" fashion.

Their finding of a correlation between plasma norepinephrine and the blood pressure fall and both phentolamine and acute clonidine could be secondary to nonspecific changes (decreased baroreceptor sensitivity, structural changes) and an increased sympathetic activation as hypertension becomes more severe. The possible importance of secondary changes is underlined by the findings of Weidemann et al.[53] that with debrisoquine, a sympatholytic agent, the fall of norepinephrine was the same in normotension, borderline hypertension, and established hypertension, but the blood pressure fall was only significant in hypertension and was more marked in established hypertension.

The role of structural vascular changes in hypertension was more directly addressed by Buhler's group.[54,55] In order to avoid activation of circulatory reflexes they infused small doses of an alpha-adrenergic antagonist directly into the forearm. Changes in forearm blood flow to phentolamine were similar in normotension and hypertension, but in the hypertensive, resting plasma norepinephrine correlated with local responses to phentolamine. This tighter relationship between norepinephrine and vascular responses in hypertension is similar to earlier quoted evidence of a closer relationship of norepinephrine and blood pressure in advancing hypertension.[41,42]

Kiowski and co-workers, however, do not believe that secondary vascular hypertrophy contributes to this sensitization of vessels to norepinephrine. Using prazosin and nitroprusside, they[55] pointed out that only the response to prazosin was altered. Their conclusion that hypertension is marked by a specific hypersensitivity of alpha-receptors is tempting but cannot be accepted unless the comparison of prazosin and nitroprusside is carried out over a wide range of dose response curves.

Philipp et al.[56] used total body responses to norepinephrine infusion.

They found that for a given level of endogenous (plasma) norepinephrine the reactivity to exogenous norepinephrine was higher in hypertension. The more severe the hypertension, the more responsive were the patients. As they have found normal responses to angiotensin, they conclude that the hyper-responsiveness is specific for sympathetic agonists. However, Weidemann et al.[53] and Meier et al.[57,58] find an increased sensitivity to both norepinephrine and angiotensin in hypertension.

The experiments with sympathetic agonists and antagonists uniformly suggest that the blood pressure in hypertension is more dependent on sympathetic drive than in normotension. The mechanism of this tighter relationship between norepinephrine and blood pressure as hypertension becomes more severe is unclear. We do not believe that the sensitivity of alpha-receptors increases. The claims for alpha-receptor hypersensitivity become more perplexing when one takes into account that the responsiveness to beta-agonists is uniformly reduced in hypertension.[31,59,60,76] It is difficult to visualize how one set of sympathetic receptors would become less and the other more sensitive in the course of hypertension. It is more likely that hypertension-induced structural changes account for these differences. In the heart such restructuring would little affect the heart rate, but on the arterioles, hypertrophy causes changed wall-to-lumen ratio,[51] and this will render the vessels hyper-responsive to pressor stimuli.

Behavorial Treatment of Hypertension

Previous paragraphs serve to underline the fact that the autonomic nervous system plays a role in the pathophysiology of hypertension, even when the hypertension is not of neurogenic origin. Blood pressure variability is increased in some cases of essential hypertension due to emotional factors. Frequent tachycardia points toward a central nervous "permissive" role of the nervous system in a large number of patients with essential hypertension. Finally, increased sensitivity to a normal sympathetic tone and a larger dependence of the blood pressure on the autonomic drive becomes more evident with increasing degrees of severity of hypertension. It follows that regardless of etiology, withdrawal of the endogenous sympathetic tone could be useful in the management of human hypertension. This should particularly be the case in very labile hypertension and, paradoxically, in more severe hypertension.

Rest and relaxation have been used in the treatment of essential hypertension for about as long as the disease has been recognized. White[61] encouraged patients to achieve "relief from all avoidable nervous and physical strain." Page[62] advised patients to rest twice a day and preserve their equanimity. Jacobson[63] advocated progressive muscle relaxation for high blood pressure in the 1920s.

About ten years ago a series of studies, some carefully done, began to demonstrate that self-regulation of autonomic physiology was possible.[64,65]

Studies on the utility of self-regulation to lower the blood pressure soon followed. There are three major approaches in this field: meditation, relaxation, and biofeedback. Each will be discussed next.

Most of the studies on meditation[66] have employed the transcendental meditation (TM) technique. This technique was introduced in the West by Maharishi Mahesh Yogi in the late 1950s. It is learned by participating in a standard 6–8 hour course offered by local TM centers[67] and involves a simple mental technique that produces a "wakeful hypometabolic state"[64] consistent with deep rest. A few other studies in this category use other mental or breathing practices.[68,69] Significant reductions in blood pressure were found by most authors. For example, Benson and Wallace[70] measured the blood pressure of 22 subjects with mild hypertension 1119 times over 4–63 weeks and found an average decrease of 9 mm systolic pressure and 6 mm diastolic pressure. This study and most of the others in this category lack a control group. Stone and De Leo[69] did employ a control; however, the patients were not randomized to the treatments.

A second group of studies have used relaxation procedures primarily based on Jacobson's progressive muscle relaxation.[63] This practice trains the patient to consciously relax individual muscle groups in a sequential manner. These studies commonly report decreases in blood pressure over 6–12 months of 9–20 mm systolic and 6–14 mm diastolic, although this is not uniform.[66] All authors asked their subjects to train regularly at home but, as with the meditation studies, we know little about compliance. The intervention in the control groups varied widely from simple bed rest to psychotherapy and placebo.

Biofeedback techniques have been employed to lower high blood pressure in many studies since the early 1970s. The methods used range from comparatively simple noncontinuous blood pressure biofeedback to elaborate machinations in the laboratory to a portable blood pressure feedback apparatus.[66] Most studies report significant decreases of systolic and/or diastolic blood pressure in the laboratory during training sessions but few report blood pressure in between sessions. Several have no initial baseline period. Notable exceptions are the study of Elder and Eustis[71] and Glasgow et al.[72] The former reported that blood pressure reductions within training sessions did not continue outside the sessions. The latter did find sustained reductions in systolic blood pressure at 18 months follow-up. The general impression from the literature is that most biofeedback techniques do not successfully lower blood pressure over the long term.

Regarding methods that combine approaches, we feel that in this new area of research for precise scientific understanding, the effectiveness of single behavorial methods should be established first. Therefore, we have not reviewed methods that combine multiple techniques, although some short-term results have been reported, particularly from the work of Patel.[73]

An overall review of the literature on behavorial treatment of hypertension allows the following generalizations:

1. On the whole, meditation and relaxation approaches appear to be more effective and certainly much more practical than biofeedback, which requires costly equipment. A simple technique that the patient can easily practice at home would be most useful clinically. These characteristics also enhance compliance.

2. Patient compliance was generally not reported in the studies, especially when patients were expected to practice the technique at home.

3. Designing a study with appropriate controls is difficult. Adequate placebo treatments have rarely been used.

4. The majority of investigations have been essentially pilot studies[66]—that is, Phase I type with small numbers of subjects during short treatment periods. Phase II studies—controlled trials with known effective agents as controls—are sparse. Large-scale Phase III studies have not yet been done but may be appropriate in the future.

5. More information is needed on the effects of these procedures on blood pressure outside the office or laboratory.

6. Long-term effects need to be assessed. What happens to the blood pressure, target organ damage, and other relevant physiological variables after practicing these treatments for many years? This question has only begun to be answered.[75]

7. In many of the studies, some subjects responded particularly well to a behavorial treatment, although the group change may have been insignificant. Efforts should be made to physiologically characterize responders so that future patients most likely to benefit may be targeted.

Considering the entire field, it seems that behavioral treatment of hypertension may well be effective, particularly in selected cases, and as a supplement to established pharmacologic therapy, yet more research is needed to further define and substantiate these points.

References

1. Kannel WB, Sorlie P, Gordon R: Labile hypertension: a faulty concept? The Framingham Study. Circulation **61:**1183, 1979
2. Watson RDS, Stallard AILMT, Flinn RM, Littler W: Factors determining direct arterial pressure and its variability in hypertensive man. Hypertension **2:**333, 1980
3. Conway J, Julius S, Amery A: Effect of blood pressure level on the hemodynamic response to exercise. Hypertension **16:**79, 1968
4. Sannerstedt R, Julius S: Systemic haemodynamics in borderline arterial hypertension: responses to static exercise before and under the influence of propranolol. Cardiovasc **6:**398, 1972
5. DeCarvalho JGR, Messerli FH, Frohlich ED: Mitral valve prolapse and borderline hypertension. Hypertension **1:**518, 1979
6. Cuddy RP, Smulyan H, Keighley JF, Markason CR, Eich RH: Hemodynamic and catecholamine changes during a standard cold pressor test. Am Heart J **71:**446, 1966

 7. Eich RH, Jacobsen EC: Vascular reactivity in medical students followed for 10 years. J Chron Dis **20**:583, 1967
 8. Brod J: Essential hypertension hemodynamic observation with a bearing on its pathogenesis. Lancet **2**:773, 1960
 9. Nestel PJ: Blood pressure and catecholamine excretion after mental stress in labile hypertension. Lancet **1**:692, 1969
10. Falkner B, Onesti G, Angelakos ET, Fernandes M, Langman C: Cardiovascular response to mental stress in normal adolescents with hypertensive parents. Hemodynamics and mental stress in adolescents. Hypertension **1**:23, 1979
11. Shapiro AP: An experimental study of comparative responses of blood pressure to different noxious stimuli. J Chron Dis **13**:293, 1961
12. Hollenberg NK, Williams GH, Adams DF: Essential hypertension: abnormal renal vascular and endocrine responses to a mild psychological stimulus. Hypertension **3**:11, 1981
13. Harburg E, Julius S, McGinn NF, McLeod J, Hoobler SW: Personality traits and behavorial patterns associated with systolic blood pressure levels in college males. J Chron Dis **17**:405, 1964
14. Sokolow M, Werdegar D, Kain HK, Hinman AT: Relationship between level of blood pressure measured casually and by portable recorders and severity of complications in essential hypertension. Circulation **34**:279, 1966
15. Brown AM: Coronary pressor reflexes. Am J Cardiol **44**:849, 1979
16. Hageman GR, Urthaler F, James TN: Neural pathways of a cardiogenic hypertensive chemoreflex. Am J Physiol **235**:H345, 1978
17. Peterson DF, Brown AM: Pressor reflexes produced by stimulation of afferent fibers in the cardiac syympathetic nerves of the cat. Circ Res **28**:605, 1971
18. Viljoeu FJ, Estafanous FG, Tarazi RC: Acute hypertension immediately after coronary artery surgery. J Thorac Cardiovasc Surg **71**:548, 1976
19. Fouad FM, Estafanous FG, Bravo EL, Iyer KA, Maydak JH, Tarazi RC: Possible role of cardioaortic reflexes in postcoronary bypass hypertension. Am J Cardiol **44**:866, 1979
20. Horwitz D, Sjoerdsma A: Some interrelationships between elevation of blood pressure and angina pectoris. (Proceedings) Council on High Blood Pressure Res **13**:39, 1964
21. Dye LE, Urthaler F, MacLean WAH, Russel RO, Rackley CE, James TN: New arterial hypertension during myocardial hypertension. South Med J **71**:289, 1978
22. Brody MJ, Fink GD, Buggy J, Haywood JR, Gordon FJ, Johnson AK: The role of the anteroventral third ventricle (AV3V) region in experimental hypertension. Circ Res **43** (Suppl I):I2, 1978
23. Brody MJ, Fink GD, Buggy J, Haywood J, Gordon FJ, Kneipfer MM, Mow M, Mahoney L, Johnson AK: Critical role of the anteroventral third ventricle (AV3V) region in development and maintenance of experimental hypertension. *In* Nervous System and Hypertension, edited by Schmitt H, Meyers P. New York, Wiley, 1978, p 76
24. Korner PI, West MJ, Shaw J, Uther JB: "Steady-state" properties of the baroreceptor-heart rate reflex in essential hypertension in man. Clin Exp Pharmacol Physiol **1**:65, 1974
25. Prior IAM, Harvey HPB, Neave MN, Davidson F: The Health of Two Groups of Cook Island Maoris. Department of Health Special Report, Series No. 26. Issued by the Medical Research Council of New Zealand

26. Julius S, Pascual AV, London R: Role of parasympathetic inhibition in the hyperkinetic type of borderline hypertension. Circulation **44**:413, 1971
27. Esler M, Julius S, Zweifler A, Randall O, Harburg E, Gardiner H, DeQuattro V: Mild high-renin essential hypertension. Neurogenic human hypertension? N Engl J Med **296**:405, 1977
28. Lund-Johansen P: Hemodynamics in early essential hypertension. Acta Med Scand **183**(Suppl 482):1, 1967
29. Korner PI, Shaw J, Uther JB, West MJ, McRitchie RS, Richards JG: Autonomic and non-autonomic circulatory components in essential hypertension in man. Circulation **48**:107, 1973
30. Ibrahim MM, Tarazi RC, Dustan HP, Bravo EL, Gifford RW Jr: Hyperkinetic heart in severe hypertension: a separate clinical hemodynamic entity. Am J Cardiol **35**:667, 1975
31. Julius S, Randall OS, Esler MD, Kashima T, Ellis CN, Bennett J: Altered cardiac responsiveness and regulation in the normal cardiac output type of borderline hypertension. Circ Res **36-37** (Suppl I):I-199, 1975
32. Sannerstedt R: Hemodynamic response to exercise in patients with arterial hypertension. Acta Med Scand **180** (Suppl 458):1, 1966
33. Paffenbarger RS, Thorne MC, Wing AL: Chronic disease in former college students. VIII. Characteristics in youth predisposing to hypertension in later years. Am J Epidem **88**:25, 1968
34. Stamler J, Berkson DM, Dyer A, Lepper MH, Lindberg HA, Paul O, McKean H, Rhomberg P, Schoenberger JA, Shekelle RB, Stamler R: Relationship of multiple variables to blood pressure—findings from four Chicago epidemiologic studies. *In* Epidemiology and Control of Hypertension, edited by Paul O. Miami, Symposia Specialists, 1975, p 307
35. Levy RL, White PD, Stroud WD, Hillman CC: Transient tachycardia: prognostic significance alone and in association with transient hypertension. JAMA **129**:585, 1945
36. Julius S, Esler M: Patterns of neurogenic involvement in borderline and essential hypertension. *In* Hypertension and Brain Mechanisms, Progress in Brain Research, Vol 47, edited by DeJong W, Provoost AP, Shapiro AP. Amsterdam, Elsevier North-Holland Biomedical Press, 1977, p 251
37. Julius S, Esler M: Autonomic nervous cardiovascular regulation in borderline hypertension. Am J Cardiol **36**:685, 1975
38. Frohlich ED, Tarazi RC, Dustan HP: Hyperdynamic β-adrenergic circulatory state. Arch Int Med **123**:1, 1969
39. Julius S: Abnormalities of autonomic nervous control in borderline hypertension. Schweiz Med Wschr **106**:1698, 1976
40. Trimarco B, Volpe M, Ricciar delli B, Picotti EB, Galva MD, Petracca R, Condorelli M: Studies of the mechanisms underlying impairment of beta-adrenoceptor-mediated effects in human hypertension. Hypertension **5**:584, 1983
41. Louis WJ, Doyle AE, Anavekar S: Plasma norepinephrine levels in essential hypertension. N Engl J Med **288**:599, 1973
42. Vlachakis ND: Blood pressure and catecholamine responses to sympathetic stimulation in normotensive and hypertensive subjects. J Clin Pharmacol **19**:458, 1979
43. Julius S: The psychophysiology of borderline hypertension. *In* Brain, Behavior and Bodily Disease, edited by Weiner H, Hofer MA, Stunkard AJ. New York, Raven Press, 1981, p 293

44. Esler M, Zweifler A, Randall O, Julius S, DeQuattro V: Agreement among three different indices of sympathetic nervous system activity in essential hypertension. Mayo Clin Proc **52:**379, 1977
45. Julius S, Conway J: Hemodynamic studies in patients with borderline blood pressure elevation. Circulation **38:**282, 1968
46. Julius S, Schork MA: Borderline hypertension—a critical review. J Chron Dis **23:**723, 1971
47. Agabiti-Rosei E, Alicandri C, Faviello R, Muiesan G: Catecholamines and haemodynamics in fixed essential hypertension. Clin Sci **57:**193s, 1979
48. Miura Y, Kobayashi K, Sakuma H, Tomioka H, Adachi M, Yoshinaga K: Plasma noradrenaline concentration and haemodynamics in the early stage of essential hypertension. Clin Sci Mol Med **55:**69s, 1978
49. Folkow B: Cardiovascular structural adaptation; its role in the initiation and maintenance of primary hypertension. Clin Sci Mol Med **55:**3s, 1978
50. Sleight P, Gribbin B, Pickering TG: Baroreflex sensitivity in normal and hypertensive man: the effect of beta-adrenergic blockade on reflex sensitivity. Postgrad Med J **32:**79, 1970
51. Folkow B: Role of vascular factor in hypertension. Contrib Nephrol **8:**81, 1977
52. Louis WJ, Doyle AE, Anavekar SN, Johnston CI, Geffen LB, Rush R: Plasma catecholamine, dopamine-beta-hydroxylase, and renin levels in essential hypertension. Circ Res **34–35** (Suppl I):I–57, 1974
53. Weidmann P, Grimm M, Meier A, Gluck A, Keusch G, Minder I, Beretta-Piccoli C: Cardiovascular pressor reactivity as related to plasma catecholamines: role in the pathogenesis of essential hypertension and in the antihypertensive mechanism of diuretic treatment. *In* Hypertension: Mechanisms and Management, edited by Philipp TH, Distler A. New York, Springer-Verlag, 1980, p 23
54. Amann FW, Bolli P, Kiowski W, Buhler FR: Enhanced alpha-adrenoreceptor-mediated vasoconstriction in essential hypertension. Hypertension **3** (Suppl I):I–119, 1981
55. Kiowski W, Buhler FR, van Brummelen P, Amann FW: Plasma noradrenaline concentration and α-adrenoceptor-mediated vasoconstriction in normotensive and hypertensive man. Clin Sci **60:**483, 1981
56. Philipp TH, Distler A, Cordes U: Sympathetic nervous system and blood-pressure control in essential hypertension. Lancet **2:**959, 1978
57. Meier A, Gubelin U, Weidmann P, Grimm M, Keusch G, Gluck Z, Minder I, Beretta-Piccoli C: Age-related profile of cardiovascular reactivity to norepinephrine and angiotensin II in normal and hypertensive man. Klin Wochenschr **58:**1183, 1980
58. Meier A, Weidmann P, Grimm M, Keusch G, Gluck Z, Minder I, Ziegler WH: Pressor factors and cardiovascular pressor responsiveness in borderline hypertension. Hypertension **3:**367, 1981
59. Bertel O, Buhler FR, Kiowski W, Lutold BE: Decreased beta-adrenoreceptor responsiveness as related to age, blood pressure, and plasma catecholamines in patients with essential hypertension. Hypertension **2:**130, 1980
60. Julius S, Esler MD, Randall OS: Role of the autonomic nervous system in mild human hypertension. Clin Sci Mol Med **48:**243s, 1975
61. White PD: Heart Disease. New York, Macmillan, 1931, p 401
62. Page IH: Hypertension: A Manual for Patients. Springfield, Illinois, Charles C Thomas, 1944
63. Jacobson E: Progressive Relaxation. Chicago, University of Chicago, 1929

64. Wallace RK, Benson H, Wilson AF: A wakeful hypometabolic state. Am J Physiol **221**:795, 1971
65. Wallace RK, Benson H: The physiology of meditation. Sci Am **226**:84, 1972
66. Julius S, Cottier C: Behavior and hypertension. *In* Biobehavioral Bases of Coronary Heart Disease, edited by Dembroski TM, Schmidt TH, Blumchen G. New York, Karger, 1983, p 271
67. Domash LH: Introduction. *In* Scientific Research on the Transcendental Program, Collected Papers (Vol I), edited by Orme-Johnson D, Farrow JT. Livingston Manor, NY, MERU Press, 1977
68. Datey KK, Desmuckh SN, Davi CP, Vinekar SL: "Shavasan:" a yogic exercise in the management of hypertension. Angiology **20**:325, 1969
69. Stone R, DeLeo J: Psychotherapeutic control of blood pressure. N Engl J Med **294**:80, 1976
70. Benson H, Wallace R: Decreased blood pressure in subjects who practiced meditation. Circulation **45–46** (Suppl II):516, 1972
71. Elder ST, Eustis NK: Instrumental blood pressure conditioning in outpatient hypertensives. Behav Res Therapy **13**:185, 1975
72. Glasgow MS, Gaarder KR, Engel BT: Behavioral treatment of high blood pressure. II. Acute and sustained effects of relaxation and systolic blood pressure biofeedback. Psychosom Med **44**:155, 1982
73. Patel CH: Twelve-month follow-up of yoga and biofeedback in the management of hypertension. Lancet **1**:62, 1975
74. Shapiro A, Schwartz G, Ferguson D, Redmon D, Weiss S: Behavioral methods in the treatment of hypertension. Ann Int Med **86**:626, 1977
75. Wallace R, Silver J, Mills P, Dillbeck M, Wagoner D: Long-term practice of the TM-Sidhi program. Effects of TM on systolic blood pressure. Psychosom Med **45**:41, 1983
76. McAllister RG, Love DS, Guthrie DP Jr, Dominic J, Kotchen TA: Peripheral beta-receptor sensitivity in patients with essential hypertension. Arch Int Med **139**:879, 1979

The Role of the Nervous System in the Etiology and Evolution of Essential Hypertension

M. Andrew Fitzpatrick and Stevo Julius

Introduction

Our understanding of the importance of the autonomic nervous system in hypertension is clouded by its changing role in various stages of the natural history of hypertension. There are many difficulties in assessing autonomic function in human beings,[1] but the recent development of specific autonomic receptor agonists and antagonists has provided new information about the net autonomic drive to various organ systems. Nevertheless, interpretation of these data remains complex as the receptor sensitivity and responsiveness must be accounted for along with specific functional and anatomic properties of the responding organs.

Studies performed in the early phases of human hypertension have been useful in identifying the mechanisms responsible for the initiation of the disease. Indeed, it is relatively easy to demonstrate a primary role of the autonomic system in transient (borderline) and very mild hypertension. However, as the disease progresses to even moderately sustained blood pressure levels, the evidence becomes more scanty and less direct. In this chapter we will review the evidence and give our views of the nature of the altered role of the nervous system in the course of human hypertension.

Hyperkinetic Borderline Hypertension

Individuals with an arterial blood pressure in the borderline range (140/90 to 160/100) have been investigated extensively. Although only one-quarter develop established hypertension,[2–4] numerous physiologic abnormalities have been observed (Table 15-1). A substantial proportion of these individuals have an elevated cardiac output,[5–8] heart rate,[8,9] and plasma catecholamines[10,11] indicative of a *hyperkinetic state* that is neurogenic in origin. Furthermore, in patients with mild hypertension and elevated plasma renin activity the evidence suggests that sympathetic overactivity exists, raising plasma renin and sustaining the blood pressure elevation.[11]

That these changes are neurogenic in origin can be most clearly demonstrated by the response of cardiac output to autonomic blockade.[9] Combined cardiac autonomic blockade with intravenous propranolol and atropine returns the elevated cardiac output and heart rate to the normal range. Propranolol alone does not normalize the cardiac output or heart rate. Thus, vagal inhibition of the sinus node appears to be reduced in these patients as well.[9] Despite blockade of cardiac autonomic efferents, the blood pressure is not normalized.[12] Logically, observation of the effects of alpha-blockade in these individuals was important in order to assess the influence of the remaining effective sympathetic drive to alpha-receptors. Blood pressure can only be normalized in those individuals with mild hypertension, high plasma renin and catecholamine levels, and an abnormal personality profile.[11] In most hypertensives, however, blood pressure can-

---

Table 15-1
Reported Abnormalities in Early Hypertension*

1. Biochemical indices of sympathetic activity elevated
2. Cardiac index increased
3. Tachycardia
4. Stroke volume—increased/decreased
5. Peripheral resistance elevated or inappropriately adjusted to flow
6. Plasma volume decreased
7. Peripheral to central distribution of the blood in capacitance vessels
8. Abnormal plasma renin activity—high or low
9. Vascular reactivity increased
10. Increased blood pressure responsiveness:
    to tilt
    to upright posture
    to mental stress
11. Abnormal beta-adrenergic responsiveness:
    in the heart
    in renin release
12. Abnormal forearm blood flow response to sodium loading
13. Abnormal regional resistance change to mental stress
14. Abnormal red cell cation transport
15. Different behavior and personality traits

---

*For references the reader is referred to a recent review.[1]

not be normalized by total autonomic blockade, suggesting that primary vascular factors or other mechanisms are important in sustaining elevated blood pressure levels.

The reciprocal relationship observed between enhanced sympathetic drive and diminished vagal inhibition just outlined are characteristic of the integrative function of the cardiovascular control center located in the medulla oblongata. Examination of the afferent inputs into this center revealed normal peripheral input from arterial baroceptors.[13,14] On the other hand, there is evidence[9,15] to suggest that input descending on the medullary centers from higher areas in the brain may be responsible for this abnormal integration of the autonomic discharge. These individuals are sensitive, submissive, and prone to harboring considerable anger they cannot express.[1]

Anger elevates blood pressure through activation of the sympathetic nervous system.[16-18] Furthermore, the response is greater when an outlet for aggression is not available.[16,19,20] It has been suggested that suppressed hostility in patients with borderline hypertension leads to chronic activation of the sympathetic nervous system and sustained hypertension. On the other hand, increased sympathetic nervous tone could be the initial event, with the physiologic and personality abnormalities following secondarily. This explanation cannot be excluded, as adrenergic mechanisms within the central nervous system may well influence mood and behavior.[21]

That the behavioral style may indeed be intricately involved in the blood pressure elevation has been documented in patients with mild established hypertension associated with high recumbent plasma renin and norepinephrine levels.[9] Such patients can be shown to have greater sympathetic drive to the myocardium as well as to peripheral vessels. These physiological changes are closely associated with a controlled, guilt-prone, and submissive personality with high levels of unexpressed anger.[9] The normalization of blood pressure by total autonomic blockade in these patients strongly supports the claim that hypertension in these patients is neurogenic in origin.

Normokinetic Borderline Hypertension

Is there evidence of abnormalities in autonomic activity in individuals with borderline hypertension without hyperkinetic circulation? In this group, stigmata of sympathetic overactivity are not present—heart rate is only slightly increased, the cardiac output is normal or decreased, and plasma norepinephrine is generally within normal limits. Despite this, we demonstrated altered cardiac responsiveness and regulation.[22] These patients had a diminished resting stroke volume but maintained a normal cardiac output with a higher heart rate. Cardiac receptor blockade caused a greater decrease in heart rate in those with normokinetic borderline hypertension than in the control group. After blockade, cardiac output and stroke volume were significantly lower in patients than controls. Thus, an increased net autonomic drive to the heart was necessary for the maintenance of a normal cardiac output. Decreased vagal inhibition also helped to maintain the cardiac output.[22]

Does hyperkinetic borderline hypertension lead to normokinetic hypertension? Epidemiological evidence suggests that the hyperkinetic state may be a precursor of hypertension. Faster heart rates are associated with higher blood pressure values in population studies.[23–25] Furthermore, in longitudinal studies a faster heart rate in youth predicts the future development of hypertension,[4,26–28] which is independent of initial blood pressure. Few longitudinal hemodynamic studies are available, but the data indicate that cardiac output declines and vascular resistance increases with the passage of time.[9,29,30] Even so, an increase in blood pressure paralleled the rise in vascular resistance in only one study.[30]

Cross-sectional comparison of groups of patients with borderline and established hypertension supports the notion of transition from a hyperkinetic to a normokinetic state in hypertension. Similar changes in autonomic drive are noted at all stages of hypertension. Decreased vagal inhibition is apparent in hyperkinetic and normokinetic borderline hypertension, as well as in patients with moderately severe essential hypertension.[31] On the other hand, sympathetic drive is enhanced in hyperkinetic but not in normokinetic borderline and moderately severe hypertension.[31] Thus, from the available evidence it would appear that the group with normokinetic borderline hypertension may be an intermediate or transitional group between those with hyperkinetic borderline hypertension and those with established essential hypertension.

How could such a transition occur? Why do the signs of increased sympathetic stimulation disappear during the evolution of sustained hypertension? With our current knowledge, these questions cannot be fully answered. An important part of the transition may well result from an alteration in the responsiveness to sympathetic stimuli. Sympathetic receptors are subject to "down-regulation" (or decreased sensitivity) when exposed to greater sympathetic tone.[32] In all likelihood a prolonged increase in sympathetic drive in patients with neurogenic borderline hypertension leads to changes in the density of beta-adrenergic receptors on the myocardium, resulting in decreased responsiveness to sympathetic drive and to isoproterenol infusions. There are two main objectives to this concept. First, hyperkinetic[14] and normokinetic[22] subjects show the same decreased chronotropic response to isoproterenol. Second, vascular alpha-receptors should also be subject to "down-regulation;" however, vascular reactivity to norepinephrine is normal or increased with sustained hypertension.[33] We believe that the decreased sensitivity of alpha-receptors is compensated for by a large increase in the responsiveness of the arterioles due to the changes in the wall to lumen ratio, as proposed by Folkow.[34]

Established Essential Hypertension

It should be emphasized that the mechanism of transition from neurogenic to sustained hypertension outlined remains hypothetical. One stumbling block for this hypothesis has been the lack of evidence for increased sympathetic drive in patients with established hypertension. Catecholamine elevation[10] is difficult to find; furthermore, personality abnormalities[1] cannot be well-documented in those with established hypertension. Not all patients with hypertension start out as the neurogenic hyperkinetic subtype. The smaller proportion with neurogenic hypertension merges with a larger pool of patients with essential hypertension of other pathophysiologies; thus, it becomes impossible to identify them from the larger group.

Although it is impossible to select out those patients with neurogenic hypertension once the disease is well established, the autonomic system plays a major role in maintaining elevated blood pressure and normal cardiac output no matter what the cause of the hypertension. First, hypertensive patients maintain a normal cardiac output at the expense of a faster heart rate. This is largely the result of diminished stroke volume due to ventricular hypertrophy and decreased myocardial compliance much like those individuals with normokinetic borderline hypertension. Investigations of cardiac autonomic blockade in hypertensive patients suggest that reduced vagal inhibition is largely responsible for the increased heart rate.[35] Second, an alteration in arterial baroreceptor properties occurs such that the pressure threshold and pressure operating range is increased. This baroreceptor "resetting" becomes more evident as hypertension progresses in intensity and duration.[36] Thus, the central nervous system plays a permissive role allowing hypertension to be sustained. Finally, there are changes in the vascular response to vasoactive substances, but these responses will be dealt with in the next chapter.

Summary

The role of the autonomic nervous system changes during the course of the natural history of hypertension. The case for a primary neurogenic role is strongest for a subgroup of patients with borderline hypertension who have a hyperkinetic circulation associated with elevated circulating catecholamines and plasma renin. There is good pharmacologic and humoral evidence that sympathetic drive is increased in these individuals, and this appears to be related to a peculiar personality trait. Epidemiologic studies suggest that some of these individuals will develop established hypertension; however, it is impossible, at that stage, to differentiate them from a larger pool of hypertensives with other etiologies. Vascular factors secondary to medial hypertrophy play a primary role in sustaining hypertension no matter what the etiology. Nevertheless, all patients exhibit autonomic changes that maintain cardiac output in the face of reduced cardiac compliance and permit the elevated arterial pressure to persist.

References

1. Julius S: The psychophysiology of borderline hypertension. *In* Brain, Behavior and Bodily Disease, edited by Weiner H, Hofer MA, Stunkard AJ. New York, Raven Press, 1981, p 293

2. Julius S, Schork MA: Borderline hypertension—a critical review. J Chronic Dis **23**:723, 1971

3. Julius S, Harburg E, McGinn NF: Relationship between casual blood pressure readings in youth and at age 40: a retrospective study. J Chronic Dis **17**:397, 1964

4. Paffenbarger RS, Thorne MC, Wing AL: Chronic disease in former college students. VIII. Characteristics in youth predisposing to hypertension in later years. Am J Epidemiol **88**:25, 1968

5. Julius S, Conway J: Hemodynamic studies in patients with borderline blood pressure elevation. Circulation **38**:282, 1968

6. Sannerstedt R, Julius S: Systemic haemodynamics in borderline arterial hypertension: Responses to static exercise before and under the influence of propranolol. Cardiovasc Res **6**:398, 1972

7. Lund-Johansen P: Hemodynamics in early essential hypertension. Acta Med Scand **183** (Suppl 482):1, 1967

8. Safar ME, Weiss YA, Levenson JA, London GM, Milliez PL: Hemodynamic study of 85 patients with borderline hypertension. Am J Cardiol **31**:315, 1973

9. Julius S, Pascual AV, London R: Role of parasympathetic inhibition in the hyperkinetic type of borderline hypertension. Circulation **44**:413, 1971

10. Goldstein DS: Plasma norepinephrine in essential hypertension: a study of the studies. Hypertension **3**:48, 1981

11. Esler M, Julius S, Zweifler A, Randall O, Harburg E, Gardiner H, DeQuattro V: Mild high-renin essential hypertension. Neurogenic human hypertension? N Engl J Med **296**:405, 1977

12. Julius S, Pascual AV, Sannerstedt R, Mitchell C: Relationship between cardiac output and peripheral resistance in borderline hypertension. Circulation **43**:382, 1971

13. Eckberg DL: Carotid baroreflex function in young men with borderline blood pressure elevation. Circulation **59**:632, 1979

14. Julius S: Neurogenic component in borderline hypertension. *In* The Nervous System in Arterial Hypertension, edited by Julius S, Esler M. Springfield, Illinois, Charles C Thomas, 1976, p 301

15. Harburg E, Julius S, McGinn NF, McLeod J, Hoobler SW: Personality traits and behavioral patterns associated with systolic blood pressure levels in college males. J Chronic Dis **17**:405, 1964

16. Cochrane R: High blood pressure as a psychosomatic disorder: a selective review. Br J Soc Psychol **10**:61, 1971

17. Hokanson JE, Burgess M: The effects of status, type of frustration and aggression on vascular processes. J Abnorm Soc Psychol **65**:232, 1962

18. Gambaro S, Rabin AI: Diastolic blood pressure responses following direct and displaced aggression after anger aroused in high- and low-guilt subjects. J Pers Soc Psychol **12:**87, 1969

19. Von Euler S: Quantitation of stress by catecholamine analysis. Clin Pharmacol Ther **5:**398, 1964

20. Elmadjian F, Hope JM, Lamson ET: Excretion of epinephrine and norepinephrine in various emotional states. J Clin Endocrinol **17:**608, 1957

21. Ketty SS: Catecholamines in neuropsychiatric states. Pharmacol Rev **18:**787, 1966

22. Julius S, Randall OS, Esler MD, Kashima T, Ellis CN, Bennett J: Altered cardiac responsiveness and regulation in the normal cardiac output type of borderline hypertension. Circ Res **36–37** (Suppl I):I–199, 1975

23. Prior IAM, Harvey HPB, Neave MN, Davidson F: The Health of Two Groups of Cook Island Maoris. Department of Health Special Report Series No. 26. Issued by the Medical Research Council of New Zealand

24. Simpson FO: Beta-adrenergic receptor blocking drugs in hypertension. Drugs **7:**85, 1974

25. Sive PH, Medalie JH, Kahn HA, Neufeld HN, Riss E: Distribution and multiple regression analysis of blood pressure in 10,000 Israeli men. Am J Epidemiol **93:**317, 1971

26. Levy RL, White PD, Stroud WD, Hillman CC: Transient tachycardia: prognostic significance alone and in association with transient hypertension. JAMA **129:**585, 1945

27. Stamler J, Berkson DM, Dyer A, Lepper MH, Lindberg HA, Paul O, McKean H, Rhomberg P, Schoenberger JA, Shekelle RB, Stamler R: Relationship of multiple variables to blood pressure—findings from four Chicago epidemiologic studies. *In* Epidemiology and Control of Hypertension, edited by Paul O. Miami, Symposia Specialists, 1975, p 307

28. Thomas CB: Developmental patterns in hypertensive cardiovascular disease: fact or fiction? Bull NY Acad Med **45:**831, 1969

29. Eich RH, Cuddy RP, Smulyan H, Lyons RH: Hemodynamics in labile hypertension: a follow-up study. Circulation **34:**299, 1966

30. Weiss YA, Safar ME, London GM, Simon AC, Levenson JA, Milliez PM: Repeat hemodynamic determinations in borderline hypertension. Am J Med **64:**382, 1978

31. Korner PI, Shaw J, Uther JB, West MJ, McRitchie RJ, Richard JG: Autonomic and non-autonomic circulatory components in essential hypertension in man. Circulation **48:**107, 1973

32. Lefkowitz RJ: β-adrenergic receptors: recognition and regulation. N Engl J Med **295:**323, 1976

33. Philipp TH, Distler A, Cordes U: Sympathetic nervous system and blood-pressure control in essential hypertension. Lancet **2:**959, 1978

34. Folkow B: Cardiovascular structural adaptation: its role in the initiation and maintenance of primary hypertension. Clin Sci Mol Med **55:**3s, 1978

35. Korner PI, West MJ, Shaw J, Uther JB: "Steady-state" properties of the baroreceptor-heart rate reflex in essential hypertension in man. Clin Exp Pharmacol Physiol **1:**65, 1974

36. McCubbin JW, Green JH, Page IH: Baroreflex function in chronic renal hypertension. Circ Res **4:**205, 1956

Chapter 16

Centrally Acting Anti-Hypertensive Drugs

Gordon P. Guthrie, Jr. and Terry W. Sherraden

Introduction

Evolution of our knowledge about the physiology of the circulation has been accompanied by the development of effective drugs for the treatment of hypertension. Many such drugs have been useful as probes for exploring mechanisms of blood pressure control, including those that owe their anti-hypertensive effect to a central action. Two of the first effective anti-hypertensive drugs were reserpine and the veratrum alkaloids, both of which acted in part through the brain. The centrally acting alpha adrenergic agonists, typified by methyldopa and clonidine, continue to be mainstay anti-hypertensive drugs, with newer agents of this class coming such as guanabenz, guanfacine, and lofexidine. The beta adrenergic antagonists with propranolol as the prototype are now widely used and effective blood pressure lowering drugs, although the major mechanism for their anti-hypertensive action remains unsettled, one theory of their action being a central effect. The proposed central mechanisms and clinical actions of each of these types of drugs are described next.

Reserpine

Extracts of the Indian climbing shrub, Rauwolfia serpentina, had long been used in primitive Hindu medicine for disorders such as insomnia. Therapeutic application to hypertension was first described in 1931, followed by the first report in Western literature by Vakil in 1949.[1] Extensive reviews of its pharmacology have been published.[2]

The major and most widely used anti-hypertensive alkaloid of the Rauwolfia root is reserpine. The principal action of this drug is to deplete stores of bioactive amines. This degree of depletion occurs in the brain, adrenal medulla, and in post-ganglionic neurons peripherally, which all contribute to its hypotensive effect. The depletion of norepinephrine in adrenergic neurons accounts for most of its anti-hypertensive action, and this depletion of norepinephrine and other monoamines occurs by inhibition of the vesicular storage mechanism for neurotransmitters via an action at the membranes of storage granules.[3]

The anti-hypertensive effect of reserpine derives from net inhibition of peripheral sympathetic activity. In normal and hypertensive animals and man it crosses the blood-brain barrier by nature of its lipid solubility and gradually lowers arterial blood pressure without an acute pressor effect. The delay in action is because of a time-dependent depletion of monoamine stores. In man the hypotensive action is associated with early reductions in both cardiac output and peripheral resistance. After prolonged treatment, however, cardiac output returns to basal levels and peripheral resistance remains reduced.[4] Little change in renal function is produced by reserpine.

Since reserpine has major effects on the monoamines of the central nervous system, its prominent central side effects are not surprising. Reserpine has pronounced sedative and tranquilizing actions. It also lowers body temperature, can produce extrapyramidal symptoms in man, and may produce from mild to profound depression. Reserpine further affects the functions of the hypothalamus and pituitary. Over the long term, pituitary ACTH stores are depleted and responses to stressful stimuli are impaired.[5] Other hormonal effects include impairment of thyroid and gonadal function and stimulation of prolactin release, and other side effects include increased gastric acidity with the promotion of ulcer formation, and diarrhea.

Reserpine is still used alone and in conjunction with other drugs, usually thiazide diuretics, to control chronic hypertension, and is effective in mild to moderately severe hypertension. Testimony to its efficacy was provided by the widely cited Veteran's Administration Multi-Clinic Cooperative Study, which found that the combination of reserpine plus hydrochlorothiazide was superior to propranolol alone, propranolol plus hydrochlorothiazide, or propranolol plus hydralazine in controlling mild hypertension.[6] The drug also has some advantages over other anti-hypertensive agents in that its cost is low and it often requires little titration of dosage (usually from 0.25 to 0.50 mg daily). However, in the minds of many, these advantages of reserpine in the treatment of essential hypertension have been overshadowed by the prominence of its adverse side effects. It certainly should no longer be used for the treatment of hypertensive emergencies, given the clear superiority of other more effective modern drugs.

Veratrum Alkaloids

The veratrum alkaloids are a family of plant products formerly used to treat hypertension, but now no longer employed for this purpose because of their relatively high incidence of adverse side effects, although they are still used in studies on the physiology of the circulation. The major compounds formerly used clinically were protoveratine A and B.

The veratrum alkaloids lower blood pressure through a central action.[7] The mechanism of this action has not been completely defined, but involves several important cardiovascular reflexes. Prominent among these is the so-called Bezold-Jarisch reflex, defined as stimulation of chemoreceptors in the coronary circulation leading to activation of cardiac afferents, and reflux efferent activation of the cardiac vagus nerve and inhibition of peripheral sympathetic tone. This reflex produces bradycardia and depressed blood pressure via chemoreceptor stimulation of the heart, and is potentiated either centrally, peripherally, or in both areas by the veratrum alkaloids. The prominence of the central action of this drug has been supported by a series of experiments in the 1950's.[8,9] Potentiation of the action of the baroreflexes has also been implicated in its action.

Treatment with the veratrum alkaloids leads to diminished sympathetic tone and bradycardia associated with the fall in blood pressure. The great limitation to its therapeutic use has involved its narrow therapeutic range. Doses of veratrum alkaloids that lower blood pressure are close to those that provoke major side effects, the most notable of them being nausea and vomiting, enhanced salivation, rhinorrhea, paresthesias, myotonia, and (rarely) apnea. These have understandably lead to its obsolescence.

Methyldopa

Methyldopa (L-alpha-methyl-3,4-dihydroxyphenylalanine) is currently one of the most widely prescribed anti-hypertensive drugs. Its anti-hypertensive properties were first demonstrated by Oates et al. in 1960,[10] although its mechanism of action was not clarified until some time later. Its anti-hypertensive action was initially attributed to the inhibition by this compound of aromatic amino acid decarboxylase. Inhibition of this enzyme by methyldopa and other derivatives of phenylalanine was initially described by Sourkes et al. and others,[11] but was soon discounted as the major anti-hypertensive action since the inhibition of this enzyme did not correlate quantitatively with its anti-hypertensive properties. Although methyldopa does reduce norepinephrine levels in peripheral tissues, such depletion is not thought to be from decarboxylase inhibition since stores of norepinephrine remain low several days after dopamine concentrations return toward normal.[12]

A subsequent hypothesis for the anti-hypertensive action of methyldopa was that this compound was metabolized to the "false transmitters" methyldopamine or methylnorepinephrine. Although such conversions were demonstrated both in vivo and in vitro, several other lines of evidence failed to support the peripheral "false transmitter" hypothesis. First, it had been assumed that the false transmitters were weaker vasoconstrictors than the natural agonist norepinephrine. However, in the cat and rat, methylnorepinephrine was found to be equally as potent as a pressor agent as norepinephine.[13] Furthermore, there is no correlation between the time course of the anti-hypertensive actions of this drug and its norepinephrine-replacing effect.[14]

The present and most widely accepted hypothesis for the mechanism of action of methyldopa involves the central nervous system as its primary site. This hypothesis was first proposed by Henning and van Zwieten,[15] who observed that infusion of methyldopa into the vertebral artery of cats produces a gradual fall in blood pressure and in brain norepinephrine levels. However, in their preparations, cardiac norepinephrine levels remain unaffected. Further studies have revealed that the hypertensive action of methyldopa in rats is inhibited by central but not by peripheral inhibitors of amino acid decarboxylase.[16] The anti-hypertensive action is, however, inhibited in renal hypertensive rats by a central inhibitor of amino acid decarboxylase.[17] These and other findings suggest that the site of the hypertensive action of methlydopa is central and that alpha-methyl-norepinephrine is likely to mediate the hypotensive effect of this drug.

Subsequent studies have confirmed that methyldopa acts through the central nervous system, most likely through stimulation of alpha adrenoceptors. Being an amino acid, methyldopa readily enters the brain by an active amino acid transport system. Heise and Kroneberg[18] found that perfusion of the third and fourth ventricles of cats with methyldopa, alpha-methyldopamine, and alpha-norepinephrine lead to decreases in blood pressure and that alpha-methyl-norepinephrine produced the greatest effect. Alpha adrenergic agonists antagonized the effects of all three drugs. Central depression of the sympathetic control of blood pressure by methyldopa occurs without significant alteration in blood pressure responses to orthostasis, supporting the low incidence of postural hypotension in man in early clinical studies.

Recent studies have expanded the view that the central nervous system is the major site of action of methlydopa, although the specific site of action remains controversial. Injections of alpha-methyl-norepinephrine into the anterior hypothalamus or the nucleus tractus solitarius (NTS) lowers arterial blood pressure in animals, suggesting that the NTS is in fact the major site of the anti-hypertensive action of methyldopa.[19] Other evidence suggests that methyldopa may exert anti-hypertensive actions through spinal sympathetic mechanisms.[20] Methyldopa administration to rats produces a marked reduction in the levels of norepinephrine and dopamine in anterior hypothalamic-preoptic nuclei implicated in catecholamine mediated cardiovascular inhibitory functions.[21] Similar actions can be seen in medullary nuclei including the nucleus tractus solitarius.

Alpha-methyl-dopamine accumulates rapidly after methyldopa administration in rats in these specific nuclear areas, as does alpha-methyl-norepinephrine. The time course for the accumulation of these amines in the NTS differs somewhat from the anterior hypothalamic preoptic nucleus and is more closely related to the time course of the anti-hypertensive action of methyldopa.[22] These data together suggest that the nucleus tractus solitarius is intimately involved in the anti-hypertensive action of methyldopa, most probably via stimulation of presynaptic alpha-adrenoceptors in this area.

Aside from lowering blood pressure through interaction with the brain, methyldopa also produces a number of side effects in man that are also clearly attributable to alteration of central nervous function. These include sedation, depression, extrapyramidal symptoms, and elevation in serum prolactin concentrations, occasionally producing galactorrhea. The production of sexual dysfunction highlighted by erectile impotence may also be from a central effect. Reduction of sympathetic tone again via its central action may also contribute to the development of diarrhea.

Several antisympathetic drugs that act through the central nervous system carry with them the risk of aggravation of hypertension following their sudden discontinuation. This has been termed the "rebound phenomenon," and is less common with methyldopa than with other central agents such as clonidine. It appears to be associated with hyperactivity of the sympathetic nervous system following sudden discontinuation of a drug that suppresses this system.

Clonidine

Clonidine hydrochloride is a drug of the imidazolidine class that is effective as an anti-hypertensive agent in patients with from mild to severe hypertension. It was originally tested as a nasal decongestant because of its vasoconstrictor properties, but was subsequently found to have the useful therapeutic property of blood pressure reduction.

Clonidine has complex effects on the circulation.[23] When given acutely by intravenous injection it causes a transient rise in blood pressure owing to its alpha agonistic properties. This is soon followed by a lasting fall in blood pressure accompanied by bradycardia and reduction in cardiac output. Numerous studies on its effects soon led to the prevalent concept that clonidine lowers blood pressure through interaction with the central nervous system. The drug is lipid soluble, and readily crosses the blood-brain barrier.

Administration of clonidine into the cerebral ventricles of the cat causes a fall in blood pressure and bradycardia, whereas intravenous injection of the same small dose produces no circulatory effects.[24] Subsequent investigations by Sattler and van Zwieten[25] produced further evidence of a central nervous system action. Low concentrations of clonidine infused into the vertebral arteries cause a fall in blood pressure and bradycardia again with no effect when given peripherally. Localization of the sites of the hypertensive action of clonidine has been made by selective section and injection techniques. In cats and dogs in which the brain stem has been cut rostral to the medulla, the hypotensive action of clonidine is maintained. However, if the brain stem is cut caudal to the medulla, no effect is seen.[26]

Further work by Schmitt[27] and others[28] has supported the hypothesis that clonidine stimulates post-synaptic alpha-2-adrenoceptors in the central nervous system, and owes its anti-hypertensive action to this effect.

Since clonidine and other alpha agonists produce their characteristic depression of blood pressure and heart rate after prior catecholamine depletion (as with alpha-methyl-tyrosine) or destruction of presynaptic neurons (as with 6OH dopamine), their action is presumed to be post-synaptic since the action is independent of presynaptic catecholamine receptors. In addition, these effects are blocked by alpha-2 antagonists such as rauwolscine.[28]

Hausler[29] has shown that the action of clonidine bears some similarity to a central activation of the baroreceptor reflex. Microinfusion of clonidine into the nucleus tractus solitarius (NTS), a center that integrates several cardiovascular reflexes including the baroreflex, reduces blood pressure and heart rate, suggesting this important site as a major locus for its effect. We have found that oral clonidine potentiates the baroreflex in patients with essential hypertension,[30] previously found as an effect of the intravenous drug by Sleight et al.[31] Other sites of the brain stem have, however, been implicated, including the ventral surface of the medulla.

The net effect of clonidine is central inhibition of peripheral sympathetic tone. The parasympathetic system is also involved in its action, implying that clonidine, in part, enhances vagal reflexes. Kobinger and Walland[32] have demonstrated that clonidine influences vagal reflexes by demonstrating that injection of norepinephrine and angiotensin cause reflex bradycardia, which is reinforced by intracisternal clonidine and blocked by phentolamine (See Chapter 2). Other mechanisms for the hypotensive effect of clonidine have been reported. Possible involvement of histamine H2 receptors has been noted, as have possible effects of clonidine in the spinal cord. Since clonidine has an effect on peripheral presynaptic alpha-receptors, the suggestion has been made that clonidine might also exert an anti-hypertensive effect via this peripheral action. Studies by Hausler and others suggest that in fact its peripheral action is not important.[33]

Long-term treatment of both man and experimental animals with and without hypertension shows persistent and sustained reductions in blood pressure accompanied by reductions in plasma and urinary catecholamines. This suppression of catecholamines, in fact, has been used as a provocative test to distinguish patients harboring a pheochromocytoma from those with similar symptoms who do not.[34] As mentioned before relative to methyldopa, sudden discontinuation of clonidine can produce increases in blood pressure to or exceeding levels prior to treatment, accompanied by signs and symptoms of sympathetic excess including sweating, tachycardia and anxiety. These symptoms of "rebound" are rarely seen in the clinical setting at doses of clonidine below 0.8 mg/day. Nonetheless, patients being removed from clonidine treatment are best advised to taper off and not suddenly discontinue the drug.

Along with its primary antihypertensive effect through the central nervous system, the major adverse side effects of clonidine are also central in origin. The most prominent of these is sedation, seen clinically at virtually all doses. Experimental evidence suggests that central alpha-adrenoreceptors are involved in the induction of sleep by clonidine, in that this effect is prevented by intracisternal alpha blockade. Clonidine overdose in man is accompanied by coma. The sedative effect in most patients diminishes with time, and can be further minimized by advising patients to take the major portion of a divided dose at bedtime. Clonidine also inhibits salivation, leading to the common complaint of a dry mouth. This effect is also centrally mediated via an action on presynaptic alpha-adrenoreceptors inhibiting cholinergic transmission and control of salivation by cholinergic nerves.

Beta-Adrenergic Blockers

Beta-adrenoreceptor antagonists were developed in the early 1960's for the treatment of cardiac arrhythmias and angina pectoris. Pritchard and Gilliam subsequently observed that the systemic blood pressure sometimes fell after prolonged treatment with these drugs. Further trials, first with pronethalol, later with propranolol, established the usefulness of beta-adrenergic blockers in the treatment of hypertension.[35] Propranolol has subsequently become the reference beta-adrenergic receptor blocker with which all others are compared, although similar anti-hypertensive efficacy has been confirmed in virtually all members of the beta-adrenergic blocker family.[36–39]

Approximately 60% of all hypertensive patients respond to treatment with a beta blocker alone.[40] Beta-adrenoreceptor antagonists have many physiologic actions that may contribute to the control of hypertension. The postulated anti-hypertensive mechanisms of the beta-adrenergic blockers have been reviewed,[41–48] and can be divided into predominant central and peripheral actions. The relative importance of each of these mechanisms in the hypotensive action of beta-adrenoreceptor antagonists has not been established, and may be different in different hypertensive diseases.

Postulated Peripheral Mechanisms of Action

In spite of the many pharmacological differences of beta-adrenergic blockers, all appear to have approximately equal anti-hypertensive effects. It seems likely that the anti-hypertensive action of beta-adrenergic blockers depends on competitive antagonism of catecholamines at beta-adrenoreceptors, thus preventing the effects of endogenous sympathetic stimulation. Such beta-adrenoreceptors are found in the heart, peripheral vasculature, the juxtaglomerular cells of the kidney, and other locations.

Many investigators have hypothesized that the anti-hypertensive effect of beta-adrenergic blocking agents is mediated through decreased cardiac output followed by a gradual fall in total peripheral resistance.[48–53] This effect cannot be demonstrated convincingly with all beta blockers.[48,54,55]

Other studies have demonstrated the importance of the inhibition of renin secretion in the control of blood pressure with beta blockers,[56–59] although this finding has been disputed.[60–67] There may be two discrete populations of hypertensive patients who respond to propranolol. The first responds to low doses of propranolol and demonstrates a concomitant fall in renin secretion. The second shows a fall in blood pressure at much higher levels of propranolol administration, postulated to be a renin-independent effect.[68]

Presynaptic beta-adrenoceptors have been proposed at sympathetic nerve endings in the heart and peripheral vasculature,[69–81] which attenuate the release of norepinephrine from the nerve endings. Plasma epinephrine levels are elevated in some patients with essential hypertension.[82,83,84] Propranolol may decrease secretion of catecholamines from neuronal sites by action at presynaptic receptors, thus decreasing alpha-receptor stimulation. The anti-hypertensive response to propranolol has been shown to parallel a decrease in alpha-adrenoceptor mediated vasoconstriction,[85] which may be a key effect.

Other possible mechanisms for the peripheral hypotensive actions of beta blockers include an increased sensitivity of the peripheral baroreflex mechanism.[45,86] The hypotensive effect may also be mediated by interaction with endogenous prostaglandins, which cause vasodilation,[87,88] although these findings are disputed.[89,90] Plasma volume has been shown to be reduced with beta blocker treatment, but does not correlate with the hypotensive effect.[91,92,93]

Postulated Central Mechanisms of Action

Several authors have suggested that beta-adrenergic blockers may reduce blood pressure and heart rate through an action of the central nervous system.[94,95,96] Evidence implicating a central nervous system mechanism for the anti-hypertensive effect of beta-adrenergic blockers is indirect, depending upon unconventional routes of drug administration in animals such as intracerebral microinjection and superfusion. It is clear that beta-receptors are present within the CNS and that pharmacologic agents can alter their effects. However, a definite correlation between CNS effect and blood pressure control in humans has not been established with all beta blockers.

Beta-adrenoceptors have been demonstrated on the membranes of many neurons in the central nervous system.[97,98] Brain tissue, when stimulated by isoprenaline, produces an increase in cyclic AMP. This increase can be blocked by beta blockers. Central nervous system homogenates also contain stereospecific beta-adrenoceptor binding sites of high affinity.[99–102] Using fluorescent labelling techniques, beta-adrenoceptors have been found in all areas of the rat cerebral cortex. Although marked variations in density and distribution pattern exist, the highest uptake is in the hippocampus.[103] Beta-adrenoceptors have been also found in the limbic forebrain, cerebellum, extrapyramidal areas, and the pineal gland.[100,104] There is also physiologic evidence for central beta-adrenoceptors. Intracerebroventricular (ICV) infusion of isoprenaline in conscious cats creates a tachycardia and variable blood pressure response, which can be abolished by prior beta blockade.[105]

High concentrations of some beta blockers have been found in the CNS after peripheral administration.[106] Because of the blood brain barrier, the CNS penetration of any drug is dependent on its physical properties, and concentrations found in the brain vary accordingly[106–111] (Table 16-1). Lipophilic beta blockers such as propranolol, metoprolol, oxprenolol, and aceprenolol show the greatest penetration into brain tissue.[112–114] Under equilibrium conditions the ratio of propranolol concentration in the rabbit brain to that in the plasma is high, approximately 15:1.[115] Similar brain: plasma ratios were seen in post-mortem studies in patients treated with prolonged intravenous infusions of D-propranolol as part of the treatment for paraquat poisioning. Atenolol, despite its lipophobic nature, can also be found in small amounts in the brain.[112,116] This may occur because of its low plasma protein binding and the possibility that lipophobic drugs may bypass the blood brain barrier in the area postrema and pituitary. Propranolol has been found to concentrate in the hypothalamus, medulla, pons,[117,118] and hippocampus.[119] Pindolol has been found concentrated mainly in the septum, while sotalol, which fails to lower blood pressure in animals, cannot be found in significant amounts in brain tissue.[119] In humans, both lipophilic and lipophobic beta blockers seem to have equivalent anti-hypertensive effects in spite of different levels of brain penetration.

Studies involving the administration of beta blockers to animals have produced variable results, including a marked pressor effect, depressor effect, or no effect on blood pressure.[120] To a large degree, such variability can be ascribed to the diverse animal models used, presence or absence of anesthesia, the particular anesthesia use, and the doses of drugs used. If

Table 16-1
Properties that Influence Central Nervous System Activity
of Beta Blockers

	Log$_{10}$ Octanol/Water Partition Coefficient	Protein Binding	pKa	Penetration into the CNS
Propranolol[3]	3.65	90%	9.45	+ +
Atenolol[1]	0.23	3–5%	9.50	Poor
Practolol[1,2]	0.79	—	—	Poor
Acebutolol[1,2,3]	1.87	—	—	Poor/+
Metoprolol[1]	2.15	10%	9.60	+
Sotalol	−0.79	0%	8.30	Poor
Nadolol	0.71	30%	—	NA
Pindolol[2,3]	1.75	57–73%	9.26	+
Timolol	2.10	10%	—	NA
Oxprenolol[2,3]	2.18	70%	9.20	+
Alprenolol[2,3]	2.16	—	—	+

1 = Cardioselective
2 = Intrinsic Sympathomimetic Activity Present
3 = Membrane Stabilizing Activity Present
NA = Not Available

high doses of beta blockers are infused centrally, the results can be clouded if there is diffusion of the drug from the central nervous system into the peripheral circulation, where it may also have an effect.[121]

An early pressor response to beta blockers can be seen in rats,[122,123] cats,[105] rabbits[124,125] and dogs,[126] followed by delayed onset of prolonged hypotension. This paradoxical response has a complex etiology involving increased peripheral vasoconstriction[123] and increased catecholamine secretion.[127,128] Early animal studies showing activity of propranolol in the central nervous system were done with selective infusions of the cerebral vasculature, or direct infusion into the cerebrospinal fluid through the lateral ventricle or the cisterna magna. Infusion of DL-propranolol into the vertebral or carotid arteries of anesthetized dogs has shown a hypertensive response.[129,130] A fall in blood pressure has also been seen with intracerebroventricular injection[126,130,131] or after administration into the cisterna magna.[130] This effect can be reproduced by D-propranolol,[132,133] which has local anesthetic but not beta-blocking properties,[134] thus indicating that the results are nonspecific. In anesthetized cats,[135] DL-propranolol, D-propranolol, DL-alprenolol, D-alprenolol, and DL-pindolol applied to the ventral surface of the brain stem produced a hypotensive response, whereas DL-practolol, DL-sotalol, and DL-atenolol were ineffective, thus correlating positively with each drugs' membrane-stabilizing properties.

Racemic propranolol, alprenolol, pindolol, practolol, atenolol, sotalol, and oxprenolol, when injected into the cerebral ventricles of normotensive conscious cats, showed an initial transient pressor response followed by a fall in blood pressure.[136,137] In conscious rabbits, DL-propranolol was given intracerebroventricularly in concentrations similar to those following intravenous infusion of propranolol at 1.0 ± 2.0 mg/kg/hr for 1-2 hours. After an initial pressor response, blood pressure was lowered and the effects of centrally administered isoproterenol were blocked, thus demonstrating central beta blockade.[138,115] In both of these conscious animal models, D-propranolol was found to reproduce the initial pressor responses but was ineffective in lowering blood pressure. Oral or subcutaneous propranolol and pindolol, when given to conscious hypertensive and normotensive rats for 14 days, reduced blood pressure and heart rate.[139]

Additional evidence for a central mechanism in the reduction of blood pressure by beta blockers has been obtained using electrical stimulation of the brain. The posterior hypothalamus of anesthetized cats when electrically stimulated produces a pressor and tachycardia response. Perfusion of the hypothalamus with DL-propranolol, L-propranolol, sotalol, practolol, or metoprolol causes a concentration-dependent inhibition of this pressor response.[140] D-propranolol and procaine have no effect. Superfusion with alpha-receptor blocking agents also impairs the pressor response to hypothalamic simulation.[141] When both alpha- and beta-blocking agents were infused together, the inhibition of the pressor response was twice that found with perfusion of either single agent. Further studies have characterized the central beta receptors as predominantly beta-1.[142,143]

Important evidence for a central mechanism of action of propranolol has also been provided by measuring the discharge activity of peripheral splanchnic and renal preganglionic efferent nerves. Lewis and Haeusler found that intravenous infusion of DL-propranolol resulted in hypotension and a decrease in splanchnic nerve activity in conscious rabbits.[144] This effect was specific to central beta-adrenergic blockade, because similar hypotension caused by vasodilators caused a reflex increase in splanchnic nerve activity. Central administration of propranolol in anesthetized cats has decreased blood pressure without changes in resting splanchnic sympathetic discharge.[145] Sympathetic efferent nerve activity decreased in anesthetized cats or rabbits after intravenous propranolol,[146] timolol,[146] pindolol,[146] and atenolol[147,148]

Effects of beta blockers on renal sympathetic nerve activity have been reported in both anesthetized[149] and conscious rabbits.[150] Intravenous propranolol lowered blood pressure without change in mean renal sympathetic nerve activity. However, the threshold of the renal baroreflex was lowered, and was attributed to a CNS effect of propranolol.

The central effect of beta-adrenoceptor blocking drugs may be mediated through changes in the baroreflex mechanisms. There are reductions in carotid sinus reflexes in dogs and cats after propranolol.[151,152] Propranolol antagonized hypertensive responses to afferent stimulation of peripheral nerves and chemoreceptor stimulation in cats.[132] In dogs, chronic but not acute propranolol administration antagonized pressor effects caused by occlusion of carotid arteries.[153] Action potentials recorded in aortic baroreceptor fibers increase in activity in hypertensive rabbits treated chronically with propranolol, an effect that increases with length of drug administration.[86] Baroreceptor reflexes have been reported to be enhanced by propranolol in normal subjects[154] and in patients with borderline hypertension.[155] Other studies, however, do not find any significant increase in baroreceptor sensitivity in hypertensive patients treated with long-term timolol or short-term propranolol.[156,157]

In anesthetized dogs with neurogenic hypertension induced by deafferentation and vagotomy, decreases in heart rate and blood pressure were obtained with intravenous injection of DL-propranolol, acebutolol, atenolol, bupranolol, oxprenolol, acebutolol, pindolol, practolol, and sotalol.[158] However, when injected into the cisterna magna, only DL-propranolol and bupranolol effectively lowered blood pressure and reduced tachycardia, whereas oxprenolol had only a bradycardic effect; all the other drugs were ineffective.[167] Therefore, a solitary central effect cannot explain the hypotensive effects of all the drugs that were effective peripherally.

When beta blockers are administered to humans, there are many side effects that may be attributed to central mechanisms. Administration of beta blockers enhances both growth hormone and ACTH responses to physiologic stimuli, suggesting that central beta receptors have an inhibitory role in these responses.[160] Changes in the electroencephalogram that were similar to those seen with vigilance-enhancing compounds and mood-elevating drugs have been found after propranolol administration.[161] Insomnia, vivid dreams, and nightmares can occur with administration of beta blockers;[162] there is also a modestly reduced ventilatory response to hypercapnia.[163,164] Performance on psychomotor and psychosensory tests is inconsistent and sometimes impaired.[107] Other side effects of beta blockers include confusion, hallucinations, depression, and delirium, and can probably be attributed to CNS effects.[165] These are much more common with the lipophilic beta-blockers such as propranolol. Substituting a hydrophilic agent such as atenolol for propranolol in patients with these symptoms reduces these CNS side effects.[166–168]

Interactions of beta blockers with other blood pressure regulatory systems have been proposed. These include effect on central serotonergic systems,[169–172] endogenous opioid systems,[173,174] a central renin-angiotensin axis,[174–176] and activity upon enzyme systems involved in central catecholamine systems.[177,178]

Thus in spite of almost twenty years of research, the predominant mechanism through which beta blockers lower blood pressure has not been conclusively established. It seems likely that the central effects outlined play some part in blood pressure control, although it is probable that the peripheral actions of beta blockers contribute to this effect as well.

References

1. Vakil RJ: Br Heart **2**:350, 1949
2. Bein HJ: The pharmacology of rauwolfia. Pharmacol Rev **8**:435, 1956
3. Kirshner N: Uptake of catacholamines by a particulate fraction of the adrenal medulla. J Biol Chem **237**:2311, 1962
4. Kissin I, Yazhako VS: Effects of reserpine, guanethidine and methyldopa on cardiac output and its distribution. Eur J Pharm **35**:253, 1976
5. Kitay II, Holub DJ, Jailer JW: Inhibition of pituitary ACTH release after administration of reserpine or epinephrine. Endocrinology **65**:548, 1959
6. Veterans Administration Cooperative Study Group on anti-hypertensive agents: Propranolol in the treatment of essential hypertension. JAMA **237**:2303, 1977
7. Benforado JM: The Veratrum Alkaloids. Physiological Pharmacology. Volume 4. New York, Academic Press, 1967, p 331
8. Taylor RD, Page IH: Further studies of the cerebral chemoreceptor buffers as influenced by vasoconstrictor and vasodilator drugs and veratrum viride. Circulation **4**:184, 1951
9. Swiss ED, Mayson GL: The site of cardiovascular action of veratrum derivatives. J Pham Exper Ther **105**:87, 1952
10. Oates JA, Gillespie L, Undenfre DS, Sjoerdsma A: Decarboxylase inhibition and blood pressure reduction by alpha-methyl-3,4-dihydroxy phenylalanine. Science **131**:1890, 1960
11. Sourkes TL: Inhibition of dihydroxyphenylalanine decarboxylase by derivative of phenylalanine. Arch Biochem Biophys **51**:444, 1954
12. Hess SM, Connamacher RH, Ozaki M, Undenfriend S: The effects of alpha-methyldopa and alpha-methyl-meta tyrosine on the metabolism of norepinephrine and serotonin in vivo. J Pharm Exp Ther **134**:128, 1961
13. Haefely W, Hurlimann A, Thoenen H: The effect of stimulation of sympathetic nerve in the cat treated with reserpine, alpha-methyldopa and alpha-methyl-meta tyrosine. Brit J Pharm **26**:172, 1966
14. Sjoerdsma A: Relationships between alterations in amine metabolism and blood pressure. Circ Res **9**:734, 1961
15. Henning M, van Zwieten PA: Central hypotensive effect of alpha-methyldopa. J Pharmaceut Pharm **20**:409, 1968
16. Henning M, Reubenson A: Evidence that the hypotensive action of methyldopa is mediated by central actions of methyl-norepinephrine. J Pharmaceut Pharm **23**:407, 1971
17. Henning M: Interaction of DOPA decarboxylase inhibitors with the effect of alpha-methyldopa on blood pressure and monoamines in rats. Acta Pharm Tox **27**:135, 1969
18. Heise A, Kroneberg G: Alpha sympathetic receptor stimulation in the brain and hypotensive activity of alpha-methyldopa. Eur J Pharm **17**:315, 1972
19. Struyker-Boudier H, Smeets G, Brouwer G, Van Rosumj M: Central nervous system alpha adrenergic mechanisms in cardiovascular regulation in rats. Arch Int Pharm Ther **213**:285, 1975
20. Baum T, Shropshire AT: Evidence for an inhibitory action of methyldopa on spinal sympathetic reflexes. Eur J Pharm **46**:259, 1977
21. Conway EL, Louis WJ, Jarrott B: Endogenous and alpha-methylated catecholamine levels in the anterior hypothalamic-preoptic and medullary nuclei

in rat brain after chronic alpha-methyldopa administration. Neuropharm **18:**287, 1979

22. Conway EL, Louis WJ, Jarrott B: Acute and chronic administration of alpha-methydopa: regional levels of endogenous and alpha-methylated catecholamines in rat brain. Eur J Pharm **52:**271, 1978

23. Hoefke W: Clonidine. Pharmacology of Antihypertensive Drugs, edited by Scriabine A. New York, Raven Press, 1980, p 55

24. Kobinger W, Walland A: Investigations into the mechanism of the hypotensive effect of clonidine. Eur J Pharm **2:**155, 1967

25. Sattler RW, van Zwieten PA: Acute hypotensive action of clonidine after infusion into the cat's vertebral artery. Eur J Pharm **2:**9, 1967

26. Shaw J, Hunyor SN, Korner PI: Sites of central nervous action of clonidine on reflex autonomic function in the unanesthetized rabbit. Eur J Pharm **15:**166, 1971

27. Schmitt H, Schmitt H: Localization of the hypotensive effect of clonidine. Eur J Pharm **6:**8, 1969

28. Kobinger W: Central blood pressure regulation. Chest **83:**297, 1983

29. Haeusler G: Activation of the central pathway of the baroreceptor reflex, a possible mechanism of the hypotensive action of clonidine. Naunyn-Schmeideberg's Arch Pharmacol **278:**231, 1973

30. Guthrie GP Jr, Kotchen TA: Effect of oral clonidine on baroreflex function in patients with essential hypertension. Chest **83:**327, 1983

31. Sleight P, West MJ: Effects of Clonidine on the Baroreflex Arc in Man. Central Action of Drugs in Blood Pressure Regulation, edited by Davies DS, Reed JL. London, University Park Press, 1975, p 291

32. Kobinger W, Walland A: Evidence for a central activation of a vagal cardiodepressor reflex by clonidine. Eur J Pharm **19:**203, 1972

33. Hauesler G: Studies on the possible contribution of a peripheral presynaptic action of clonidine and dopamine to their vascular effects under in vivo conditions. Naunyn-Schmeideberg's Arch Pharmacol **295:**191, 1976

34. Bravo EL, Terazi RC, Fouad FM, Vidt DG, Gifford RW Jr: Clonidine suppression test: a useful aide in the diagnosis of pheochromocytoma. N Engl J Med **3–5:**623, 1981

35. Prichard BNC, Gillam PMS: Use of propranolol (inderal) in the treatment of hypertension. Brit Med J **2:**725, 1964

36. Wilcox RG: Randomized study of six beta blockers and a thiazide diuretic in essential hypertension. Brit Med J **2:**383, 1978

37. Simpson FO: β-adrenergic receptor blocking drugs in hypertension. Drugs **7:**85, 1974

38. Morgan TO, Sabto J, Anavekar SN, Louis WJ, Doyle AE: A comparison of beta adrenergic blocking drugs in the treatment of hypertension. Postgrad Med J **50:**253, 1974

39. Louis WJ, Rand MJ, McNeil JJ, Drummer O, Jarrott B: Clinical pharmacology of adrenergic blocking drugs. Cardiology **64**(Suppl. 1), 96, 1979

40. Veterans Administration Cooperative Study Group on Antihypertensive Agents. JAMA **237:**2303, 1977

41. Lewis P: The essential action of propranolol in hypertension. JAMA **60:**837, 1976

42. Prichard BNC: β-adrenergic receptor blockade in hypertension, past, present and future. Brit J Clin Pharmacol **5:**379, 1978

43. Scriabine A: β-adrenoceptor blocking drugs in hypertension. Ann Rev Pharmacol Toxicol **19:**269, 1979

44. Buckingham RE, Hamilton TC: β-adrenoceptor blocking drugs and hypertension. Gen Pharmacol **101:**1, 1979

45. Prichard BNC, Owens CWI: Beta adrenergic blocking drugs. Pharmacol Ther **11:**109, 1980

46. Prichard BNC, Owens CWI: Mechanism of the antihypertensive action of β-adrenergic blocking drugs. Cardiology **66**(Suppl 1):1, 1980

47. Prichard BNC: Propranolol and β-adrenergic receptor blocking drugs in the treatment of hypertension. Brit J Clin Pharmacol **13:**51, 1982

48. Man in't Veld AJ, Schalekamp MADH: Effects of 10 different β-adrenoceptor antagonists on hemodynamics, plasma renin activity, and plasma norepinephrine in hypertension: the key role of vascular resistance changes in relation to partial agonist activity. J Cardiovasc Pharmacol **5:**S30, 1983

49. Conway J: The antihypertensive action of beta adrenoceptor blocking agents. Arch Int Pharmacodyn Ther Supplement 1980, p 83

50. Tarazi RC, Dustan HP: Beta adrenergic blockade in hypertension. Am J Cardiol **29:**633, 1972

51. Hansson L, Zweifler AJ, Julius S, Hunyor SN: Hemodynamic effects of acute and prolonged β-adrenergic blockade in essential hypertension. Acta Med Scand **196:**27, 1974

52. Tarazi RC, Dustan HP, Bravo EL: Hemodynamic effects of propranolol in hypertension: a review, Postgrad Med J **52**(Suppl 4), 92, 1976

53. Dreslinski GR, Messerli FH, Dunn FG, Suarez DH, Reisin E, Frohlich ED: Hemodynamics, biochemical and reflexive changes produced by atenolol in hypertension. Circulation **65:**1365, 1982

54. Atterhog J-H, Duner H, Pernow B: Experience with pindolol, a beta receptor blocker, in the treatment of hypertension. Am J Med **60:**872, 1976

55. Svensson A, Gudbrandsson T, Sivertsson R, Hansson L: Mode of action of β-adrenoceptor blocking agents in hypertension. A comparison between metoprolol and pindolol with special reference to peripheral vascular effects. Acta Med Scand Suppl **665:**103, 1982

56. Michelakis AM, McAllister RG: The effect of chronic adrenergic receptor blockade on plasma renin activity in man. J Clin Endocrin Metabol **34:**386, 1972

57. Buhler FR, Laragh JH, Baer L, Vaughan ED, Brunner HR: Propranolol inhibition of renin excretion. A specific approach to diagnosis and treatment of renin-dependent hypertensive disease. New Engl J Med **287:**1209, 1972

58. Laragh JH, Buhler FR: Propranolol, renin and hypertension: a review. Postgrad Med J **52**(Suppl 4):109, 1976

59. Buhler FR: Antihypertensive β-blockade and the renin-angiotensin system. Cardiology **66**(Suppl 1):12, 1980

60. Amery A, DePlaen JF, Fagard R, Lijnen P, Reybrouck T: The relationship between beta-blockade, hyporeninaemic and hypotensive effect of two beta-blocking agents. Postgrad Med J **52**(Suppl 4):102, 1976

61. Bravo EL, Tarazi RC, Dustan HP, Lewis JW: Dissociation between renin and arterial pressure responses to beta-adrenergic blockade in human essential hypertension. Circ Res **36**(Suppl 1):241, 1975

62. Leonetti G, Mayer G, Morganti A, Terzoli L, Zanchetti A, Bianchetti G, DiSalle E, Morselli PL, Chidsey CA: Hypotensive and renin suppressing activities of propranolol in hypertensive patients. Clin Sci Mol Med **48:**491, 1975

63. Morgan TO, Roberts R, Carney SL, Louis WJ, Doyle AE: β-Adrenergic receptor blocking drugs, hypertension and plasma renin. Brit J Clin Pharmacol **2**:159, 1975
64. Zweifler AJ, Esler M: Dissociation of fall in blood pressure, renin activity and heart rate during propranolol therapy. Circulation **54**(Suppl 2):87, 1976
65. Frohlich ED, Tarazi RC, Dustan HP, Page IH: The paradox of beta-adrenergic blockade in hypertension. Circulation **37**:417, 1968
66. Stokes GS, Weber MA, Thornell IR: Beta-blockers and plasma renin activity in hypertension. Brit Med J **1**:60, 1974
67. Weber MA, Thornell IR, Stokes GS: Effects of beta-adrenergic blocking agents on plasma renin activity in the conscious rabbit. J Pharmacol Exp Ther **188**:234, 1974
68. Hollifield JW, Sherman K, Vander Zwagg R, Shand DG: Proposed mechanisms of propranolol's antihypertensive effect in essential hypertension. New Engl J Med **295**:68, 1976
69. Mylecharane EJ, Raper C: Prejunctional actions of some β-adrenoceptor antagonists in the vas deferens preparation of the guinea pig. Brit J Pharmacol **39**:128, 1970
70. Adler-Graschinsky E, Langer SZ: Possible role of a β-adrenoceptor in the regulation of noradrenaline release by nerve stimulation through a positive feedback mechanism. Brit J Pharmacol **53**:43, 1975
71. Stjarne L, Brundin J: Dual adrenoceptor-mediated control of noradrenaline secretion from human vasoconstrictor nerves: facilitation by β-receptors and inhibition by α-receptors. Acta Physiol Scand **94**:139, 1975
72. Stjarne L, Brundin J: β$_2$-adrenoceptors facilitating noradrenaline secretion from human vasoconstrictor nerves. Acta Physiol Scand **97**:88, 1976
73. Ablad B, Carlsson E, Dahlof C, Ek L: Some aspects of the pharmacology of β-adrenoreceptor blockers. Drugs **11**(Suppl 1):100, 1976
74. Rand MJ, Law M, Story DF, McCulloch MW: Effects of β-adrenoreceptor blocking drugs on adrenergic transmission. Drugs **11**(Suppl 1):134, 1976
75. Yamaguchi N, De Champlain J, Nadeau RA: Regulation of norepinephrine release from cardiac sympathetic fibers in the dog by presynaptic α- and β-receptors. Circ Res **41**:108, 1977
76. Langer SZ: Presynaptic receptors and their role in the regulation of transmitter release. Br J Pharmacol **60**:481, 1977
77. Starke K: Regulation of noradrenaline release by presynaptic receptor systems. Rev Physiol Biochem Pharmacol **77**:1, 1977
78. Celuch SM, Dubocovich ML, Langer SZ: Stimulation of presynaptic β-adrenoceptors enhances (^{3}H)-noradrenaline release during nerve stimulation in the perfused cat spleen. Brit J Pharmacol **63**:97, 1978
79. Langer SZ, Cavero I, Massingham R: Recent developments in noradrenergic neurotransmission and its relevance to the mechanism of action of certain antihypertensive agents. Hypertension **2**:372, 1980
80. Majewski H, McCulloch MW, Rand MJ, Story DF: Adrenaline activation of prejunctional β-adrenoceptors in guinea pig atria. Brit J Pharmacol **71**:435, 1980
81. Majewski H, Tung LH, Rand MJ: Adrenaline-induced hypertension in rats. J Cardiovasc Pharmacol **3**:179, 1981
82. Franco-Morselli R, Elghozi JL, Joly E, Di Ginilio S, Meyer P: Increased plasma adrenaline concentrations in benign essential hypertension. Brit Med J **2**:1251, 1977

83. Bertel O, Buhler FR, Kiowski W, Lutold BE: Decreased beta-adrenoreceptor responsiveness as related to age, blood pressure and plasma catecholamines in patients with essential hypertension. Hypertension **2:**130, 1980

84. Buhler FW, Kiowski W, van Brummelen P, et al.: Plasma catecholamines and cardiac, renal and peripheral vascular adrenoceptor-mediated responses in different age groups of normal and hypertensive subjects. Clin Exp Hypertens **2:**409, 1980

85. Amann FW, Bolli P, Hulthen L, Kiowski W, Buhler FR: Decrease in alpha-adrenoceptor-mediated vasoconstriction parallels the antihypertensive response to propranolol in patients with normal renin essential hypertension. Clin Sci **61**(Suppl 7):4455, 1981

86. Angell-James JE, Bobik A: Modification of blood pressure and aortic baroreceptor activity in propranolol treated hypertensive rabbits. (Proceedings) J Physiol **278:**16P, 1978

87. Durao V, Rico JMGT: Modification by indomethacin of the blood pressure lowering effect of pindolol and propranolol in conscious rabbits. Eur J Pharmacol **43:**377, 1977

88. Durao V, Prata MM, Goncalves LMP: Modification of antihypertensive effect of β-adrenoceptor blocking agents by inhibition of endogenous prostaglandin synthesis. Lancet **2:**1005, 1977

89. Graham RM, Campbell WB, Jackson EK: Effects of short term beta blockade on blood pressure, plasma thromboxane B_2 and plasma and urinary prostaglandins E_2 and $F_{2\alpha}$ in normal subjects. Clin Pharmacol Ther **31:**234, 1982

90. Pitkajarvi T, Ylitalo P, Metsa-Ketela T, Vapaatalo H: The effects of a $beta_1$-blocking agent, atenolol, on blood pressure, plasma renin activity and prostaglandin $F_{2\alpha}$ excretion in patients with essential hypertension. Acta Med Scand **206:**107, 1979

91. Tarazi RC, Frohlich ED, Dustan HP: Plasma volume changes with long term beta adrenergic blockade. Am Heart J **82:**770, 1971

92. Julius S, Pascual AV, Abbrecht PH, London R: Effect of beta-adrenergic blockade on plasma volume in human subjects. (Proceedings) Soc Exp Biol Med **140:**982, 1972

93. Gordon RD: Effects of β-adrenoreceptor blocking drugs on plasma volume. Renin and aldosterone as components of their hypertensive action. Drugs **11**(Suppl 1):156, 1976

94. Day MD, Roach AG: Central adrenoceptors and the control of arterial blood pressure. Clin Exp Pharmacol Physiol **1:**347, 1974

95. Dollery CT, Lewis PJ: Central hypotensive effect of propranolol. Postgrad Med J **52**(Suppl 4):116, 1976

96. Conway J, Greenwood DT, Middlemiss DN: Central nervous actions of β-adrenoreceptor antagonists. Clin Sci Mol Med **54:**119, 1978

97. Iverson LL: Catecholamine sensitive adenylate cyclases in nervous tissue. J Neurochem **29:**5, 1977

98. Kakiuchi S, Rall TW: The influence of chemical agents on the accumulation of adenosine 3'5'-phosphate in slices of rabbit cerebellum. Mol Pharmacol **4:**367, 1968

99. Nahorski SR: Association of high affinity stereospecific binding of ^{3}H propranolol to cerebral membranes with β-adrenoceptors. Nature (London). **259:**488, 1976

100. Alexander RW, Davis JN, Lefkowitz RJ: Direct identification and characterisation of β-adrenergic receptors in rat brain. Nature (London). **258:**437, 1975

101. Byland DB, Snyder SH: Beta adrenergic receptor binding in membrane preparations from mammalian brain. Mol Pharmacol **12:**568, 1976
102. Sporn JR, Molinoff PB: β-adrenergic receptors in rat brain. J Cyclic Nucleotide Res **2:**149, 1976
103. Melamed E, Lahav M, Atlas D: β-adrenergic receptors in rat cerebral cortex: histochemical localization by a fluorescent β-blocker. Brain Res **128:**379, 1977
104. Kebabian JW, Zatz M, Romero JA, Axelrod J: Rapid changes in rat pineal β-adrenergic receptor: alterations in L-[^{3}H]alprenolol binding and adenylate cyclase. (Proceedings) Nat Acad Sci (USA) **72:**3735, 1975
105. Day MD, Roach AG: Central α and β-adrenoceptors modifying arterial blood pressure and heart rate in conscious cats. Brit J Pharmacol **51:**325, 1974
106. Schneck DW, Pritchard JF, Hayes AH Jr: Studies on the uptake and binding of propranolol by rat tissues. J Pharmacol Exp Ther **203:**621, 1977
107. Patel L, Turner P: Central actions of β-adrenoceptor blocking drugs in man. Medicinal Res Rev **1**(4):387, 1981
108. Cruickshank JM: The clinical importance of cardioselectivity and lipophilicity in beta blockers. Am Heart J **100:**160, 1980
109. Weerasuriya K, Patel L, Turner P: β-adrenoceptor blockade and migraine. Cephalagia **2:**33, 1982
110. Middlemiss DN, Buxton DA, Greenwood DT: β-adrenoceptor antagonists in psychiatry and neurology. Pharmacol Ther **12:**419, 1981
111. Taylor EA, Jefferson D, Carroll JD, Turner P: Cerebrospinal fluid concentrations of propranolol, pindolol and atenolol in man: evidence for central actions of β-adrenoceptor antagonists. Brit J Clin Pharmacol **12:**549, 1981
112. Neil-Dwyer G, Bartlett J, McAinsh J, Cruickshank J: β-adrenoceptor blockers and the blood brain barrier. Brit J Clin Pharmacol **11:**549, 1981
113. Day MD, Hemsworth BA, Street JA: The central uptake of β-adrenoceptor antagonists. J Pharm Pharmacol **29:**52P, 1977
114. Street JA, Hemsworth BA, Roach AG, Day MD: Tissue levels of several radio-labelled β-adrenoceptor antagonists after intravenous administration in rats. Arch Int Pharmacodyn Ther **237:**180, 1979
115. Myers MG, Lewis PJ, Reid JL, Dollery CT: Brain concentration of propranolol in relation to the hypotensive effect in the rabbit with observations on brain propranolol levels in man. J Pharmacol Exp Ther **192:**327, 1975
116. van Zwieten PA, Timmermans PBMWM: Comparison between acute hemodynamic effects and brain penetration of atenolol and metoprolol. J Cardiovasc Pharmacol **1:**85, 1979
117. Bakke OM, Dollery CT, Lewis PJ, Myers MG, Reid JL: Regional brain concentration of propranolol and its hypotensive effect in the conscious rabbit. Brit J Pharmac **51:**148P, 1974
118. Bianchetti G, Elghozi JL, Gomeni R, Meyer P, Morselli PL: Kinetics of distribution of DL-propranolol in various organs and discrete brain areas of the rat. J Pharmacol Exp Ther **214:**682, 1980
119. Garvey HL, Ram N: Comparative antihypertensive effects and tissue distribution of β-adrenergic blocking drugs. J Pharmacol Exp Ther **194:**220, 1975
120. Buckingham RE, Hamilton TC: β-adrenoceptor blocking drugs and hypertension. Gen Pharmacol **10:**1, 1979
121. Anderson WP, Korner PI, Bobik A, Chalmers JP: Leakage of DL-propranolol from cerebrospinal fluid to the bloodstream in the rabbit. J Pharmacol Exp Ther **202:**320, 1977

122. Sweet CS, Wenger HC: Central antihypertensive effects of propranolol in the spontaneously hypertensive rat. Neuropharm **15:**511, 1976
123. Yamamoto J, Sekiya A: On the pressor action of propranolol in the rat. Arch Int Pharmacodyn **179:**372, 1969
124. Reid JL, Lewis PJ, Meyers MG, Dollery CT: Cardiovascular effects of intracerebroventricular D-, L- and DL-propranolol in the conscious rabbit. J Pharmacol Exp Ther **188:**394, 1974
125. Dollery CT, Lewis PJ, Meyers MG, Reid JL: Central hypotensive effect of propranolol in the rabbit. Brit J Pharmacol **48:**343P, 1973
126. Srivastava RK, Kulshrestha VK, Singh N, Bhargava KP: Eur J Pharmacol **21:**222, 1973
127. Sugawara K, Takami N, Maemura S, Niwa M, Ozaki M: β-adrenoceptor blocking agents release catecholamines from rat adrenal medulla. Eur J Pharmacol **62:**287, 1980
128. Myers MG, Lewis PJ, Reid JL, Dollery CT: Central noradrenergic mechanisms and the cardiovascular effects of intracerebroventricular (+)- and (−)-propranolol in the conscious rabbit. Neuropharmacol **14:**221, 1975
129. Stern S, Hoffman M, Braun K: Cardiovascular responses to carotid and vertebral artery infusions of propranolol. Cardiovasc Res **5:**425, 1971
130. Carter JK, Mitchell HW, Poyser RH: Comparison of some hemodynamic changes between central and intravenous administration of (+)-propranolol in anaesthetized dogs. Brit J Pharmacol **51:**146P, 1974
131. Klevans LR, Kovacs JL, Kelly R: Central effect of beta-adrenergic blocking agents on arterial blood pressure. J Pharmacol Exp Ther **196:**389, 1976
132. Kelliher GJ, Buckley JP: Central hypotensive activity of dl- and d-propranolol. J Pharm Sci **59:**1276, 1970
133. Offerhaus L, van Zwieten PA: Comparative studies on central factors contributing to the hypotensive action of propranolol, alprenolol and their enantiomers. Cardiovasc Res **8:**488, 1974
134. Barrett AM, Cullum VA: The biological properties of the optical isomers of propranolol and their effects on cardiac arrhythmias. Brit J Pharmacol **17:**605, 1978
135. Bousquet P, Feldman J, Bloch R, Schwartz J: Is the hypotensive effect obtained by application of drugs to the ventral surface of the brain stem due to a membrane stabilizing mechanism? A study with beta-blockers. Neuropharmacol **17:**605, 1978
136. Day MD, Road AG: Cardiovascular effects of β-adrenoceptor blocking agents after intracerebroventricular administration in conscious normotensive cats. Clin Exp Pharmacol Physiol **1:**33, 1974
137. Day MD, Roach AG: β-adrenergic receptors in the central nervous system of the cat concerned with control of arterial blood pressure and heart rate. Nature New Biology **242:**30, 1973
138. Reid JL, Lewis PJ, Myers MG, Dollery CT: Cardiovascular effects of intracerebroventricular D-, L- and DL-propranolol in the conscious rabbit. J Pharmacol Exp Ther **188:**394, 1974
139. Garvey HL, Ram H: Centrally induced hypotensive effects of β-adrenergic blocking drugs. Eur J Pharmacol **33:**283, 1975
140. Philippi A, Kittel E: Presence of beta-adrenoreceptors in the hypothalamus: their importance for the pressor response to hypothalamic stimulation. Naunyn-Schmiedeberg's Archives of Pharmacology **297:**219, 1977

141. Philippi A: Hypothalamic adrenoceptors and blood pressure. Recent Advances in Hypertension, edited by Milliez P, Safar M. **2**:7, 1975

142. Philippi A, Stroehl U: Beta-adrenoreceptors of the posterior hypothalamus. Clin Exp Hypertension **1**:25, 1978

143. Montastruc JL, Montastruc P: Effect of intracisternal butoxamine, a beta-2 adrenoceptor blocking agent, on blood pressure and heart rate in the dog. Arch Int Pharmacodyn **243**:132, 1980

144. Lewis PJ, Haeusler G: Reduction in sympathetic nervous activity as a mechanism for hypotensive effect of propranolol. Nature **256**:440, 1975

145. Clark B: Pharmacology of beta-adrenoceptor blocking agents. β-Adrenoceptor Blocking Agents, edited by Saxena PR, Forsyth RP. Amsterdam, North-Holland Publishing Company, p 45, 1976

146. Friggi A, Chevalier-Cholat AM, Torresani J: Hemodynamic and baroreceptor responses to β-adrenoreceptor blocking agents in rabbits with cardiopulmonary bypass. Eur J Pharmacol **45**:295, 1977

147. Scott EM: The effect of atenolol on the discharge of sympathetic efferent nerves in the anesthetized cat. Brit J Pharmacol **64**:394P, 1978

148. Friggi A, Chevalier-Cholat AM, Brodard H: Effects of a beta-adrenergic blocking drug, atenolol, on the efferent nerve activity in rabbits. Experientia **33**:1207, 1977

149. Dorward PK, Korner PI: Effect of DL-propranolol on renal sympathetic baroreflex properties and aortic baroreceptor activity. Eur J Pharmacol **52**:61, 1978

150. Korner PI, Dorward PK, Blombery PA, Frean GJ: Central nervous β-adrenoceptors and their role in the cardiovascular action of propranolol in rabbits. Circ Res **46**(Suppl I):I–26, 1980

151. Booker WM, West WL, Hyde AJ, May-Cole M: Alteration of the carotid sinus reflex response by propranolol and by alphamethyldopa. Circulation **40**(Suppl 3):48, 1969

152. Korczyn AD, Goldberg G: Inhibition of hypertensive reflexes by propranolol. Res Commun Chem Pathol Pharmacol **7**:145, 1974

153. Dunlop D, Shanks RG: Inhibition of the carotid sinus reflex by the chronic administration of propranolol. Brit J Pharmacol **36**:132, 1969

154. Pickering TG, Gribbin B, Petersen ES, Cunningham DJC, Sleight P: Effects of autonomic blockade on the baroreflex in man at rest and during exercise. Circ Res **30**:177, 1972

155. Takeshita A, Tanaka S, Nakamura M: Effects of propranolol on baroreflex sensitivity in borderline hypertension. Cardiovasc Res **12**:148, 1978

156. Simon G, Kiowski W, Julius S: Antihypertensive and β-adrenoceptor antagonist action of timolol. Clin Pharmacol Ther **23**:152, 1978

157. Krediet RT, Dunning AJ: Baroreflex sensitivity in hypertension during beta-adrenergic blockade. Brit Heart J **41**:106, 1979

158. Baisset A, Besombes JP, Montastruc P, Tran MA: Effets compares de quelques beta-bloquants adrenergiques sur trois types d'hypertension experimentale chez le chien. Therapie **31**:517, 1976

159. Montastruc JL, Montastruc P: Antihypertensive effects of intracisternal beta-blocking agents in dogs with acute neurogenic hypertension. Arch Int Pharmacodyn **237**:275, 1979

160. Johnstone EC, Ferrier IN: Neuroendocrine markers of CNS drug effects. Brit J Clin Pharmacol **10**:5, 1980

161. Itil TM, Itil KZ: Central mechanisms of clonidine and propranolol in man. Quantitative pharmaco-EEG with antihypertensive compounds. Chest **83**(Suppl):411, 1983

162. Jefferson JW: Beta-adrenergic receptor blocking drugs in psychiatry. Arch Gen Psychiat **31**:681, 1974

163. Campbell SC, Lauver GL, Cobb RB: Central ventilatory depression by oral propranolol. Clin Pharmacol Ther **30**(6):758, 1981

164. Patrick JM, Pearson SB: Beta-adrenoceptor blockade and ventilation in man. Brit J Clin Pharmacol **10**:624, 1980

165. Turner P: β-blockade and the human central nervous system. Drugs **25**(Suppl 2):262, 1983

166. Mattiasson I, Henningsen NC: Side effects during treatment with lipid-soluble beta-adrenergic blocking substances (Abstract). VIIIth World Congress of Cardiology, Tokyo, September 1978

167. Fleminger R: Visual perceptual disorders and other central nervous system side effects: a comparison between propranolol and atenolol (Abstract). VIth Scientific Meeting of the International Society of Hypertension, Gothenburg, June 1979

168. Fraser HS, Carr AC: Propranolol psychosis. Brit J Psychiat **129**:508, 1976

169. Kuhn DM, Wolfe WA, Lovenberg W: Review of the role of the central serotonergic neuronal system in blood pressure regulation. Hypertension **2**:243, 1980

170. Montastruc JL, Montastruc P: Effect of intracisternal 5,7-dihydroxytryptamine on the acute antihypertensive action of propranol in the sino-aortic denervated anesthetized dog. Brit J Pharmacol **72**:411, 1981

171. Middlemiss DN, Blakeborough L, Leather SR: Direct evidence for an interaction of β-adrenergic blockers with 5-HT receptor. Nature (London) **267**:289, 1977

172. Simon W, Schaz K, Ganten U, Stock G, Schlor KH, Ganten D: Effects of enkephalins on arterial blood pressure are reduced by propranolol. Clin Sci Mol Med **55**(Suppl 4):237s, 1978

173. Moore RH III, Dowling DA: Effects of intravenously administered leu- or met-enkephalin on arterial pressure. Regul Peptides **1**:77, 1980

174. Severs WB, Summy-Long JY, Kell LC: The brain renin-angiotensin system. Drug Dev Res **2**:231, 1982

175. Simon W, Schaz K, Mann JFE, Ganten U, Johnson AK, Unger TH, Raschler W, Ganten D: The effects of beta-adrenoreceptor blockers on blood pressure responses to central angiotensin II. Neuropharmacol **20**:719, 1981

176. Nahmod VE, Finkielman S, Benarroch EE, Pirola CJ: Angiotensin regulates release and synthesis of serotonin in brain. Science **202**:1091, 1978

177. Denoroy L, Heimburger M, Renaud B, Affara S, Wepierre J, Cohen Y, Sassard J: Effects of chronic β-blockers treatment on catecholamine synthesizing enzymes in spontaneously hypertensive rats. Biochem Pharmacol **30**:2673, 1981

178. Raine AEG, Chubb IW: Long term β-adrenergic blockade reduces tyrosine hyroxylase and dopamine β-hydroxylase activities in sympathetic ganglia. Nature (London) **267**:265, 1977

Index